I Didn't Know

I Didn't Know

Avoidable Deaths and Harm Due to Medical Negligence

Aubrey Milunsky, MD, D.Sc.

Printed by Createspace, an Amazon.com Company

ISBN-13: 978-1981289714
ISBN-10: 1981289712

Library of Congress Number: 2017919700

PRAISE FOR I DIDN'T KNOW, *I DIDN'T KNOW*

"Dr. Aubrey Milunsky has written an important book that deals with subject matter near and dear to my heart, as my own daughter died due to the negligence of not one, but many, providers. I agree entirely with Dr. Milunsky's emphasis on the preventable nature of most medical errors, and if medical providers would listen more carefully to their patients and communicate more effectively with both their patients and their colleagues, we would see a substantial reduction in the devastating effects of medical error."

Naomi Kirtner, mother to Talia Goldenberg* (1990 - 2014)
Founder of Talia's Voice: Projects for Patient Safety

*See Chapter 17

"This new book by Dr. Milunsky – one of the world leaders of human genetics and personalized medicine – exposes the "open secret" of organized medicine: that doctors are fallible and their actions account for a significant proportion of suffering and death within our health care system. Despite the oft-quoted "God Complex", physicians are human like everyone else and subject to the same fallibilities – in their case amplified by the high stakes, chronic overwork, and the near impossibility of keeping up with the pace of new discoveries. Modern health care is indeed miraculous, but there is a dark underbelly of ignorance, incompetence, denial and outright malfeasance, exposed by this book, that we ignore at our peril. Fortunately, Dr. Milunsky draws lessons from the shocking and tragic real-life cases he passionately describes that we – both patients and medical professionals – can use to protect ourselves and avoid mistakes. For modern medicine, it is truly 'the best of times and the worst of times.'"

Wayne W. Grody, M.D., Ph.D.
Professor, UCLA School of Medicine
Past President, American College of Medical Genetics and Genomics

"This most distinguished physician and geneticist relates the poignant stories of many patients and their families who were victims of medical errors, from firsthand knowledge as an expert witness in almost all of the cases described. He poses the question: "Why have we been so passive in the face of 250,000 annual deaths due to medical negligence?", and proceeds to examine the root causes that result in the tragedies. He further advocates far reaching remedies aimed at avoidance and prevention. He argues effectively for instituting mandatory risk management certification requirements in medical school and in medical practice.
This is a book for all who will become patients as well as for all healthcare providers. It really is a book like none other in its balanced and novel approach to this recurring, tragic, and often preventable problem.

Stuart Z Grossman Esq.
GROSSMAN ROTH YAFFA COHEN
Trial Lawyers, Coral Gables, Florida.

"Dr. Milunsky's book puts emphasis on the need for clear interdisciplinary communication amongst medical professionals. This builds on his long and successful track record of providing a superb educational forum conducive for enhanced communication among the medical and legal professions."

Mary D'Alton, MD
Willard C. Rappleye Professor of Obstetrics and Gynecology
Chair and Director, Department of Obstetrics & Gynecology
Columbia University Medical Center
New York, NY

Member, National Academy of Sciences Institute of Medicine

"Dr. Milunsky's latest book is a fascinating picture of the interface between genetics and medical negligence. His background in both fields and his ability to explain complex medical concepts gives him a unique perspective on situations that affect hundreds of thousands of Americans every year, and will hopefully lead in improvements in both medicine and law."

Bruce G. Fagel, MD, JD
Bruce G. Fagel and Associates
Beverly Hills, CA

"Reading the cases in the book focuses the reader's mind on one biological reality and two clinical realities. The biological reality: Causation of adverse outcomes is complex. The first clinical reality: Medical knowledge almost always has a dimension of uncertainty. The second clinical reality: Physicians have the professional responsibility to manage this uncertainty to reduce preventable risks of adverse outcomes. An organizational culture of safety is essential for achieving this goal. Patients need to trust that their physicians are committed to safety. Like President Reagan and the (now defunct) Soviet Union, patients can also verify by asking a simple question of their physicians: What are your safety practices?"

Laurence B. McCullough, Ph.D.
Distinguished Emeritus Professor
Center for Medical Ethics and Health Policy
Baylor College of Medicine
Houston, Texas

PRAISE FOR DR. MILUNSKY'S PREVIOUS TRADE BOOKS

"Important reading . . . The book stands as a rich and valuable source to be recommended to all adults – potential parents or not."

The Kirkus Reviews

"Thoughtful, sensitive . . . Milunsky writes with pleasing clarity and simplicity . . . eventually everyone should know his genes."

Los Angeles Times

"The sheer quantity of useful information here makes this book required reading."

Publishers Weekly

"Pediatricians are fortunate to have Benjamin Spock to explain child health to parents. As geneticists, we are lucky to have Aubrey Milunsky to explain genetic health to people."

The American Journal of Human Genetics

"Dr. Milunsky's book is carefully written and thoughtful. It provides valuable information to prospective parents and answers many of the questions that concern them both before and after childbirth."

David G. Nathan, MD
Professor and Chairman
Dept. of Pediatrics, Harvard Medical School,
Physician-in-Chief, Children's Hospital, Boston

"This fine book was written by a leading expert in genetics and obstetrics . . . As he says, 'Not knowing does not remove the chances – it removes the choices' . . . This will be an enormous help for couples who have had or might have difficulties in conception or pregnancy."

T. Berry Brazelton, MD
Chief, Division of Child Development, Children's Hospital
Harvard Medical School
Author of **Infants and Mothers**

"The best and most comprehensive . . . guideline to a successful pregnancy and a healthy baby that I have ever seen, written by one of America's top authorities."

Louis Gluck, MD,
Professor of Pediatrics and Obstetrics
University of California, Irvine

"This lucid and authoritative discussion of clinical genetics and its implications should be welcomed by all who are curious about the nature of heredity and the risks of inheritable disease."

Mary Ellen Avery, MD
Chair, Dept. of Pediatrics
Harvard Medical School

"Dr. Milunsky has provided us the extraordinary gift of a health literate translation of the complex and evolving science of genetics and how this understanding is a critical component of our pursuit of optimal health. This book should be required reading for all professionals and families."

Richard Carmona, MD, MPH, FACS
17th Surgeon General of the United States

"Dr. Milunsky's book is a welcome guide for individuals, families, and health professionals trying to navigate through the vast and ever-growing body of genetic information available today. I recommend this book for all. It should help to improve the health literacy of our populations. "

Louis W. Sullivan, MD
US Secretary of Health and Human Services, 1989-1993
President Emeritus, Morehouse School of Medicine

Books by Aubrey Milunsky, M.D., D.Sc.

Know Your Genes
Choices, Not Chances
How to Have the Healthiest Baby You Can
Heredity and Your Family's Health Your
Genetic Destiny
Your Genes, Your Health: A Critical Family Guide That Could Save Your Life

and

Medical Texts (as Author, Co-author, or Editor)

The Prenatal Diagnosis of Hereditary Disorders
The Prevention of Genetic Disease and Mental Retardation
Coping with Crisis and Handicap
Clinics in Perinatology
Advances in Perinatal Medicine (5 Editions)
Genetics and the Law (3 Editions)
Genetic Disorders and the Fetus: Diagnosis, Prevention, and Treatment (7 Editions)

To the memory of the many patients who died or were injured as a consequence of medical negligence

Knowledge is proud it knows so much, wisdom is humble it knows no more

William Cowper (1731-1800)

Law seeks justice while science seeks truth

Howard A. Denemerk

CONTENTS

PREFACE

You, like all of us, have been or will eventually become a patient. It is therefore distressing to read that a 2016 Johns Hopkins study concluded that the third most common cause of death in the United States is medical negligence, third only to heart disease and cancer. That translates to approximately 250,000 deaths per year, or, to comprehend the depth of this staggering reality, the equivalent of 12 jumbo jet crashes per week killing all travelers. One does not have to speculate about the number of patients who were harmed, but survived. Serious harm is estimated to be 10 to 20 fold more common than lethal harm as a consequence of medical care.

Recognizing this toll of lives lost and patients harmed, one would think that a national emergency would be sparked.... no, a national crisis! An outraged populace up in arms? A government declaring a state of emergency? This would be worse than the 9/11 losses occurring every week. I pause for a moment to consider that multiples of that number of patients are harmed, but are alive.

But have you noticed any uprising, anger, or indignation? Calls for urgent action by any physician organization or any government action? Would one notice that we are in the midst of a national crisis? Some may quibble with the figure of 250,000 deaths as estimated by the Johns Hopkins researchers, led by Professor Martin Makary, who first developed the life-saving operating room checklist. Would you settle for 200,000? 150,000?

Why have people been so passive in the face of such heartless statistics? Are we oblivious of the need to secure the health and survival of our loved ones and ourselves? Is it because of the crucial need that we all have to implicitly trust and believe in our doctors? After all, a doctor's work is guided by a defined code of conduct that conveys expectations with which we are all familiar. These include expectations of selflessness, particular skill that incorporates knowledge and expertise, and of course, trustworthiness, sensitivity, and empathy.

As patients, we need to believe, trust, and depend on our physicians. Fortunately, the overwhelming majority of physicians are caring, good, and competent, providing medical care with wisdom coupled with the comfort we all crave when sick. Physicians are fallible, as we all are, and subject to mistakes. Contrary to what many patients think, it is these good and usually competent doctors that as a group commit most medical errors and constitute most defendants in lawsuits, yours truly being no exception. The Institute of Medicine 1999 report that estimated up to 98,000 deaths annually, was appropriately titled "To Err is Human". Well, tell that to the family that has just lost a loved one due to medical malpractice.

I have had the uncommon opportunity to witness and participate in a broad range of specialty medical practice in three countries (South Africa, England, and the United States), given that I am board-certified as a specialist in Pediatrics, Clinical Genetics (both in the United States), and in Internal Medicine and Pediatrics by the Royal College of Physicians in England. For much of my professional life, I have focused on the all-encompassing field of clinical genetics. This includes genetic disorders of the fetus, the newborn, children, and adults. Prenatal genetic diagnosis has, for many decades, been a primary interest, reflecting the first book ever written on the subject and the seven subsequent editions of a major textbook[1] written and edited thereafter.

In line with my life-long dedication to both learning and teaching, I established a continuing medical and legal continuing education course for physicians, lawyers, midwives, risk managers, and other healthcare providers. This became the longest running and most successful postgraduate course in the long history of Boston University School of Medicine, when we left over five years ago. Now as a faculty member at Tufts University School of Medicine the course has continued, and we have completed the 34th successful year.

Unexpectedly, my experience with genetic disorders and the dramatic technological advances in human genetics dovetailed with the need for plaintiff and defense lawyers in preparing their medical negligence cases. As a consequence, I have provided expert testimony equally on both sides of the bar, weighing in always with the facts and the truth. The painful and poignant cases discussed in this book are culled from my experience in reviewing close to 2,000 claims of medical malpractice and appearing in over 100 trials, equally for both plaintiffs and defense

---

(1) Milunsky, A, Milunsky JM. Genetic Disorders and the Fetus: Diagnosis, Prevention and Treatment 2015, Wiley: UK.

At least 1500 of these cases were claims of medical negligence that caused brain damage to babies or infants. My role in all but a handful of cases (prior court decisions and those in published media) was to determine if the cause of the brain damage was due to a genetic disorder or not. As a consequence many of the sad cases described in this book were pregnancy-related, but the lessons learned are applicable to all medical specialties. Every couple who plan to have a child without brain-damage or a genetic disorder would be well-advised to absorb the salutary lessons conveyed in many chapters. Since there are between 21,000-22,000 genes, thousands of catalogued genetic disorders, over 7,000 rare genetic disorders, with about 1 in 12 affected, my task has always been challenging, intriguing, fascinating and inevitably, distressing, given the frequent sad outcomes.

Given the dramatic technological advances in human genetics and the huge challenge physicians face in keeping up-to-date while in active medical practice, current information about the "new genetics" is seeded throughout the case discussions.

One critically important and commonly encountered issue is a patient's perception of risk. This is an arena of practice in which I have been immersed for many decades. Genetic risk assessment occupied the attention of virtually every patient seen for a genetics consultation. The perception of risks is wildly variable and dependent upon the circumstances. You might be concerned about a personal risk of being affected by a genetic disorder, the risk of being a carrier of a fatal flaw, the risk of conceiving or having an affected child, the risks of aborting a pregnancy, and the risks of various procedures, all carrying a range of issues and questions that are usually addressed in such consultations. What one person, for example, sees as "only" a 25% risk of a bad outcome, another's view is that there is a 75% chance all will be well, and that 25% is "not such a high risk."

The cases I have culled from an extensive experience, focus on the pathogenesis of error, that is, how and why medical errors were made and how they could have been avoided or prevented. My main purpose, however, is to derive lessons from avoidable and demoralizing failures that could help stem the carnage and to urge all patients to be alert to the possibility of harmful errors. We all need to be fully aware of the treatment, arrangements, plans and their reasons, and to make no assumptions, even about the simplest of matters (see Chapters 11 and 28).

I have selected cases that are instructive, invariably tragic, and which provide sharp insights into the nature of errors made. Professor James Reason of the University of Manchester in England, a world authority on safety and human error, has pointed to two main paths leading to error. The first, despite an adequate plan, slips occur due to attentional failures, while lapses result from failures of memory. The second follows an imperfect plan resulting in failures of intention for either not following rules or making knowledge-based mistakes. These two paths invoke failures at the level of execution. Slips, lapses, trips or fumbles, Professor Reason emphasizes, occur mostly during "automatic performance," or routine care or procedures. That is where we physicians are vulnerable, always trying to avoid distraction and preoccupation. Error knows no boundary and recognizes no specialty.

This book is for you, the non-physicians. All of us will become patients, aside from unexpected sudden death. My aim is to provide knowledge and insight that enables you to be prepared, proactive, and able to take preventive actions. Yes, the book is also for you, the physician and the nurse, to inform and remind you both of the many pathways to error that can be anticipated and avoided. The lessons from the cases I described are also of vital importance, especially to young physicians, pointing to the pitfalls in practice, and encouraging anticipatory care, caution, and foresight. In the epilogue I have distilled my recommendations based on these lessons so painfully learned from an experience with many litigated cases. Undoubtedly more could be added, but I venture to say that incorporation of all these recommendations would significantly reduce the epidemic of medical negligence.

All but two of the chapters open with the history of an individual or family that led to a claim of medical negligence, and is followed by a discussion of pertinent medical facts, the questions that arise, and commentary on the case. In order to protect the privacy of the families involved, I have changed the names of individuals and have not named hospitals, doctors, or states, except for those published in the media. While many of the histories are embellished or disguised for privacy reasons, the medical facts are absolute. My intent is not to cover the genetic or other disorders discussed in their entirety. Rather, it is to provide a solid factual base for the reader to understand the medicine and the issues involved. All of the cases described and not in the popular press have had my involvement, either in review, consultation, deposition, or as expert witness for trial testimony. Because of the often egregious, but very instructive nature of the published cases of medical negligence, and the valuable lessons they teach, I have taken the liberty of including a few of them with full appellation.

My aim is not to deride those of us involved in the practice of medicine, but rather to focus on the need for patient safety measures. Following the Institute of Medicine (now the National Academy of Medicine) report "To Err is Human," there has been an eruption of safety-directed research, and the creation of a whole string of agencies and organizations dedicated to patient safety goals. One recognizable effect has been the development of a safety- culture especially in hospitals. The "success" of all these efforts and huge associated expenditures is now self-evident. About 250,000 people die each year due to medical negligence!

Regulatory, credentialing, licensing and legislative efforts and actions have systematically aimed at tort reform that ultimately seeks to limit litigation, to cap damage awards, and to effectively deprive the harmed and their families of due redress. Worse still, to punish the victims of negligence. Desperately absent are informed programs that focus on the root causes of error, the anticipated limitations we all have, the necessary formal, early, and continuing education in medical school on risk recognition and management, and the untried remedies.

My hope is that the lessons learned from the many sad events described will serve to instruct and guide those engaged in the complex practice of medicine. From the medical literature and personal practice of medicine, I can report that the problem of medical errors is universal. While we Americans are regarded the world over as litigious, few pause long enough to recognize that our system provides the freedom to seek redress, even if poor. In the vast majority of countries, patients without money are unable to sue. One important consequence of a paucity of litigation and the use of ICD disease codes, is that, in most other countries, they have no idea of the number of deaths or injured due to medical negligence.

I can safely predict the refrain as you read about the cases and consequences of medical negligence. 'I can't believe this happened?' 'How did this happen?' 'Why did this happen?'. It did. It does. And the carnage will continue unless there is new and well-conceived concerted action on many levels.

Most of the doctors and nurses involved in the cases described didn't know, they didn't know. But after reading the histories of the patients and families and the errors they fell victim to, you will know. And to know is to care.

ACKNOWLEDGMENTS

Overwhelming sadness, grief, and anger inevitably cascade over the family of a deceased or harmed member due to actual or claimed medical negligence. I have borne witness to this grief in appearing in over 100 trials and reviews of close to 2,000 negligence claims. This extensive experience moved me to write about the harmed families described in this book. The express aim is to inform all who will become patients (that is all of us except for sudden death) about the pitfalls, mishaps, and errors in medical care that in many cases can be avoided or prevented. I acknowledge first the insights that I have gained from the pain these families have suffered. But, I also acknowledge that the vast majority of care providers are good physicians.

The poignant stories of harmed families that populate every chapter serve to inform about avoidance and prevention. Too late for many, including Naomi Kirtner and Jeff Goldenberg MD, whose daughter Talia, they lost due to medical negligence. I am grateful to them for sharing the details of their daughter's illness and the awful end. I am also indebted to Mike Baker and Justin Mayo at *The Seattle Times* for providing me with many details on their sterling investigative reporting about Talia's care.

I would be remiss in not acknowledging the outstanding teaching and training I received from remarkable teachers (including a Nobel Laureate) at the University of Witwatersrand School of Medicine in Johannesburg, South Africa, from which I graduated so many decades ago.

I have followed about forty journals per month for many decades. I am grateful to the many researchers, physicians, and scholars from whose work I have learned so much. All of the chemical and scientific facts in this book have appropriate sources. It was not feasible, however, to have an endless list of references. I therefore have included many sources of information relevant to specific chapters, even though many apply to a number of different chapters.

I am fortunate to have had the outstanding help of a very talented, superbly organized, interpersonally skilled assistant in her final college year. Rachel Andreas is a gem, with a bright future whose work brought only pleasure and admiration.

My son, Jeff Milunsky MD, whom I had the privilege of teaching and training, also became a full Professor of Pediatrics, Genetics, and Genomics. He is triple-boarded in Pediatrics, Clinical Genetics, and Molecular Genetics, Co-Director of our nonprofit Center for Human Genetics, and the Senior Director of Molecular Genetics. I am grateful to him for reviewing this manuscript and providing wise counsel. I have been blessed in being able to work with him now for almost 25 years. We are now faculty members at Tufts University School of Medicine.

My wife, Laura Becker, PhD, unreservedly contributed not only her grammar and language skills, but also critical thinking in many thought provoking discussions. I am very grateful to her for her help and editorial guidance, and also for supporting and enabling me to take the time committed to this book.

INTRODUCTION

"Your wife needed augmentation for her slow progress in labor, so an intravenous infusion with a drug to stimulate the uterus was given. After an hour she complained of a terrible pain on the right side of her abdomen, and the fetal heart rate plunged to sixty-six beats per minute. An emergency Cesarean section followed, and your baby was found floating free in your wife's abdomen due to a large tear in her womb. We were unable to stem her bleeding in time, and she died. We are desperately sorry. Your baby son is doing well and was taken to the intensive-care unit."

"I didn't see this small shadow in the lung on the x-ray."

"No, I didn't notice that your son's head was growing too fast."

"No, I didn't see the lab report."

"I thought the other specialist had taken care of this medication."

"Labor was progressing well, when Maria's blood pressure suddenly shot up. She became confused and then had a seizure. We now know that she has had a stroke. It's so sad; she's only seventeen years old. I'm so sorry."

All of these incidents ended with death or severe permanent injury. Other authors have pointed to the fact that nearly all patients will experience a diagnostic error in their lifetime, sometimes with devastating consequences. We will all become patients, excepting sudden death. While diagnostic errors rank at or near the top of medical-negligence claims, desperately simple failures of omission and slips or lapses account for many adverse outcomes. The toll for all of us is mind numbing.

In 1999, the Institute of Medicine (now the National Academy of Medicine) published their estimate of forty-five thousand to ninety-eight thousand deaths annually in the United States due to medical errors. That report was based on 1984 and 1992 data from reviews of medical records. Many felt that these figures were a significant underestimate of the actual number of patients dying as a consequence of medical malpractice. Professor Martin Makary, lead author of the 2016 Johns Hopkins School of Medicine report, estimated that in the United States, over 250,000 die each year due to medical negligence.

A report of *inpatient* deaths in the Medicare population between 2000 and 2002 had an estimate of 575,000 deaths due to medical error, that is, about 195,000 deaths a year. The US Department of Health and Human Services Office of the Inspector General, again on *inpatients*, reported in 2008 that medical error caused 180,000 deaths a year among Medicare beneficiaries. Yet another study of hospital admissions estimated that there were over 400,000 deaths a year.

Very worrisome is the realization that all of these studies were on inpatients, including the original one by the Institute of Medicine. Deaths due to medical negligence that occurred in nursing homes, at home, or as outpatients have not figured in any of these estimates. A 2007 study of closed claims of pediatric malpractice, from the Physicians Insurers Association of America, showed that 43 percent of the incidents occurred in doctors' offices, not in the hospital.

For some perspective, pause for a moment. The Korean War saw 36,574 battle deaths, and the Vietnam War saw 58,220 battle deaths (Department of Veterans Affairs). Drunk drivers in 2014 killed 9,967 people in the United States (National Highway Traffic Safety Administration).

Sadly, the truth is that the number of deaths due to medical negligence is huge, and no *effective* nationwide alarm bells were sounded in 1999—or now. Yes, there have been studies aplenty. Safety cultures have been rejuvenated and more guidelines promulgated. The results after eighteen years can be summarized thus: about 250,000 deaths per year!

The common and egregious acts of malpractice reflected in the histories of patients recorded in this book are startling and serve as a reminder of the gravity of the problem. It is not comforting to know that the medical literature is replete with reports of medical negligence from all continents but is seriously underrecognized. Medical malpractice is a universal problem, but its frequency is grossly underestimated in at least 117 countries because of the ICD coding system used that does not record all types of medical error. In May 2016, the BBC reported that in England there were fourteen hundred "mistakes" per week (seventy-two thousand per year) in maternity units.

Errors occur in every branch of medicine, and as physicians, we all face the real and deep complexities in the practice of medicine. Efforts to second-guess a physician's decision making can be perilous. Decisions made (or not) or actions taken (or not) must be tempered with a patient's comprehension (complicated by languages and cultures), compliance, understanding of the severity of the illness, consent, perception of risk, concern about a physician's competence, the desire for a second opinion, and on and on.

A patient's memories of discussions under conditions of anxiety often lack clarity after an adverse outcome following a surgery or a stormy birth. Awareness of this anxiety block enshrines the value and importance of the doctor's notes in the file. In England, the National Health Service Litigation Authority handles all malpractice claims. Remarkably only 4 percent of claims actually reach court. One can only guess that claimants face financial burdens if claims are pursued. An estimate published in 2002 pointed to a possible eighty thousand US hospital deaths annually due to misdiagnosis. Moreover, about 5 percent of autopsies in a 2003 report revealed lethal diagnostic errors for which treatment could have averted death.

A Johns Hopkins University School of Medicine study reported in 2013 an analysis of 350,706 paid claims over a twenty-five-year period (1986–2010). Diagnostic errors led the pack, accounting for 28.6 percent of the total and for the highest proportion of all payments. Diagnostic errors more often resulted in death compared with other allegations and were the leading cause of claims-associated death and disability.

Since we are all subject to making mistakes and recognize our fallibility, can the errors that occur in medicine be avoided and prevented? When errors do occur, we don't have the equivalent of the National Transportation Safety Board to come and investigate to determine the cause so that next time changes made can prevent and avert another catastrophe. We do have root-cause analysis, but this is not a formal, mandatory requirement. Many unexpected deaths occur without a thorough review, let alone a deep analysis of the events that preceded the untimely end.

The National Association of Insurance Commissioners has recognized a nine-point graded severity of injury scale, which I summarize as follows:

- Death

- Grave: quadriplegia, severe brain damage, lifelong care, or fatal prognosis

- Major permanent: paraplegia, blindness, loss of two limbs, brain damage

- Significant permanent: deafness, loss of limb, loss of eye, loss of one kidney or lung

- Minor permanent: loss of fingers, loss or damage to organs, nondisabling injuries

- Major temporary: burns, surgical material left in the body, medication side effects, recovery delayed

- Minor temporary: infections, misset fractures, recovery delayed

- Insignificant: lacerations, contusions, minor scars, rashes, no delay in recovery

- Emotional: no physical harm, but fright or worry

The Physicians Insurance Association of America (PIAA) has a data-sharing project that was initiated in 1985. It is the largest independent database of legal professional-liability claims worldwide. By the end of 2012, over 278,000 closed malpractice claims had been reported, and they had paid out about 81,000 claims totaling nearly $25 billion. Note, however, that historically only 2–4 percent of patients who have suffered from alleged negligent care file a malpractice claim. A study in the *New England Journal of Medicine* ten years ago concluded that courts had failed in 25 percent of cases by either awarding monetary damages to patients where there was no medical negligence or not providing compensation when negligence was the cause of injury. About 27 percent of the time, claims had been resolved through out-of-court settlement.

According to Michael C. Stinson of the PIAA, writing in the *Health Lawyer* published by the American Bar Association, the most common categories of medical error between 2003 and 2012 by data collected from PIAA are as follows:

- Improper performance of procedures
- Errors that included vicarious liability, consent issues, breach of contract or warranty, and billing and collection issues
- Diagnostic errors, especially involving the abdomen and the pelvis, and particularly for chest pain and cancers of the breast and lungs
- Failures to supervise or monitor a case
- Failure to recognize a complication of treatment

The most prevalent claims for procedural errors originated in the failures in diagnostic interviews, evaluation or consultations, prescription medications, and physical examination.

One way to examine the nature and type of errors and negligence is to examine those cases in which failure has occurred. The hope is that lessons would be learned and incorporated into practice, which may avert future tragedy. As patients, we would like to think that medical students would specifically and repeatedly be taught about the pathogenesis of error and how mistakes can be avoided. After many decades of teaching, this has not been my experience.

Physicians are not immune to the many factors that lead us humans to make mistakes. Sadly, such errors are too often fatal. The eternal challenge is to be constantly aware, to be able to anticipate serious potential pitfalls, and to have in place practical systems with well-thought-out backups that enable avoidance of tragic errors. Once a serious error has occurred, taking responsibility is important and is the first step taken to learn from that mistake. Disclosure of the medical error to a patient or family should be accompanied by an apology. This is easier said than done. Unfortunately, many physicians are unwilling to disclose their error or apologize, and some lawyers advise against disclosure. Two obvious overriding concerns relate to reputation and the fear that a lawsuit would likely follow.

All medical institutions are required by law to report all claims of malpractice to the National Practitioner Data Bank (NPDB). Review of the accumulated information by the NPDB (for the period from 2003 to 2012) reveals a significant decrease in the number of medical-malpractice payments made over that period. Nevertheless, for 2012 (the most recent figures available), 9,194 physicians had payments made for medical malpractice. In addition, adverse-action reports about physicians and dentists totaled 6,063 for 2012. Those action reports included reinstatements, restorations, state-licensure actions, clinical-privilege actions, professional society membership actions, Medicare and Medicaid exclusions, Drug Enforcement Agency actions, and exclusions by the Office of the Attorney General. While the number of payments made on behalf of physicians and dentists dropped significantly over this ten-year period, there was a marked escalation of malpractice payments made on behalf of professional nurses. Over the same ten- year period, there was also a steep increase in the number of adverse-action reports concerning physicians and dentists as well as Drug Enforcement Administration actions.

My hope is that the patients' experiences recorded here light the fire of indignation into meaningful action. All of us as present and future patients should demand actions that will prevent avoidable failures that result in death and injury. The responsibilities devolve on many and include Congress, state legislatures, the Joint Commission on Hospital Accreditation, governors, Boards of Registration in Medicine, deans of medical schools, CEOs of hospitals, boards of trustees, the American Hospital Association, the American Healthcare Association, the American Medical Association, and all medical professional colleges and societies.

Many attempts have been made to cap payments to victims of medical negligence. Thirty-five states have imposed caps on such payments. Unfortunately, this step has had the effect of further punishing the injured and families of the dead, doing nothing to prevent future medical negligence.

Punishment and lawsuits are not the answer. Discussions of tort reform have had no effect on mortality and morbidity rates due to medical negligence. A very much greater stringency will be required if there is to be any progress in significantly changing these mortality rates. Since so many lives are lost through medical negligence, would you be willing to consider the following?

- A law that makes physicians who, after a final court judgment, are found to have not met the expected standard of care that resulted in the death of more than one patient, have their license to practice medicine revoked. Would your opinion be more than two deaths? Or three deaths? (Read chapters 21 and 22 before you decide.)

- The recidivists who cause personal injury, according to a jury verdict, be required to redo one year of full-time residency training and three subsequent years of probation with oversight.

- CEOs of hospitals or health-care systems found to be the root cause of avoidable deaths or injury be held accountable and dismissed from their posts. (See chapters 17, 21, and 22.)

- Physicians who write untrue letters of reference be disciplined by a state's Board of Registration in Medicine.

- To obtain a license to practice medicine, every physician should be required to pass a risk-management examination, with every biennial renewal.

What restrictions are sufficient to prevent 250,000 deaths? A rap on the institutional knuckles of reputation? Naming and shaming? Dismissal of the CEO? Lawsuits against the boards of trustees that have fiduciary responsibilities? Cessation of payments by the Centers for Medicare and Medicaid Services (which has been done) that effectively makes a hospital nonfunctional? Would these actions prevent future catastrophes? Longtime patient-safety advocates Lucian Leape, MD, and Donald Berwick concluded that advances in securing patient safety "must come from outside the health industry." They considered how public outrage had failed to effect change and how limited regulation had been. They did point to the potential value and importance of financial disincentives and incentives on hospitals and doctors regarding unsafe practices. Minnesota, for example, ceased paying hospitals for serious preventable adverse events. The trouble is we haven't found an effective remedy to prevent medical negligence. The *combined* application of *all* the abovementioned actions and other punitive steps, with long-term *required* early-medical-school and continuing-postgraduate risk-management training, has never been used. Is this approach unreasonable? Other than World Wars I and II, when did we last lose 250,000 citizens?

In a thorough Stanford and Harvard paper published in the *Journal of the American Medical Association* in 2014, the highly accomplished authors focused on nontraditional approaches to medical liability reform. I can summarize these as follows:

- *Communication and resolution programs:* The idea is that physicians and institutions discuss adverse outcomes with patients (including resolution, apology, and restitution for maloccurrence), discussion about whether or not the standard of care was breached, and finally the matter of compensation.

- *Mandatory presuit notification laws:* The proposal was to promulgate laws that require plaintiffs to give advance notice of one to six months before they file a lawsuit. The purpose would be to enable time to investigate what happened and allow sufficient time to settle the case before a lawsuit is filed.

- *Apology laws:* The proposal is to establish laws that protect physicians who make statements of apology, regret, or fault that could later be used in malpractice lawsuits.

- *State-facilitated dispute-resolution laws:* This proposal is for laws that allow voluntary filing of complaints to a state agency that would then assist all parties through a communication and resolution process including mediation.

- *Safe harbors:* The proposal is for laws that enable physicians and health-care providers a defense against malpractice claims as long as they can demonstrate that specific guidelines or protocols were followed.

- *Judge-directed negotiations:* This proposal would require all litigants to meet early and often in a case with a judge to seek a settlement. That judge would retain responsibility should the cases proceed to trial.

- *Administrative compensation systems:* This proposal requires laws that have medical-malpractice claims enter an alternative adjudication process using highly qualified experts, evidence-based guidelines, and compensation standards.

Few could launch meaningful objections to these carefully considered nontraditional approaches to medical liability reform. These proposals lean heavily in the direction of defending errant physicians and would likely do little to diminish the frequency of medical malpractice. The range of legislative tort reforms that have been proposed aim primarily to reduce the number and dollar amount of claims, cut the costs of professional-liability premiums, decrease the frequency and costs of litigation, and lessen the costs of practicing defensive medicine. These steps would do little, if anything, to significantly decrease the frequency of medical error. In this publication and the vast majority of published materials, there is a failure to recognize the fundamental cause of medical malpractice. While system errors are an indisputable contributor to medical errors, the key culprit is us humans. Just as most automobile crashes involve the driver, *the majority of medical errors are committed by individual and usually good physicians.* That is a truism no amount of tort reform will change. In my opinion, it is not laws that will ultimately make the difference in reducing medical errors.

The Lucian Leape Institute at the National Patient Safety Foundation in 2010 made recommendations for "reforming medical education to focus on quality and safety." The goal they expressed was that medical schools and teaching hospitals *should* create "learning cultures that emphasize patient safety," teach professionalism, enhance collaboration, and encourage transparency. The extant failure we now witness lies in the ineffective *should*. I firmly believe that all of these and other educational goals must be *required* and fulfilled by examination in order to graduate from medical school *and* to complete residency training.

Required CME risk-management credits awarded for attending lectures or grand rounds have failed to decrease the carnage. A written, even online, examination should be a standard requirement for maintaining a medical license. This would be a test that *teaches* practical risk management and could be preceded by a required webinar. There should be mandatory education and training in risk management, despite the fact that many states require *risk-management credits*. I propose lifetime required biennial risk-management certification for license renewal. Such certification could be overseen by Boards of Registration in Medicine appropriately funded by each state. I would add that this certifying process begin and be required in the third and fourth years of medical school and continue through each year of residency training in any specialty. This seemingly draconian measure needs to be considered mindful of the incredible 250,000 deaths per year and multiples of that number being harmed.

Intuitively I know my physician colleagues will be muttering angrily about my proposal. I have, however, had the privilege of having physicians as my patients and can safely relate common and unfortunate experiences they or their families have been subject to. Physicians are not immune to suffering errors in their own care. As a group, we are battered by paperwork, time spent, and problems with the electronic medical record, as well as endless aggravations with insurance companies. So forgive me for adding to these burdens, but it is because I care.

Both before and since the Institute of Medicine report, major efforts have been made to establish a culture of safety in hospitals and health systems. Only the World Health Organization Surgical Safety Checklist (originated by Professor Martin Markay of Johns Hopkins University School of Medicine) has clearly improved operative outcomes. While there is a greater awareness of the need to reduce the mortality and morbidity rates, efforts thus far point to largely ineffective methods.

Humans are fallible, but when we or our families are at serious risk, we seem less forgiving about this common limitation. What we need is training for our doctors and nurses to anticipate the *possibility of error* and establish prompt warning signals (checklist, task list, follow-up list, office rules), automatic checks for decisions, medications, and key arrangements making "assurance doubly sure." This would require physicians and their practice or hospital staff to meet regularly, to consider and review literally everything they do in the context of risk management, to question how and what error could possibly be made, and then to establish safeguards. We know that courts look poorly at those who forget to use reasonable precautions. To paraphrase Professor Mark Grady of Northwestern School of Law, if a physician forgets to notice risk, it is often because he or she forgot to take the precaution of looking for it. A lack of knowledge, arrogance, and hubris are much more difficult to manage and will require serious disciplinary responses.

Lawyers too will find real value in more fully comprehending the complexities and challenges physicians face in the practice of medicine. This book is not a road map to litigation. Quite the contrary. The aim is to avoid death and harm from medical malpractice. Lawsuits clearly do not accomplish that goal. There is a desperate need for collective action from our elected representatives at all levels of government and from all credentialing organizations, all patient-safety organizations, and especially all medical schools and hospitals that teach and train physicians. Professional associations, specialist colleges, associations in all health-care fields, and all accrediting agencies finally need to recognize the continuing carnage and take long overdue action. To err is human, but it is also human to think, to anticipate, to prevent, and to care.

If you were to suffer the death or permanent injury of a loved one due to medical negligence, beyond litigation, what policy changes would you demand? Do you have to wait for a personal loss to make your voice heard? The physicians involved in the tragic cases accounted for in this book mostly didn't know they didn't know.

EYES OF THE BEHOLDER

Casey was blind and pregnant. At twenty-six years of age, she knew only that she had become blind as a toddler. She thought she remembered what trees looked like, but not much else. She was adopted and grew up in a loving family. She attended a local school for the blind, learned Braille, and graduated high school.

Subsequently, Casey met her future husband, Jim, a kind and gentle but tough man who worked in a construction company. Soon after her marriage, she found herself with an unplanned pregnancy. She felt very unprepared for the challenge, and, together, they decided on early pregnancy termination.

A couple of years later, with family support, Casey and Jim decided to try for another pregnancy. A few short months later, they succeeded. Casey received her obstetrical care from an obstetrician recommended by a family friend. Routine care was provided, but he never asked about the cause of her blindness. After an uneventful pregnancy, Casey delivered a beautiful baby girl whom they named Irene.

All was well as Irene reached her developmental milestones. However, at nine months of age, Jim noticed that there was something odd in the way Irene looked at objects. Seemingly she did not look directly at a toy being held out to her and did not initially reach for the toy. Looking closely at her, Jim thought he saw a whiteness behind the pupil of one eye. Their family doctor had difficulty examining the eyes of an uncooperative infant and promptly referred them to an ophthalmologist. Worried and suspicious about Casey's blindness (who had no idea why she was blind), he proceeded with his examination. A drop into each of Irene's eyes allowed the ophthalmologist to see, through the dilated pupils, a ball of white tissue at the back of the eye (the retina) behind each pupil. The diagnosis was bilateral retinoblastoma, a cancer of the eyes. He immediately realized that Irene had inherited this cancer from her mother. Casey's adoptive parents had been told that she had tumors in her eyes, resulting in their surgical enucleation (removal), when she was a toddler, but that she was then healthy. Casey's adoptive mother died some years later.

Within weeks of the diagnosis, and with unspeakable agony, Casey and Jim gave permission for the required surgery—enucleation of both of Irene's eyes. Surgery was followed by chemotherapy, a painful healing, and what would be a lifetime of blindness.

Casey and Jim sued the obstetrician for his negligent care and for depriving them of the chance to avoid having a blind child and, because of a delayed diagnosis, the opportunity for prompt treatment, which could have saved her sight.

Pertinent Medical Facts

Retinoblastoma is a heritable eye cancer, which has been known for hundreds of years, the culprit gene having been identified in 1986. This tumor occurs in both eyes 40 percent of the time. It is an autosomal dominant disorder, meaning that an affected person has a 50 percent risk of transmitting this disorder to each of his or her children. This eye cancer is estimated to occur in one in fifteen thousand to one in twenty thousand live births. The precise diagnosis is made by DNA analysis of the retinoblastoma gene (*RB1*) (sequencing or deletion analysis of the gene seeking tiny deleted areas of the genome). In 7 percent of patients with bilateral retinoblastoma, a microscopically visible piece of DNA—a tiny microdeletion (see chapter 38) in the long arm of one chromosome 13 (13q14)—will facilitate the diagnosis. Those with a microdeletion often have developmental delay and other birth defects, possibly because other contiguous genes have also been deleted. Irene did not have this exact chromosomal abnormality.

Guidelines for infants known to harbor an *RB1* gene mutation (as should have been the case for Casey and Irene) require eye examination under anesthesia every three to four weeks until the age of six months and then less frequently until the age of three years. Thereafter, eye examinations are required (without anesthesia) every three to six months until the age of seven years and then annually and eventually biannually for life! Gene analysis can of course also be done for the purpose of prenatal diagnosis as early as eleven weeks of pregnancy.

The expectation is for the parents and siblings of an affected person to be tested for defects in the retinoblastoma gene. Where there is no family history of retinoblastoma, which is commonly the case, a brand-new mutation may have occurred in either the testes or ovary of either parent. However, once an affected person has developed retinoblastoma from this brand-new mutation, he or she has a 50 percent risk of transmitting this cancer to each of his or her offspring. Apparently, Casey's parents were not affected.

A range of treatments is available and includes enucleation (surgical removal of one or both eyes), cryotherapy (freezing), laser therapy, chemotherapy, and radiation therapy.

Unfortunately, survivors with a mutation in the retinoblastoma gene have a significantly increased risk of developing other malignancies, especially of bones and soft tissues, as well as melanomas. This risk is increased to over 50 percent in those who have received radiation therapy.

There are over seven thousand known rare genetic disorders with about one in twelve people affected, unwittingly or not. Practicing physicians are not expected to know these rare disorders. However, the expected standard of care is to confer with or refer to a clinical geneticist or a specialist on the organ system involved (e.g., the heart or nervous system).

Questions

- Why did Casey's obstetrician never ask her why she was blind?

- Why didn't he refer her to an ophthalmologist?

- Why didn't he simply call an ophthalmologist and ask if there was an important diagnosis he needed to consider for his blind, pregnant patient?

- Why did he not realize that, since there was no history or signs of trauma, a serious diagnostic explanation existed that could be of genetic origin or due to a cancer?

- Why did he not simply call or refer to a clinical geneticist or an oncologist?

Commentary

How is it possible for a physician to be so uncaring as to not ask, "Why are you blind?" All he had to do was confer or refer to an ophthalmologist or a clinical geneticist. This could have enabled Casey to have a blood test that would have shown that she carried the characteristic gene abnormality that resulted in retinoblastoma. Counseling would have followed, with the information that Casey and Jim would have a 50 percent risk of having a child who would also develop retinoblastoma. However, they would have had the option of prenatal diagnosis or preimplantation genetic diagnosis. If the fetus in early pregnancy carried this genetic flaw, they would have been able to terminate the pregnancy, a step they had taken once before. Moreover, early diagnosis of retinoblastoma enables the saving of eyes and sight in almost all patients.

The obstetrician testified that he had never heard of retinoblastoma and that the eyes were not "his organ of interest." Moreover, he stated that the major textbook on obstetrics (*William's Obstetrics*) had no mention of this disorder!

Who knows what thoughts crossed through this doctor's mind after receiving notice of the lawsuit. It is well known that physicians feel guilty after making a serious mistake. Worse still, they may avoid the harmed patient who in fact may be especially needy. Guilty physicians may experience fear of losing their license, ruining their reputation, and damaging their livelihood.

The emotions experienced by physicians pale when compared with those of the harmed patients and families. Sadness and anger may predominate initially. Fear of further harm or lack of care if they complain (and certainly if they sue) can become a preoccupying concern. Guilt by a family member(s) for "not being there" or "not intervening" or "not having him transferred to a teaching hospital" is real and frequently expressed. Lack of trust in physicians is an early and serious casualty.

One can only imagine Jim's feeling of guilt for not having accompanied Casey to her early appointments with her obstetrician and for not having pressed for an answer about the cause of Casey's blindness. About the need for another opinion. About the risk of having a child who would also be blind. Questions, questions, and recriminations. All too late.

Casey herself would also have experienced grief and anger. But having lived almost all her years being blind, her reactions are likely to have been complex. Realization that she had unwittingly passed on the gene mutation that caused Irene's blindness was a heavy burden to bear. Yet having to abort a pregnancy knowing that the fetus possessed her genetic flaw would be facing her own "extinction." She would never have been born. Would never have met Jim. Would never have had Irene to cuddle and sing lullabies to.

All these concerns invoke deep emotional conflicts. The overriding concern, however, should have been for Casey and Jim who sadly had trusted their doctor who totally failed them. He failed (1) to recognize that her blindness could be genetic, (2) to recognize that they might have an increased risk of having a blind child, (3) to confer with an ophthalmologist or a clinical geneticist, (4) to refer to one of these specialists, (5) to consider the possibility of prenatal diagnosis, (6) to offer a genetic study on Casey, and (7) to discuss prenatal diagnosis contingent upon a precise molecular diagnosis being made on Casey.

These were the standards of care required of this physician. The very least he could have done was to telephone either an ophthalmologist or a geneticist and simply ask if there was a genetic disorder that could have led to ocular enucleation. Beyond everything else, a physician must care! This doctor's lack of caring compounded by ignorance resulted in a lifetime of grief and handicap. He didn't know, he didn't know!

The case was settled.

A BLEEDING SHAME

Claire was twenty-three when she delivered her first baby, Cliff, by Cesarean section. Pregnancy was uneventful, as was the delivery. However, shortly after birth, Cliff was noted to have tiny hemorrhagic spots on his skin (called "petechiae"). An immediate blood count revealed that his white blood cells and red blood cells were normal but that the accompanying tiny cells called "platelets" were strikingly insufficient. Promptly admitted to the neonatal intensive-care unit, because of his low platelet count (called "thrombocytopenia"), the attending specialist, Dr. Vary Ominous, ordered a transfusion of platelets and, because of a heart murmur, an ultrasound of his heart as well. The imaging study revealed a serious cardiac abnormality, called "hypoplastic left heart syndrome," and the doctor arranged for Cliff to be transferred to a major teaching hospital.

Prior to transfer, Dr. Ominous considered the possibility that Claire harbored antibodies that were destroying Cliff's platelets, a condition called neonatal alloimmune thrombocytopenia (NAIT). Even though he ordered the blood test for antibodies on Claire, he failed to inform her obstetrician, Dr. Loop Hazard. Since Claire was Dr. Hazard's patient, the blood-test result was expected to appear in her obstetrics chart and not in Cliff's pediatric chart. Dr. Ominous did not bother to see the result and was satisfied by being informed by a nurse that the report was negative. Even though the expectation was for the report to be placed in the obstetric chart of Dr. Hazard, that never occurred. The hospital could not explain why this vital lab report, generated from outside the facility, was never transmitted to Dr. Hazard. Dr. Hazard was neither informed by Dr. Ominous nor did he see the report.

Cliff was promptly transferred to the teaching hospital, and no communication was made about the original suspicion Dr. Ominous had when he ordered the test on Claire to determine whether she had platelet antibodies.

Needless to say, Cliff's parents, Claire and Steve, were never informed of these test results, nor were they given any warning about the potential implications of the results on any future pregnancies. As it is, their attention was fixed on Cliff's congenital heart defect and the need for surgery. Soon after the platelet transfusion, Cliff's platelet level improved, and he was able to undergo heart surgery without a bleeding problem. Claire and Steve were never informed about the cause of Cliff's very low platelet count. They were told at the teaching hospital that the low platelets were of no known cause, despite Dr. Ominous's original concern about NAIT.

At the teaching hospital, Cliff was seen in the neonatal intensive-care unit by the attending neonatologist, Dr. Noall. Cliff was examined initially by the pediatric resident, Dr. Soo Newby, whose original *plan* was to check Claire's antiplatelet antibodies. A few hours later, the neonatal fellow, Dr. See Yu, also wrote a progress note with the same intention to check Claire's antiplatelet antibodies. Later, Dr. Noall also wrote a note about the *plan* to check Claire's antiplatelet antibodies and also to consider a consultation with the hematologist.

With a shift change, the new attending neonatologist, Dr. Mira Kal, formally requested a consultation with the pediatric hematologist, Dr. Lyse Fibrin. Dr. Fibrin's note stated that a blood sample should be obtained from both Claire and Steve to check for antiplatelet antibodies. She was unaware, of course, that any such blood test had already been done at the direction of Dr. Ominous in the referring hospital. Dr. Mira Kal subsequently wrote in her progress note that the consulting pediatric hematologist, Dr. Fibrin, had recommended the antibody platelet tests on both parents. However, none of these doctors actually issued an order to test the parents. Subsequently, two other physicians decided, without explanation or evidence, that Cliff's platelet problem did not appear to be NAIT.

Following heart surgery and recovery, Cliff was discharged from the teaching hospital, and there was no further reference to the problem with his platelets. Over the next two years, Claire saw Dr. Hazard intermittently for unrelated gynecological issues. He never inquired about Cliff's condition, and there was never a discussion about low platelets immediately after his birth. Nor was there any discussion about potential implications for any future pregnancy.

About two years after Cliff's birth, Claire again attended for obstetrical care for her second pregnancy, again with Dr. Hazard. The routine history taking at the beginning of this pregnancy made no reference to the thrombocytopenia that had affected Cliff. Because of Cliff's congenital heart defect, Dr. Hazard referred Claire to a maternal-fetal-medicine specialist, Dr. June Wonder, requesting a full evaluation. When filling out the intake form, Claire indicated that her first child had been born with low platelets and had required a platelet transfusion. Dr. Wonder, given this information, did not initiate any blood test for platelet antibodies, assuming that such studies had been done and had been negative. She did not, however, document that thought process in the chart, nor did she seek a copy of the laboratory test originally ordered by Dr. Ominous.

Claire delivered Ian by Cesarean section following an uneventful pregnancy. Within one hour of his birth, Ian was found to have an extremely low level of platelets. He was immediately admitted to the neonatal intensive-care unit, where the plan was to start a platelet transfusion immediately. This, however, took an inexplicable eleven hours to initiate. Even after that, his platelet count dropped precipitously again. Curiously, Dr. Ominous ordered an antibody test on Claire again, not remembering that he had done that once before (and never gotten the result). The results were promptly returned as positive for platelet antibodies once again, and Ian was transferred to the teaching hospital. An ultrasound of his brain revealed a major bleed in his left temporal lobe. This large hemorrhage occupied much of his left temporal lobe. Expert neurologists testified that this bleed must have occurred at least a week before Ian's birth.

The hemorrhage and damaged brain tissue slowly resolved, becoming a large cyst, which in turn became the source of serious seizures. Neurosurgery was done at eighteen months of age to alleviate the seizures that had become a life-threatening issue. Unfortunately, Ian's brain injury left him with a severe expressive aphasia, with a near total inability to communicate verbally and impairing his ability to learn.

Pertinent Medical Facts

Our tiny platelets have a major role in blood clotting. When the platelet count is very low, a serious to fatal hemorrhage can occur. On the surface of the platelets are very specific and different proteins (antigens), of which there are twenty-four. If a fetus inherits a particular antigen (the most common one is found in 80 percent of whites) that the *mother* does not possess, her body's immune system *fights* the *foreign* antigen by making antibodies. These antibodies are already functional toward the end of pregnancy and, as a consequence, even before birth, and certainly after birth, may destroy fetal platelets, resulting in serious to fatal hemorrhage.

This could happen in a mother's first pregnancy but is mostly not severe. However, the mother's antibodies remain ready to attack the platelets of a subsequent child, and this time the effect can be disastrous without preventive treatment of the disorder termed neonatal alloimmune thrombocytopenia (NAIT).

As a fetus, Cliff inherited his father's specific platelet antigen, which his mother's immune system recognized as *foreign*, with her antibodies mounting an attack. Fortunately, it takes time to develop a formidable antibody force, so Cliff was born with tiny skin hemorrhages (petechiae) due to his lower than normal platelet count. However, when Ian was a fetus, his mother's antibodies were able and ready and quickly moved to destroy his platelets, resulting in a profound bleed in his brain.

Recognition of NAIT in Cliff after birth would have led to treatment of his mother with intravenous immunoglobulin and steroids during her pregnancy with Ian. This treatment would have given Ian at least an 80 percent chance of avoiding his brain bleed and a lifetime of handicap.

The diagnosis of NAIT in Cliff meant a risk of 100 percent for a future sibling and an 80 percent risk of a hemorrhagic stroke for Ian. Moreover, the severity of NAIT increases with each pregnancy, so both parents have to be carefully counseled, tested, and informed if tragedy is to be avoided. NAIT is not rare and occurs in one in one thousand to fifteen hundred births.

Without warning, Cliff was born with hypoplastic left heart syndrome. Congenital heart defects are common, occurring in about 1 in 120 babies born. The hypoplastic left or right heart syndrome occurs in close to 1 in 3,000 births. Cause is mostly unknown and results in abnormal development of the left or right side of the heart. It often includes underdevelopment of the aorta and may also have abnormalities of the heart valves. While Cliff was born without immediate obvious heart complications or heart failure, the undeveloped ventricles quickly failed. Hence, his transfer for heart surgery. Surgery for this abnormality, however, is complicated and requires repeated operations, which, not unexpectedly, is associated with a high mortality rate. Another important, but hard to achieve, option is cardiac transplantation. Without the latter option, the long-term prognosis for survival and quality of life is seriously limited. This heart abnormality can be diagnosed by high-resolution ultrasound (fetal echocardiography) between eighteen and twenty-two weeks of pregnancy. The only option at that point, unfortunately, is pregnancy termination.

Questions

- Why did Dr. Ominous, who originally ordered the antiplatelet antibody tests, not make sure he *saw* the report?

- How could he have relied on an inexperienced nurse to interpret a complex laboratory report?

- How could a hospital have such a cockamamy system that allowed a vital lab report to not reach the physicians who were supposed to care for both mother and baby?

- Why was the obstetrician, Dr. Hazard, so ignorant and uncaring as not to recognize the grave implications of NAIT?

- Why was the leadership in the neonatal intensive-care unit at the teaching hospital so pathetic, resulting in total failure by nine physicians talking and writing about the possibility of NAIT, without any one actually ordering this critical test?

- Why did the maternal-fetal-medicine specialist, Dr. June Wonder, assume that the antibody platelet test had yielded a negative result, without bothering to obtain and see the laboratory report herself?

- Why did physicians in both hospitals not explain the results of the antibody test and its grave implications for a subsequent pregnancy?

Commentary

Few realize the frequency of stroke around the time of birth (perinatal) and during the first week of life. Rates of perinatal stroke (thrombosis or hemorrhage) are greater than one in thirty-five hundred live births. NAIT is relatively rare but devastating, especially when causing intracranial hemorrhage, as it did in Ian. NAIT may also cause serious to fatal bleeding in fetuses or newborns at sites other than the brain, including the eyes, intestines, spinal cord, lungs, and kidneys, all of which have been reported. Although NAIT occurs in one in one thousand to one in fifteen hundred live births, this disorder ranks among the most important causes of low platelet disorders in newborns.

Since NAIT can be accurately diagnosed, treated, and corrected by platelet transfusions, there is no excuse for failing to predict a recurrence and to provide timely intervention.

The standard of expected care would hold that a physician who orders a test would see the result. Moreover, if that result is of such importance as to ultimately have life-threatening implications, it is absolutely mandatory that the result be obtained and communicated to those at risk. Teams of physicians in hospital wards or intensive-care units work under considerable stress. They need clear and defining leadership that ensures correct and proper implementation of specialist recommendations, as was made by the hematologist, Dr. Lyse Fibrin. The ignorance displayed by nine physicians, which resulted in the catastrophe that befell Ian, is troubling in the extreme. A combination of lack of knowledge, poor decision making, uncaring practice, and systems failure was unforgivable. I testified under oath for this family and stated that, in my large and long experience, I could not recall a case in which the care rendered by so many physicians revealed a combination of ignorance and incompetence across the board. They didn't know; they didn't know, didn't care, and took no action when it was so important.

Claire and her husband were profoundly unlucky in having both sons so severely impaired, especially when one could have been spared by proper anticipatory management.

Compounding the lack of leadership and hospital systems failure was the pervasive ignorance of the physicians, their collective inaction, and their shameful lack of caring. The settlement award could never replace the normal life that was stolen from Ian.

THE POWER OF WORDS

For a few years, Andrew and Clara lived together, while they completed their studies. Andrew became a chemical engineer, and Clara, a Hungarian immigrant, obtained a degree in fine arts. They both found good jobs and decided to marry and begin a family. Clara soon became pregnant, and they both reveled in the thought of having a family and buying a house.

Pregnancy was uneventful, as were labor and delivery. Yvette was a beautiful baby girl, weighing six pounds ten ounces, whose smile eventually captured the heart of all who saw her. She was healthy, reaching all of her milestones even earlier than expected, sitting at five months, taking steps at ten months, and becoming verbal in the months soon after her first birthday.

At twenty months of age, Yvette caught a cold that developed into an upper-respiratory infection with fever. Without warning, she had a major seizure, with jerking limbs and loss of consciousness. Andrew and Clara rushed her to the emergency department at the local hospital, where they found that she had fully recovered, was alert, and was communicative. They did think that she was rather floppy but concluded that the lack of muscle tone reflected the postseizure recovery. On returning home, Andrew and Clara noticed that Yvette tended to twitch or have jerks in her arms or legs, but not have an actual seizure.

During the ensuing weeks, they became increasingly worried when they noticed that Yvette was having some difficulty walking and that her lack of balance and coordination while holding a spoon or toy was obvious. Moreover, the few words that she had already accomplished had mostly disappeared. They returned to their pediatrician for further evaluation, and a series of appropriate and complex biochemical and genetic tests were done on an inpatient evaluation. Those studies included analyses of Yvette's blood, urine, and cerebrospinal fluid. Imaging by an MRI of her brain revealed no abnormality. No specific diagnosis was made despite Yvette's progressive deterioration, accompanied by long, continuous episodes of seizures. At one point, her doctors thought that she had had a stroke, since her eyes did not seem to be able to focus and that one side of her body seemed weaker and to move less than the other side. The seizures became more frequent and more difficult to control despite the best-available treatment. While things could hardly get worse, Yvette had another chest infection with fever that caused intractable seizures for which she was hospitalized. This was at twenty-three months of age, when, during that admission, liver failure became evident, as she lapsed into a coma and died.

The clinical suspicion was that she might have a mitochondrial disorder (see discussion below), but none of the biochemical and DNA studies available at the time enabled a definitive diagnosis. Moreover, the autopsy also concluded without recognition for a clinical cause of Yvette's disorder and demise.

Distraught by the loss of their beautiful little girl, Andrew and Clara sought genetic counseling. They confirmed that they were both healthy; that there were no birth defects, intellectual disability, or known genetic disorders in their families; and that they were not related. Andrew's ancestry was English and Irish, while Clara had Hungarian roots. Absent any definitive diagnosis, the geneticist counseled that the disorder could be of autosomal recessive origin, implying that they each possibly harbored a defect (mutation) in the same gene. If that were true, they would have a 25 percent risk of having a second child with the same disorder. Another potential concern was the transmission of a gene mutation directly from Clara. This would have been a mitochondrial mutation that would invariably mean a 100 percent likelihood of having Yvette's disorder recur in every single pregnancy in the future. The likelihood of that scenario was very remote, given that Clara was completely healthy. Nevertheless, absolute certainty could not attach to that possible explanation.

A year later, and still grief-stricken, they decided to try again to have another child. They realized that no prenatal genetic diagnosis would be possible, given no known precise diagnosis for Yvette. They thought long and hard about their potential 25 percent risk of recurrence but decided to go ahead anyway.

Clara soon became pregnant, and following an uneventful, but extremely anxious, pregnancy, she delivered a healthy boy they named Timothy. He was a bundle of joy, and they were ecstatic to hear his infectious laugh. At twelve months of age, Tim developed an upper-respiratory infection with fever. The following morning, when Clara went to change his diaper and feed him, she found him having continuous seizures in his crib. They rushed him to the hospital, where only after great difficulty were they able to control his seizures. Following discharge from the hospital, without a definitive diagnosis, but a suspected unproven mitochondrial disorder, they watched in dismay Tim's regression. He lost his ability to walk, stand, or sit and could no longer mouth the few words he had achieved. Intractable seizures supervened again; he became drowsy, was admitted to a hospital, lapsed into a coma, and died at seventeen months of age.

At a consultation with a geneticist, they again revisited the potential autosomal recessive mode of inheritance associated with a 25 percent risk of recurrence. With the loss of Yvette and Tim in mind, the discussion turned to other options should they decide to try and have another child. Since the plan would be to avert a gene contribution from either Andrew or Clara, the first option was to have a sperm donor. Andrew, however, was strenuously opposed to that plan and insisted that he wished to have his genes in a future child. The second option was to obtain a randomly chosen egg donor. This choice would remove the theoretical question that Clara was transmitting a mitochondrial disorder or a recessive gene. At that consultation, the geneticist discussed all of the issues, including a lack of a definitive diagnosis and that by choosing a random egg donor, their future risk for having a child affected like Yvette or Tim would be negligible.

Many months later, they chose the egg-donor option and were fortunate to be the recipients of a healthy donor who had a normal, disease-free history and was in good health. Using in vitro fertilization with the donor egg and Andrew's sperm, pregnancy was achieved, and a healthy seven-pound-eight-ounce girl was delivered after an uneventful pregnancy. Their daughter, Alexandra, thrived and achieved her milestones throughout her first ten months of age. At eleven months, she developed a slight fever and tested positive for influenza type A. Within twenty-four hours, Alexandra developed intractable seizures and was rushed to the pediatric intensive-care unit at the local hospital. The seizures were controlled, and a suspected diagnosis of viral encephalitis was considered, but not confirmed. During the hospitalization, Alexandra quickly lost her ability to stand, to sit, or to reach out for a toy. Andrew and Clara were overwhelmed with the incredible thought that they were confronting tragedy yet again. However, Alexandra recovered and was able to sit again and put toys in her mouth, smiling and laughing at interactions with her parents and strangers, and they felt relieved. Biochemical and genetic studies, even more extensive than the ones for Yvette and Tim, were done but again failed to provide a clear diagnosis. A mitochondrial disorder was again thought likely, but not able to be confirmed. Imaging studies of her brain were originally normal, and repeat imaging revealed mildly abnormal changes in Alexandra's gray matter of her brain, the findings of which were considered to possibly result from her intractable continuous seizures at the time.

Over the ensuing weeks, Alexandra remained floppy and had to be supported with pillows when sitting. It also became difficult to feed her, and there was the need to insert a nasogastric tube into her stomach for one week, after which she began eating solids again. However, after she developed a cough with a slight fever, generalized continuous seizures began again. In hospital, she rapidly deteriorated, developed liver failure, became comatose, and died. The autopsy revealed the cause of death to be liver failure but did not determine the fundamental cause of the disorder. Liver tissue was immediately frozen for DNA studies. At this time, advances in human genetics enabled the analysis of other mitochondrial genes. Analysis of Alexandra's DNA revealed that she had inherited a gene mutation in the *POLG1* mitochondrial gene from her father and, incredibly, a mutation in the same gene from the egg donor!

Andrew and Clara sued the geneticist for misleading them by describing their future risk of recurrence as negligible.

Pertinent Medical Facts

Mitochondria are tiny organelles, each containing thirty-seven genes, that float around in the liquid (cytoplasm) surrounding the nucleus in all of our cells. In addition, as many as two thousand or more mitochondrial genes are located *within* the nucleus of every cell. Generally, mitochondria are responsible for the production of the energy that the cell needs to survive and fulfill a key role in the body's chemistry. A defect in the mitochondria results in the body's inability to properly turn food into energy. Since mitochondrial genes, whether they are in the cytoplasm or in the nucleus, are so vital to the chemical function of every cell in the body, mild to fatal illness can occur if certain mutations are present. Occurrence and severity depend mainly upon the mutation present, the mode of inheritance, and the action of modifying genes (e.g., from a partner).

Mitochondria in the cytoplasm come directly from the mother and will be present in every one of her children. Hence, there is 100 percent risk that each one of her children will be affected if she is affected, even mildly. Nuclear mitochondrial genes with their mutations are transmitted just like other genes, according to the hereditary pattern: dominant, recessive, or sex-linked. Someone who harbors a dominant *single* gene with a mutation has a 50 percent risk of transmitting it to each of his or her offspring. Andrew and their egg donor each carried a gene mutation that was silent alone but together combined as a recessive disorder that led to Alexandra's death. In sex-linked disorders, the usual situation is that a female is a carrier of a specific gene mutation. Then there is a 50 percent risk a son will be affected and a 50 percent risk that a daughter will be a usually unaffected carrier, just like the mother. Mitochondrial disorders typically cause multisystem disease.

Yvette and Tim tragically inherited an undetermined mutation in the *POLG1* gene from both Andrew and Clara. No test for this gene mutation was available at the time. Genetic advances had occurred around the time of Alexandra's illness and death, which led to the discovery of a mutation in the *POLG1* gene from both her father and the randomly selected egg donor.

Today, DNA analysis allows for straightforward diagnosis of the mitochondrial disorder that killed these three beautiful children.

As many as 1 in 70 people of European ancestry may carry one of at least twenty-four mutations in the *POLG1* gene. This would mean that the randomly chosen egg donor possibly had about a 1-in-70 risk of being a carrier, and that, combined with Andrew's mutation, there was a 1-in-560 risk that an affected offspring would be conceived—a 0.36 percent risk.

Certain mutations in the *POLG1* gene act as a dominantly inherited disorder, where a carrier of a single mutation has a 50 percent risk of transmitting the condition to each of his or her offspring. The mutation subsequently found in Andrew and Clara, as well as the egg donor, was recessive, not a dominantly transmittable one.

Questions

- Was the geneticist culpable of medical negligence in stating that Andrew and Clara's risk of having an affected third child was *negligible*?

- Was the geneticist responsible in any way for them choosing to have a third child, when the risk was low, but not zero?

Commentary

Communicating genetic information to couples who have an increased risk of having a child with a genetic disorder requires careful choice of words and attention to body language. A strong, positive emphasis that there is a 75 percent likelihood of a healthy outcome can influence a couple's strong desire to have a child despite the actual risk of 25 percent for an autosomal recessive disorder. Raised eyebrows, a grimace, and other body language by the geneticist may also influence a couple's thinking and have unintended consequences. Descriptors for risks such as "low" or "high," "uncertain," or "unlikely" may serve to confound decisions by prospective parents. None of us have negligible risks when it comes to childbearing. How risk is perceived varies greatly. I have had patients who thought that they had a 50 percent risk of having an affected child but were relieved that their risk was *only* 25 percent! Others, who thought they had no risk, felt overwhelmed to hear that their risk was *only* about 10 percent.

The standard of expected care was for the geneticist to inform the parents that the cause of the illness that took the lives of Yvette and Tim was unknown and was possibly recessive, with a 25 percent risk of recurrence, and that there were no available tests at the time to determine their carrier status or to provide prenatal genetic diagnosis. This he did and with a clear explanation. Given that all couples have a 3–4 percent risk of bearing a child with a major birth defect, intellectual disability, or a genetic disorder, was it negligent for him to have described their future risks as negligible, when their actual *additional* risk approximated 0.36 percent? Remarkably, the court decided that 75 percent of the responsibility in this case would be apportioned to the parents and 25 percent to the geneticist. I doubt that neither the physicians nor the judge didn't know they didn't know.

THE PRESCRIBER

Alice did not really know what happened. She vaguely recalled sitting in class and feeling light-headed. Her next memory was waking up in the hospital with a needle in her arm and a fluid dripping through into her vein from the suspended container. At her bedside was her mother, who explained to the teenager that her teacher had reported Alice having a major convulsion. Her friends told her mother that Alice had fallen to the floor from her desk, her arms and legs shaking and twitching, and that she had wet herself. They could not wake her immediately, while they waited for the emergency medical services.

During the few days in the hospital, an extensive battery of tests were done and ordered, including brain imaging and an electroencephalogram (EEG) to study her brain waves. All the tests done then and subsequently yielded no clues to the cause of her seizure, including brain imaging and genetic tests, except for slight abnormalities found in her brain waves. Her physicians concluded that she had *idiopathic* epilepsy, being unable to determine any definitive cause for her seizures. In particular, she had no family history of epilepsy, intellectual disability, or known genetic disorder. Carefully considered was the fact that Alice was born premature at thirty-five to thirty-six weeks of pregnancy, was small for her gestational age (three pounds fourteen ounces), and her mother was subject to a long labor. Alice had spent her first week of life in the neonatal intensive-care unit.

Subsequently, Alice thrived, grew well, gained weight, and participated in sports. Early on, she needed glasses and was found to have a mild learning disability for which she was given additional attention in school. The anticonvulsant medication she received was discontinued after two years, during which she had no seizures. She completed high school and went to work in a retail store. However, not long after starting her new job, Alice had another major seizure. The decision, this time, was to keep her on continuous anticonvulsant treatment for her epilepsy. Repeated tests again showed nothing more than a mildly abnormal EEG.

Soon after Alice's nineteenth birthday, she met and married Colin, a coworker. She continued to see her neurologist every four to six months, continuing the antiepileptic medication (valproic acid/Depakote) that seemed to keep her seizure free. About eighteen months after their wedding, they decided to start a family. Her closest friend from high school recommended her own obstetrician. Alice promptly made an appointment, at which time she filled out the necessary medical information, indicating that she had seizures. She also provided the name of her neurologist. Her obstetrician did a physical and genital examination, declared her healthy, and wished her good luck. In particular, he was encouraging that epilepsy was no bar to healthy pregnancy. He promised that when she became pregnant, he would monitor her blood pressure, blood sugar, and urine to be sure that all went well.

Alice returned three months later, having missed two menstrual periods and having tested herself to confirm that she was indeed pregnant. Alice did tell her obstetrician that in the past three months, she had had another grand mal seizure and that her neurologist had increased her dose of Depakote (valproic acid). Her obstetrician retorted that he was leaving the treatment of her epilepsy to her neurologist. The ultrasound study that he did on her first visit revealed that she was between ten and eleven weeks pregnant and that everything looked good. Alice declined maternal serum screening, specifically for disorders like spina bifida (called "neural tube defects") or Down syndrome because "she would not abort her pregnancy." He recommended she start taking a daily prenatal multivitamin.

At about thirty-four weeks along in her pregnancy, Alice noted that her womb had become much bigger than expected. During her next visit, an ultrasound showed an excess of the amniotic fluid surrounding the developing fetus. To her dismay, however, the ultrasonographer immediately told her that the fetus had a lump protruding from the lower back, which was probably a birth defect called spina bifida. Her obstetrician concurred, and she rushed home in tears, not even hearing him talk about the need for spine surgery directly after birth. Alice was completely inconsolable and in so much fear and distress that she could not return to work. Some ten days later, her membranes ruptured prematurely, and she went into labor, delivering their son, whom they named Bruce.

Immediately after birth, the lump on Bruce's back was covered with a sterile pack, and he was taken

directly to surgery. The purpose was to repair the defect and close the leak, which was cerebrospinal fluid.

The nurses told Alice and Colin that Bruce was not moving his legs.

Less than three months after the surgical closure of Bruce's spina bifida, his pediatrician noticed that his

head circumference was progressively becoming larger. Alice described that horrible weekend when

Bruce began vomiting, becoming drowsy, and his soft spot (anterior fontanel) seemed to be bulging. They

rushed him to the hospital, where it was immediately recognized that the pressure in his head had risen

precipitously. Imaging of his brain showed that his cerebral ventricles were markedly dilated and that he had

the diagnosis of hydrocephalus. Urgent neurosurgery was called for, and a tube was inserted into his brain

and threaded down into his abdomen (called a ventriculo-peritoneal shunt) that enabled decompression of

his brain. The neurosurgeon warned Alice and Colin that the V-P shunt would have to be replaced as Bruce

grew and that there was a risk that infection could complicate management in the future. Sure enough, when

Bruce was almost two years of age, infection of his shunt supervened, and he

developed meningitis, which required extensive treatment and hospitalization. Fortunately, he recovered

but later was found to have developed some hearing impairment as well as a learning disorder.

The original nurse's observation about Bruce's legs was accurate. Bruce was paraplegic, being unable to

move his legs at all, with markedly impaired sensation and no control of his bladder and bowel.

Alice and Colin sued both the neurologist and the obstetrician for their negligent care before Bruce was

conceived.

<u>Pertinent Medical Facts</u>

The brain and spinal cord develop together in the early embryo. The brain growth dictates the

development and size of the skull. If there is a failure of brain growth, the skull hardly forms, a condition

called anencephaly. The spine develops as a flat tissue that quickly folds into a tubelike structure

enclosing the spinal cord. This neural tube closes between twenty-six and twenty-nine days after conception. A failure to close anywhere along its length leaves an opening in the spine that allows spinal nerves to protrude and form a sac with cerebrospinal fluid on the back. The lower back is involved most often. The skin is stretched over the sac and may crack, allowing cerebrospinal fluid to leak out (called open spina bifida). If the gap in the spine is not closed immediately, infection almost invariably occurs and results in meningitis and possible death. Often, the surgical closure of the gap leads to accumulation of cerebrospinal fluid in the brain (called hydrocephalus), resulting in increased pressure and possible brain damage, if not promptly relieved.

The fetal liver produces a particular protein called alpha-fetoprotein (AFP), which exists at much higher concentrations in the fetus compared to the mother. If there is any leak from the fetal blood or spinal fluid, AFP enters the mother's bloodstream. Her AFP level then rises and can be detected by a test around sixteen weeks of pregnancy, called the maternal serum AFP screen. This is the screen that Alice declined. An elevation in that protein level would have immediately led to ultrasound imaging, which would have revealed the spina bifida. The options, however, at that point in pregnancy would have been termination of pregnancy or continuation until near term, at which time the possibility of high-risk surgical closure while the fetus was still in the womb was possible. At that time, there was little experience with that approach, which is much improved today.

In 1989, we published a seminal paper in the *Journal of the American Medical Association* showing that women who took folic-acid supplements during the three months prior to becoming pregnant and for the first three months after conception had a 70 percent protection against this birth defect developing. That study was heralded by the *New York Times* in November 1989, with a front-page heading about our study, which involved almost twenty-four thousand pregnant women. Subsequently, a few years later, the Medical Research Council in England confirmed our original observations. Since that time, women the world over are advised to take folic-acid supplements when *planning* a pregnancy. In our study, we also showed that sitting in a hot Jacuzzi or using a sauna in the first six weeks of pregnancy leads to a two to three times greater risk of having a child with spina bifida. The risk for a mother on Depakote having a child with a birth defect approximates 11 percent. The risk of autism is up to five times higher than those

mothers not on medication.

The cause of spina bifida or anencephaly is regarded as a birth defect in which multiple genes interact

with environmental factors such as folic acid or where the mother has severe uncontrolled diabetes. The

recurrence rate in a subsequent pregnancy is 3–5 percent.

The complications and consequences of being born with spina bifida can be devastating. Follow-up

studies up to the age of thirty-eight years have revealed a very sad outcome for many. In a group of 117

with spina bifida, 21 percent had died by the age of one year, 41 percent had died by the age of sixteen,

and 48 percent had died by the age of twenty-five. The treatment of hydrocephalus by ventriculo-

peritoneal shunting had been required by 87 percent, 6 percent were blind, 32 percent had intellectual

disability, 17 percent had epilepsy, 75 percent were incontinent of urine and 30 percent incontinent of

feces, 51 percent were wheelchair bound, 48 percent needed lifelong continuous care, 46 percent had

chronic pressure sores, and 33 percent of survivors developed obesity. Only 7 percent had little or no

disability and were able to walk. Sadly, researchers in Seattle noted the remarkable rate of abandonment

by the parents of children with spina bifida. That is an awful commentary on our ability to care for the

handicapped. It also points to how simple omissions in the care of patients may have disastrous and

lifelong consequences.

Questions

- Why did both the neurologist and the obstetrician not inform Alice about the risk of birth defects
  due to the Depakote if she became pregnant?
- Why did the obstetrician not communicate with the neurologist about their shared patient and the
  treatment and administration of a drug with potentially serious consequences for fetal
  malformation?

- Why did the obstetrician not prescribe folic-acid (vitamin B) tablets to be taken daily just in case an unplanned pregnancy occurred?

Commentary

The standard of expected care for the prescribing neurologist was to warn a woman in her reproductive years of the potential birth-defect risks related to any prescribed medication should she become pregnant. That communication should have been documented in the patient's record. Alice's obstetrician, knowing she was taking this medication prior to her becoming pregnant, should have also warned her of the potential risks. He could also have pointed out that an ultrasound study at sixteen to eighteen weeks of pregnancy would have enabled the detection of most serious structural defects of the fetus. His lack of insistence about this was likely tempered by Alice's clear statement that she would not terminate a pregnancy.

Alice was not advised to take the daily folic-acid tablets (0.4–0.8 mg/day). It is still uncertain, however, if folic acid taken by a pregnant patient on Depakote would provide any protection against the development of spina bifida. At present, it is wise for all women to take folic acid daily if there is any possibility of pregnancy. Physicians are typically wary of prescribing medications that have the potential of causing birth defects. An uncommon, but real, pitfall is providing prescription medications that have the potential to cause birth defects in women who are not pregnant or who insist they have no plan to become pregnant or are teenagers. Almost always, physicians will warn of the risks to the fetus due to the effects of the medication. The problem, however, is that 50 percent of pregnancies are unplanned. One study of 1,144 women with epilepsy reported that 78.9 percent had at least one unintended pregnancy.

Physicians who prescribe these teratogenic medications need to document, in the patient's record, that they have provided the necessary warnings. None of the anticonvulsant medications are risk-free, but a few have much lower risks than Depakote. Women with epilepsy who plan their pregnancy need to change their medication, if necessary, prior to becoming pregnant. Making a change during pregnancy risks precipitating seizures that could be harmful to the fetus and the mother. Taking a single anticonvulsant is safer than two drugs. Depakote alone is associated with about three times the average risk of having a child with birth defects.

Two additional examples serve to illustrate the wider problem.

Women who have had a deep vein thrombosis, most commonly in the leg, receive an anticoagulant, most often in the Coumadin (Warfarin) group of drugs. This particular medication has an affinity for developing cartilage in the fetus, including cartilage that forms the nose. One consequence of fetal exposure is the child being born with a single nostril. Other abnormalities may occur and include defects of the bones, brain, and eyes. For the most part, treatment may last for six weeks to three months, but if the thrombosis is recurrent, the prescription may last for a much longer period to avoid the potential fatal pulmonary embolism (a clot in the lungs that may cause death).

Another medication, used as a cream for the treatment of acne, is isotretinoin (Accutane). Absorption of this medication through the skin is sufficient to damage the early developing fetus. Results may include tiny, malformed, or even absent ears; some facial abnormalities; as well as heart and brain defects. Instances are known when a teenager has borrowed the medication from her friend after seeing the excellent results it had in resolving the friend's facial acne. Needless to say, the borrowed item never came with the warning from the physician not to use du ring pregnancy. Teenage pregnancy is not a rarity.

Intercommunications between physicians and other health-care providers have become more complex and demanding. One large study of Medicare claims revealed that a typical primary-care doctor coordinates the care of patients with 229 other physicians. Communications during shared care between physicians is vitally important but recognized as often lacking. The use of the electronic medical record is unlikely to remedy this deficiency. Interpersonal direct communication remains the surest and safest way when patient care is shared.

Alice and Colin were left to care for their severely disabled son. Both the doctors, who may have cared, didn't know, they didn't know. They were both found to have been negligent and guilty of medical malpractice.

In 2017, France banned the prescription of Depakote for women of childbearing age or when pregnant. In Paris, the association of "Depakote victims" has filed a class-action suit against the pharmaceutical giant company Sanofi-Aventis France. A compensation fund has been established by France's National Office for Medical Accidents Compensation that projects payments for at least 10,290 affected children.

MURDER?

Patricia and David Stallings had eagerly awaited the birth of their son, Ryan. They had planned to move into their new house a few weeks before his birth. Pregnancy was uneventful, as were labor and delivery. Ryan was a beautiful baby, and happiness ruled. Within days of Ryan's birth, he vomited up his bottle-fed formula but then seemed to improve. This pattern continued for about three months. Then one morning they found him listless in his crib, breathing heavily and staring. Patricia and David quickly rushed off to the hospital with Ryan, and the nightmare began.

Multiple tests were done in the emergency department, and the report of one key test for toxins revealed that Ryan had high levels of ethylene glycol (a component of antifreeze) in his blood. Guided by legal requirements, the pediatrician receiving the results, called the Missouri division of Family Services, reporting his conclusion that Ryan appeared to have been poisoned. Family Services, given that warning, took custody of Ryan and placed him with a foster family after discharge from the hospital. Patricia and David were devastated. Patricia was allowed to visit her son once a week and give him his bottle. Subsequently she learned that three days after feeding Ryan, he had been hospitalized again but knew nothing else. Without warning, police materialized at her home, handcuffed her, and placed her under arrest. Only when she reached the police station was she told that Ryan had died. Patricia was then charged with the murder of Ryan due, they said, to her having poisoned him during her last visit. Again, they said that ethylene glycol was found on his baby bottle that she had used to feed him while he was in foster care. She remained in jail for the next seven months, while the legal process grinded on.

While in jail, Patricia discovered that she was pregnant again and was beside herself with sadness. Meanwhile, the newly appointed prosecuting attorney, George B. McElroy III, found a half gallon of antifreeze in the basement of the couple's home. Two independent laboratories had confirmed high levels of ethylene glycol in Ryan's body. An autopsy also showed crystals in Ryan's brain, further suggesting

that he had succumbed to ethylene-glycol poisoning.

Patricia's attorney was not able to find any expert witness to testify on her behalf. Nor did he depose any

of the state's experts. Prosecutor McElroy instructed the jury not to be concerned about motive but rather

focus on the fact that there was no rational explanation for the laboratory results except deliberate

poisoning. As a consequence, the jury verdict was first-degree murder. The judge sentenced Patricia to

spend the rest of her life in prison without the possibility of parole. You can imagine the emotional

devastation felt by Patricia upon hearing that verdict.

Patricia gave birth to her son, David Jr., in prison, and he was promptly placed in foster care. Press reports

began to circulate that David Jr. had a rare biochemical genetic disease called methylmalonic acidemia

(MMA). McElroy obviously became aware of this information.

About six months later, McElroy made a remarkable move by asking the judge to retry Patricia's case,

stating that Patricia's defense was seriously inadequate. The judge was startled by this precedent-setting

motion by a prosecutor recognizing the ineffective defense that Patricia had experienced. The prosecuting

attorney had paid attention to press reports that had focused on Patricia's second son, David, and his

diagnosis of MMA.

In the interim, one of the original toxicology laboratories provided a small sample of Ryan's blood to

biochemical geneticists at St. Louis University, where one of my colleagues, Professor William S. Sly,

professor and chairman of the Department of Biochemistry and Molecular Biology, got involved. There

was considerable argument and discussion within that department about whether the original results were

valid. Most of the senior staff members concluded that Ryan had probably been poisoned. However,

Professor Sly, who had other tests performed on the stored blood sample, concluded that there was no

ethylene glycol in Ryan's blood. He did find high levels of organic acids, confirming the diagnosis of methylmalonic acidemia and pointed out that those chemical compounds could be confused with ethylene glycol in the method (gas chromatography) that was used.

To the credit of the prosecuting attorney, he sought further expertise by consulting with an outstanding biochemical geneticist who at that time was at Yale University. Dr. Piero Rinaldo, internationally known for his expertise in biochemical genetics, confirmed the findings of Professor Sly. It was then realized that Ryan had died from MMA and not from ethylene-glycol poisoning. Dr. Rinaldo went on to blast the chemistry laboratories for their incompetence and to criticize the pathetic defense that failed to find experts to challenge the position of the prosecuting attorney. Additionally, he went on to criticize the hospital staff, who had incorrectly treated Ryan for his MMA. In fact, his view was that the treatment actually contributed to Ryan's death! He also explained that the crystallization that had occurred in Ryan's brain was almost certainly the direct result of the intravenous treatment the hospital physicians had used to treat Ryan for his alleged ethylene-glycol poisoning. Thereupon, Prosecutor McElroy, recognizing the grievous error made in the prosecution of Patricia, immediately sought her dismissal and release from prison.

Patricia and David were left to care for their surviving son, David Jr., facing the considerable difficulty in managing his biochemical genetic disorder. They filed a wrongful-death lawsuit against the hospital and the laboratories involved, as well as against the doctors who erred in the care of their deceased son, Ryan. At that time, I was contacted by an attorney of behalf of the commercial laboratory involved to determine whether I could lend my expertise in this case. Given my insufficient expertise about the chemical methods and their limitations used to demonstrate the presence of the alleged poison, I declined involvement.

Patricia and David's second son, David Jr., was quickly returned to them from foster care where he had been placed after his birth. He continued to need his treatment for MMA, but after a protracted struggle, he died at twenty-three years of age.

Pertinent Medical Facts

Methylmalonic acidemia (MMA) is a serious biochemical genetic disorder that results from the transmission of a mutation in a single gene contributed by each parent equally. The mode of inheritance for almost all affected is autosomal recessive, carrier parents having a 25 percent risk in every pregnancy of having a child with MMA. It occurs in about one in twenty thousand newborns. MMA interferes with the body's ability to digest specific fats and proteins, resulting in a toxic accumulation of methylmalonic acid in the blood and potentially fatal levels of ammonia. Within weeks to months after birth, a multitude of symptoms and signs may become evident, including feeding difficulties, vomiting, development of anemia, recurrent infections, failure to gain weight, developmental delay, kidney failure, seizures, respiratory distress, stroke, coma, and death. Children who respond to vitamin B_{12} treatment and a very low-protein diet may survive but also may have intellectual disability. However, kidney failure is common in the first ten years of life. In unresponsive patients whose lives hang in the balance, kidney or liver transplantation can result in long-term survival.

Three genes have been recognized as having mutations that cause this disorder. Once a mutation is recognized, future prenatal diagnosis or preimplantation genetic diagnosis is possible. Patricia and David, deprived of the opportunity to discover Ryan's disorder, unwittingly had a 25 percent risk of having a second child affected. Prenatal therapy has also been successful in cases responsive to vitamin B_{12} administered by intramuscular injection or given by mouth to the mother. There are reports where prenatal therapy was provided in a timely fashion, and infants were born with the disorder but were healthy and appeared to develop normally.

Questions

- Was it really necessary for the pediatrician to report his suspicion about child abuse and poisoning to the Missouri Family Services, which began this catastrophic chain of events?

- Did the prosecuting attorney do due diligence in pursuing Patricia Stallings and charging her with murder, relishing the spotlight, only to apologize later about his error?

- Why did McElroy not find Dr. Piero Rinaldi and Professor William Sly *before* ruining the lives of Patricia and David Stallings?

- Were the hospital physicians culpable of medical negligence by treating Ryan for ethylene-glycol poisoning and thereby causing or hastening his death?

- What happened to the laboratory whose results ultimately led to Ryan's incorrect diagnosis, inappropriate treatment, and death?

- Why did the defense attorney for Patricia Stallings do such a pathetic job and not reach these experts who were subsequently found by the relenting prosecuting attorney?

- Was it possible to have the life of their first son saved, and would he have been normal and healthy with appropriate treatment?

Commentary

The pediatrician who reported his suspicion of ethylene-glycol poisoning of Ryan was required by law to report his suspicion directly to the state Family Services. This required reporting system arose after it had become clear that some cases of child abuse and neglect went unreported and children died. However, there is another psychiatric disorder, termed "Munchausen syndrome by proxy," which is always considered in cases of possible child abuse. This term usually applies to a mother or caregiver who lies and exaggerates health issues in the children under their care, aiming to gain attention or sympathy for themselves. This thought process was a concern in the early stages of this case.

McElroy was a young, inexperienced prosecutor, but given the weight of the office he occupied, he had the wherewithal to fully investigate and find the true experts who could have blown this case apart and who subsequently did. One wonders how much he relished the spotlight, which in turn blinded him from the awful reality of his case against an innocent mother. McElroy later ran for election in a Democratic primary, only to be defeated by his opponent, who received a $10,000 donation from Patricia Stallings!

No satisfactory excuse can be proffered for the hopeless effort by Patricia's defense attorney. He too could have found the true experts by simply calling professors of biochemistry around the country. Was he under the false assumption that he understood and could interpret the results, given that he had an undergraduate degree in biochemistry?

The judge in this case is also not beyond reproach. He ruled as inadmissible the fact that Ryan's *brother* had MMA and that Ryan had a one-in-four risk of also having this diagnosis. The lack of knowledge judges have of science and especially genetics is well recognized (see commentary in chapter 18). A major effort to remedy this deficiency came with the initial *Daubert* ruling in June 1993. That decision established criteria for federal courts to follow in admitting scientific evidence or excluding it from consideration by juries. That case hinged on the use of a medication (Bendectin) used for the treatment of morning sickness in pregnancy. The claim made was that this drug caused birth defects even though by then some thirty-three million pregnant women had used the drug over twenty-seven years. By that time, there had been thirty published epidemiologic studies that indicated that 130,000 women had taken Bendectin in early pregnancy, without any demonstrating a statistical association with birth defects. Even though the defendant pharmaceutical company Merrill Dow never had to pay, they withdrew the drug from the market because of the extraordinary cost of defending endless lawsuits.

The quintessential purpose of this ruling was to ensure that a judge was the gatekeeper who assured the scientific reliability and relevance of the evidence, including scientific methodology and knowledge, and allowed the judge access to independent experts for additional guidance. For this case, the judge did not seek independent scientific counsel.

The hospital physicians simply accepted the laboratory diagnosis and instituted treatment with ethanol that hastened or caused Ryan's death. It was incumbent for them to consider a differential diagnosis and do additional tests. That was exactly what Professor Sly did to make an accurate diagnosis of MMA. Practicing physicians continue to rely heavily on results of tests they order, including biochemical, imaging, and genetic test reports. The admonition to treat the patient, not the laboratory test, is even more pertinent today with so many advances, especially in genetics. Other sad examples are explored later in subsequent chapters.

The commercial laboratory that produced, interpreted, and reported the results of ethylene glycol in the submitted sample was eventually closed. The conclusion they made that the sample showed ethylene glycol was later demonstrated to be propionic acid! They never did apologize for the inaccuracy of their analytic method or for the grievous harm they vicariously inflicted on an innocent child and family.

The Stallings filed a wrongful-death suit against the laboratories, physicians, and hospital. They sought actual and punitive damages and claimed that these defendants knew *before trial* that Ryan's younger brother, David Jr., had MMA and refused to test Ryan for this disorder. Because of the defendant's incompetence, Ryan suffered and died; Patricia faced criminal prosecution for murder; and they lost custody of both children, had huge medical and legal expenses, lost earnings, and suffered damage to their reputations.

The abysmal actions of the laboratory, physicians, prosecuting attorney, defense attorney, *and* the judge were a profound reflection of systemic incompetence. None of these actors had any idea that they didn't know, they didn't know.

On the day the Stallings' wrongful-death suit was scheduled for trial, a settlement in the millions was reached. McElroy later stated that it was impossible to make restitution for what happened to Patricia Stallings. Amen!

THE ORDER

Sam and Josie were the proud parents of two lovely daughters, and they felt their family was complete. Nevertheless, after Josie suddenly missed two menstrual periods, they realized that an unplanned pregnancy was in progress. The little concern they had related to the family history of cystic fibrosis in one of Sam's nieces. With this information, his doctor ordered a cystic-fibrosis carrier test, the result of which showed that Sam was a cystic-fibrosis gene-mutation carrier. This result led directly to his doctor's recommendation that he and Josie go for a genetics consultation.

At that consultation, following genetic counseling, the geneticist obtained a blood sample for DNA analysis, which quickly showed that Josie too was a cystic-fibrosis gene-mutation carrier. This meant that they had a 25 percent risk of having an affected child with this chronic, life-threatening disorder.

Sam and Josie were close to Sam's sister, whose daughter had cystic fibrosis. They had watched her continuing battle with chronic lung infections, multiple hospitalizations, intravenous antibiotics, constant pill-taking, and severely limited energy. They needed very little description of the disorder and its implications for an affected child and his or her parents.

The availability of prenatal genetic diagnosis for cystic fibrosis was explained by the geneticist. By that time, Josie had reached sixteen weeks of pregnancy, and they elected to have prenatal studies via amniocentesis. The geneticist referred them to an experienced obstetrician in a local hospital with the specific request that an amniocentesis be done for prenatal genetic studies for cystic fibrosis. The procedure was done without eventuality, and the sample of amniotic fluid was sent to the genetics laboratory.

After the amniotic-fluid cells had grown in cell culture, the cells were harvested, and the chromosomes were analyzed. Three weeks later, the geneticist called the referring doctor's office to report that the chromosome analysis and the alpha-fetoprotein test (for spina bifida) were normal. The doctor's nurse called Josie to tell her that the prenatal test results were *normal.*

Some six months later, the geneticist received a very angry telephone call from an extremely upset Josie. I was the geneticist! How was it possible, she asked, that Ariel's doctors were telling her that her newborn daughter has cystic fibrosis, after I had specifically recommended the prenatal studies and reported a normal result? Her daughter had been born about two weeks prematurely and had meconium ileus (the very first bowel movement is called meconium and, in cystic fibrosis, can be extremely tough and sticky, resulting in total obstruction of the bowel). Staggered by Josie's call, I asked her to remain on the line while I retrieved the medical chart. It only took a few minutes for me to return to the call with the file in hand. My heart was pounding, my mind was racing, and my thoughts were focused on the anguish these parents must have been experiencing. I also reflected momentarily and wistfully that an impeccable record lasting many decades was about to be trashed.

I opened the file and read the requisition order to Josie on the telephone. The test ordered was a chromosome analysis and alpha-fetoprotein assay (for spina bifidia). There was no order to perform the cystic-fibrosis gene analysis. In the clinical information section, there were a few words that simply stated family history of cystic fibrosis. Josie was speechless. She reminded me that I had sent her to the specialist obstetrician who had extensive experience with the amniocentesis procedure, while she continued with her regular obstetrician for routine care. I confirmed that the normal chromosome report was sent to the obstetrician who performed the amniocentesis, as well as to her regular obstetrician. Josie asked why we did not perform the cystic-fibrosis test, given that the words "family history of cystic fibrosis" appeared on the requisition form. I responded that the laboratory staff simply followed the physician's order to perform chromosome analysis and the alpha-fetoprotein test. It was not unusual for families to have a prenatal test without committing to terminating a pregnancy or simply decide not to have the test at all despite the family history. It was purely logical for the chromosome study to be done, given the maternal age of thirty-five.

The next communication I received was from Sam and Josie's lawyers with the notice that I and the

nonprofit Center for Human Genetics laboratories had been sued for medical negligence.

Pertinent Medical Facts

Cystic fibrosis is a multisystem, chronic, and life-threatening disease that is inherited as an autosomal

recessive disorder. This means that each parent carries a mutation in the cystic-fibrosis gene (*CFTR*) and

that there is a 25 percent risk that each offspring will receive a mutation from each parent and therefore be

affected. About one in twenty-five whites, one in forty-six blacks, and one in sixty-five Asians carry a

mutation in the cystic-fibrosis gene. Between one in twenty-five hundred and one in three thousand

whites are born with this recessive disorder. Cystic fibrosis primarily involves the lungs, the digestive

system (including the pancreas, intestine, and gallbladder), and the genital system in males. Lifelong

treatment is required, often with frequent hospitalizations and antibiotic treatment. Because of the

associated malabsorption of food, pancreatic-enzyme supplements are required to be taken with every

meal. Chest physiotherapy is a constant need. Males with cystic fibrosis are almost always infertile, but

not sterile. The vas deferens (the tube that transports sperm from the testes out via the penis) is poorly

developed or obstructed. The condition is termed "congenital bilateral absence of the vas deferens." Males

with this disorder can still sire children, but since they are likely to harbor two cystic-fibrosis gene

mutations, sequencing of the entire gene of their partner is mandatory. Sperm can be recovered by

needling the testes (a process called epididymal sperm aspiration).

More than two thousand mutations have been reported in the *CFTR* gene. Based initially on a specific

gene mutation, a pharmacogenetic approach has led to the discovery and use of two new drugs that

facilitate the transfer of ions across cell walls and alleviate some of the lung problems. Side effects are a

nuisance, and the cost is staggering ($300,000 per year). Long-term efficacy is still to be determined.

Questions

- How was it possible that a maternal-fetal-medicine specialist, to whom a patient had been

  referred for an amniocentesis specifically to determine whether the fetus had cystic fibrosis, did

  not order the required test on the requisition form that accompanied the sample?

- Why did the nurse who knew, or should have known, about the reason for the prenatal test inform

  Josie that the fetus was normal, without mentioning cystic fibrosis?

- Why did the obstetrician, who did the amniocentesis and who received the laboratory report of

  normal chromosomes, not recognize that the reason for the amniocentesis, cystic fibrosis

  exclusion, was not reflected in the normal chromosome report?

- Why did Josie's regular obstetrician not recognize that the normal chromosome report that he

  received did not refer to cystic fibrosis?

Commentary

Sam and Josie, filled with anguish and anger, filed a wrongful birth lawsuit on behalf of their daughter. They named both obstetricians, the laboratory, and me. The sad trail of carelessness combined with ignorance became clear on legal discovery.

As part of the procedure of amniocentesis, a careful ultrasound is performed to check on the structural integrity of the fetus as well as the location of vital parts and the placenta. The ultrasonographer did the ultrasound, which was followed by, and under ultrasound guidance, the amniocentesis itself. The procedure was impeccable, the amniotic fluid was clear, and the tube was appropriately labeled. The ultrasonographer completed the requisition form and ordered the chromosome and alpha-fetoprotein tests (to detect spina bifida). Even though she knew that the amniocentesis was being done for cystic fibrosis, she forgot to order the test. The obstetrician failed to look at the requisition form, which was then dispatched with the sample to our nonprofit Center for Human Genetics laboratory.

Upon receipt of the amniotic-fluid sample in the genetics laboratory, the coordinator responsible for allocating an accession number for the sample, as well as logging it into the computer system, was unaware that these patients had been seen for genetic counseling. She noted the family history of cystic fibrosis but simply followed the written order to perform only chromosome and alpha-fetoprotein analysis. Later, she said that it was not very unusual for couples to have a prenatal test simply to be prepared for what may come, but not be interested in pregnancy termination.

The analysis was duly performed, and the result was reported to the obstetrician who performed the amniocentesis. The precise and critical message delivered to the obstetrician's office was taken by a nurse, who received the report that the chromosome and alpha-fetoprotein studies were normal. She, in turn, called Josie with the "good news" that the prenatal tests were *normal*. She never mentioned the words "cystic fibrosis." Shortly thereafter, the formal printed laboratory report, showing normal chromosomes and alpha-fetoprotein concentration, was sent to the obstetrician who performed the amniocentesis, as well as the patient's regular obstetrician.

Neither of the two doctors who received the printed report noticed that the words "cystic fibrosis" did not appear in the report. Worse still were the statements they both made in legal depositions that they thought a normal chromosome result would automatically exclude a diagnosis of cystic fibrosis! (This recessive disorder is a single-gene disease, not determinable by whole chromosome analysis.)

The painful lessons that emerged from this very sad saga were unfortunately not novel, in that once again, more than a single error occurred, with devastating consequences. Who knows why a very competent ultrasonographer was distracted, or had a break in concentration, and failed to fill in the requisition form appropriately? Why did the laboratory coordinator not think it necessary to enquire about the absence of a test order for cystic fibrosis? Assumptions made about life-threatening matters need concentrated thought. Especially worrisome in this case, however, was the sheer ignorance of the two obstetricians who had no idea that a normal chromosome report had nothing to do with cystic fibrosis and not diagnostic by that type of analysis.

Required continuing medical education is the only recourse that hopefully enables doctors to remain up to date given the enormous and continuing advances in medicine. All that it would have taken in this case beyond the knowledge required was a brief glance at the requisition form by the maternal-fetal-medicine specialist, which would have prevented a lifetime of suffering for Ariel. Just caring enough to *remind* the ultrasonographer about the purpose of the test would have been enough. Over and over again, the simplest errors have led to catastrophic consequences.

Maintenance of Certification examinations are required to be taken by physicians in most specialties. The purpose is to assess their medical knowledge, competence, diagnostic reasoning, and clinical judgment. These programs require physicians to also demonstrate professionalism, to participate in quality-improvement activities, and to promote lifelong learning.

The obstetricians sadly didn't know, they didn't know. The case against the two obstetricians was settled. The laboratory, registered as a public charity, was required to pay a nominal settlement. After two upsetting years, I was dismissed from the case.

THE CONNECTION

They watched in disbelief as their precious little Joey, who stood and took his first steps soon after nine months, seemed unable to stand without holding on at one year of age. Some weeks later, they told his pediatrician that even though he sat up unsupported just before he was six months of age, they now needed to provide support for him even while sitting; otherwise he would topple over. The physical examination showed him to be floppy and weak and confirmed his inability to stand, although he seemed able to sit unsupported. Compared to his sister, his mother said, Joey's development was much slower. He did not say "dada" or "mama," nor did he respond to his name. He had difficulty holding his bottle and was unable to use a pincer grasp to pick up a small toy piece. His doctor, reassuring his parents, said that the development of boys "was slower than girls," was very variable, and that he would "catch up." When they returned three months later, Joey had made very little progress. Joey's mother insisted that he should be seen by a neurologist.

On examination by the neurologist, Joey's weakness, lack of muscular tone, and weak to absent knee and elbow reflexes were painfully obvious. A blood sample was drawn and sent to a laboratory for measurement of a muscle enzyme called *creatine phosphokinase*. Joey's level was very high, confirming the neurologist's clinical diagnosis of muscular dystrophy. He promptly referred Joey to a clinical geneticist. That referral quickly led to DNA tests, which revealed that Joey had a deletion in the *Duchenne muscular dystrophy* (*DMD*) gene on his X chromosome. The terribly sad consultation that followed outlined the likely course of this genetic disorder.

Although Joey learned to walk, his weakness slowly became progressively worse, ascending from his legs upward. In addition, by three years of age, it was clear that he had significant intellectual disability as well as typical signs found in the autism-spectrum disorder. He had considerable self-stimulatory and self-abusive behavior, including hitting himself on the head to the point of developing bruises and cuts.

He tended to hit his head on the floor or walls and would bite his hands. He demonstrated many perseverative behaviors, which included tongue clicking and echolalia. Curiously, one unusual behavior he had was to cry when he heard someone cough.

His muscle weakness progressed throughout his childhood, leaving him wheelchair bound by the age of nine. The ensuing four years were marked by his suffering from complications that included contractures of his knees and ankles, curvature of his spine (scoliosis), sleep apnea, breathlessness at night, choking, and, at the age of twelve, the advent of seizures. He was profoundly thin and weak and, by fourteen years of age, required oxygen at night and had to wear a diaper. At fifteen years of age, he had difficulty taking enough calories, and a gastrostomy tube was placed into his stomach through his abdomen (G-tube). This was also when he had his first bout of pneumonia.

Complications continued to mount, including the development of pressure sores on his buttocks. At seventeen, with chronic respiratory failure, the decision was made to perform a tracheostomy and to connect him to a portable ventilator. Discussions with his parents at this time included consideration of a *do-not-resuscitate* order, which meant that if he stopped breathing, they would not resuscitate him. At this time, his scoliosis was extremely severe, leading him to be completely bent over. He was also having two or three seizures per month.

At nineteen, he tended to turn blue at night because of insufficient oxygen reaching his lungs despite the ventilator. His mother was taught to use an oximeter to assess his oxygen saturation and to perform chest compressions (CPR) when his oxygen levels dropped. She continued to consider the *do-not-resuscitate* order. At twenty, he was in awful condition, on a portable ventilator and G-tube dependent. Soon after his twentieth birthday, he went to the hospital to have attention to his G-tube, around which there was inflammation. When he was transferred from the waiting room to the procedure room, he was suddenly noticed to be blue and unresponsive. His nurse, who had accompanied him from home, suddenly realized that he had become disconnected from his ventilator when he was moved into the procedure room.

Because of the oxygen deprivation to his brain, repetitive seizures (called status epilepticus) began. Even after they were controlled by intravenous medication, Joey remained in the hospital and was unresponsive for the next six days, effectively in a coma, until his parents decided to withdraw his care. He was provided with morphine and died soon after.

Pertinent Medical Facts

DMD occurs in about one in forty-seven hundred live male births. Typical early signs, which Joey manifested, are often difficulties in sitting and standing. If a boy with DMD is already walking, he invariably develops a waddling gait and has difficulty climbing stairs. In fact, he may have difficulty standing up from sitting on the floor. The muscle weakness is progressive, and virtually all affected boys are wheelchair dependent by the age of thirteen. Involvement of the heart muscle becomes obvious by the age of eighteen, and heart failure or heart-rhythm abnormality may lead to death. More likely, because of the ascending weakness and involvement of the diaphragm, breathing becomes more difficult, and pneumonia may supervene. Many die by the age of twenty, and extremely few survive beyond thirty.

The mode of inheritance of DMD is sex-linked. About two-thirds of the time, mothers are carriers of the mutation in the *DMD* gene. The risk of having an affected boy when a mother is a carrier is 50 percent, and the risk of having a girl who would be a carrier of the gene mutation is also 50 percent. The culprit gene is responsible for making a protein called dystrophin, which curiously functions not only in muscle but also in the brain. In about 60–70 percent of cases, there is a tiny deletion (which Joey had) within the very large *DMD* gene, or, in 5–10 percent, there is a tiny duplication within that same gene. As a consequence of the malfunctioning muscle due to the abnormally made dystrophin from the defective *DMD* gene, an enzyme called *CPK* (*creatine phosphokinase*) leaks out of the muscle cells into the bloodstream, where it is measurable and markedly elevated in the vast number of affected boys and at least 50 percent of carrier females.

The sisters of a carrier mother should all be tested to determine their carrier status. Women who are carriers are also at risk of heart-muscle involvement, leading to heart failure or a potential fatal rhythm disturbance of the heart. They should be seen annually by a cardiologist. They may also notice calf-muscle weakness and complain of muscle cramps. To prevent a range of potential different complications, huge efforts are necessary over the lifetime of an affected boy that include attention to lungs, heart, nutrition, muscles, bones, and the psychological issues, which weigh heavily on both the affected boy and his parents and siblings.

Unfortunately, just as with Joey, intellectual disability in affected boys with DMD is common and varies from mild to moderate. Moreover, there is an increased frequency of autism-spectrum disorder, as was the case with Joey. Problems with memory and executive function affect most. About 6 percent of boys with DMD also have seizures.

Sadly, despite huge efforts, a real, safe, and effective treatment that clearly extends the life-span of those with DMD has yet to be discovered. Corticosteroids have proven to be very helpful, and many other clinical trials are in progress.

All the necessary supportive care is vital to survival. This is especially the case when a tracheostomy is done, as was the case for Joey, and connection made to a portable ventilator. Recent reports indicate that treatment on a ventilator may prolong life by more than fifteen years, but not the quality of life.

Questions

- Did his ventilator not have an alarm?
- In transporting Joey into the examination room, wasn't special care required to ensure that no disconnection occurred between him and his ventilator?
- Was the hospital responsible, through their staff, for failing to provide appropriate care?

Commentary

There was an alarm on the ventilator, which was either not heard or not paid attention to by the home health nurse involved in transporting him into the procedure room. The alarm was subsequently shown to be in working order. Joey was in the end stage of this awful muscle disease, and his parents were fully aware of the likely outcome. No specific treatment could have saved him at that point.

The hospital sought a decision from the court for a summary judgment aiming to have the case dismissed. Based on Joey's health status, the hospital claimed that there was no merit in a lawsuit brought by Joey's parents claiming professional negligence. The hospital insisted that treatment provided for Joey was appropriate and met the standard of expected care. The hospital further maintained that if there was actually professional negligence, four elements were necessary for proof. (These are the elements required to succeed in any claim of medical negligence.) These four elements included:

1. The duty of the professional to use such skill, prudence, and diligence that other members of his or her profession commonly possess and exercise

2. Breach of that duty

3. A proximate causal connection between the negligent conduct and the resulting injury

4. Actual loss or damage resulting from the professional negligence

As long as these elements coexist, they constitute actual negligence. Moreover, absence of or failure to prove any one of them may sink the claim.

Joey's loving parents, exhausted emotionally and physically, had given their all in caring for a physically and intellectually disabled son. Even in his late stage of illness, they could not bring themselves to decide on a *do-not-resuscitate* order. They viewed life as precious, even though they knew that the end was near. Their actions remind us that in the care of our sick and elderly, attention to detail and caring are not only necessary but also required.

Withstanding all legal arguments, effort to seek a summary judgment failed, and the case was settled.

DOCTOR KNOWS BEST

They were immigrants from Southeast Asia. Zhi and Leoni met at a wedding of a mutual friend. Zhi was a primary-care doctor, and Leoni worked as a laboratory technologist. With a shared background culture and food tastes, they soon became inseparable. A year after meeting, they married and planned to have a family as soon as possible.

Leoni knew that in "the old country," she had lost her younger brother, who had been diagnosed with the hereditary disorder called β-thalassemia (a serious, often fatal, anemia).

After a few months of trying, Leoni achieved a pregnancy and made an appointment to see an obstetrician after she had missed two menstrual periods. Her doctor, upon hearing about her deceased brother with thalassemia, promptly ordered a DNA carrier test for Leoni. That test result showed that Leoni was indeed a carrier of a gene mutation for β-thalassemia. She was immediately referred to a genetic counselor because of the potential risk of having an affected child.

Zhi accompanied her to the appointment with the genetic counselor. Although they seemed to already know, the counselor explained the autosomal recessive mode of inheritance for β-thalassemia. This meant that, only if both carried a mutation in the gene that leads to thalassemia, they would have a 25 percent risk of having an affected child. The counselor therefore recommended that Zhi be tested immediately to determine his carrier status. Zhi, however, stated that as a doctor, he knew all about β-thalassemia and that he had previously been tested and was not a carrier. The counselor emphasized that couples who are carriers have the option of prenatal genetic diagnosis and the option to terminate a pregnancy should the fetus be affected. Since he was not a carrier, Zhi stated that there was no need for prenatal studies. About six months later, they delivered a son following an uneventful pregnancy.

The first six months of Shiva's life were unremarkable, except for some feeding difficulties that began around four months of age. They noted then that he was not gaining weight and by six months of age seemed rather pale. From being a happy, smiling baby, he became cranky and had bouts of fever and episodes of diarrhea. The primary-care doctor treated him repeatedly for what he thought were recurrent infections, until he noticed that Shiva's belly seemed to be enlarged. At that point, he determined that the spleen and liver were enlarged and that Shiva was seriously anemic. Referral to a specialist hematologist very quickly led to a diagnosis of β-thalassemia.

Clearly, Zhi was a carrier of a gene mutation for β-thalassemia. He later said that he had felt certain his own doctor had told him he was not a carrier.

Pertinent Medical Facts

The thalassemias are the most common single-gene disorders in the world. β-thalassemia is one of the hereditary anemias that occur with variable severity. Shiva had β-thalassemia major and was destined to develop serious and severe complications even with appropriate treatment. Incredibly, between one in eight and one in ten individuals in places like Cyprus, Sardinia, the Middle East, and Southeast Asia are affected by various forms of thalassemia. The structure of the iron-bearing protein called hemoglobin is defective in this disease and tends to crumble within the bone-marrow cells that manufacture the hemoglobin. An affected individual accumulates crumbling pieces of the defective hemoglobin, which in turn interferes with their manufacture of red blood cells that break up prematurely, causing anemia. The spleen and liver step in to manufacture blood cells that the failing bone marrow is unable to accomplish, each enlarging as a result. The symptoms described above, which Shiva experienced, are typical.

Treatment of the anemia is effective via repeated blood transfusions, which are given every two to three weeks. However, the many transfusions necessary progressively lead to an accumulation of iron in the body. Iron overload and anemia in children result in growth retardation and failure of sexual maturation. In adulthood, involvement of the heart (resulting in heart failure), the liver (causing cirrhosis), and the hormone-producing glands (resulting in diabetes and less commonly involvement of other hormone-producing glands) is inevitable. Enlarging spleens begin to gobble up other blood cells that could result in recurrent infections and bleeding. Additional complications include thrombosis in veins as well as the development of osteoporosis.

The treatment of iron overload employs the use of certain drugs called chelators that are given every five to seven days by twelve-hour continuous infusions under the skin via a portable pump. Needless to say, there are potential complications from these drugs that involve vision and hearing, cause growth retardation, and even cause kidney failure and pneumonia. Even with treatment, the quality of life is severely compromised, and mortality rates are high. Life expectancy using transfusions and medications rarely exceeds thirty years of age.

Before embarking on the demanding schedule of blood transfusions, it is absolutely necessary to provide hepatitis B vaccination. Recruitment by the body of bone marrow all over the body to help restore the rapidly disintegrating red blood cells leads to considerable bony deformations. The most characteristic changes result in so-called chipmunk face with up-slanting eyes, prominent forehead, flat nasal bridge, and prominent upper and lower jaw exposing the upper-front teeth.

A valuable, but not often available, mode of treatment is a bone-marrow transplant from an identically matched sibling. Even then, if the transplantation is successful, iron overload may still continue but can be managed by repeated phlebotomy (bloodletting). In these circumstances, disease-free survival can exceed 90 percent, as long as the liver is not already irreparably damaged and iron deposits are not excessive. Unfortunately, even under the best circumstance, there is about an 8 percent rejection of the donated bone marrow.

For couples who already know their precise mutations, prenatal diagnosis or preimplantation genetic diagnosis is available that enables avoidance or prevention of this chronic fatal disease.

Leoni made her first appointment for pregnancy care after she had missed two menstrual periods. This is a continuing pattern of care, which should optimally be changed through education in high school. All genetic and most environmental (medications, infections, etc.) effects have already damaged or affected the development of the embryo or fetus by eight to ten weeks (two missed periods) of pregnancy. For example, the spinal canal closes by twenty-nine days after conception. Failure to close completely results in the birth defect spina bifida (see chapter 4). Care should begin *prior to* conception if birth defects and genetic disorders are to be avoided.

Questions

- Was the genetic counselor, who worked for the obstetrician, negligent for not testing Zhi, a physician, to determine his carrier status?

Commentary .

Blaming the victim is an approach that never helps. Zhi, who was both patient and physician, should have known on what basis he was determined *not* to be a carrier for β-thalassemia. The genetic counselor who documented Zhi's statement that he was not a carrier should have insisted on him providing a copy of the report, thereby enabling either the necessary reassurance or the option of prenatal diagnosis. Notwithstanding the aforegoing, Zhi and Leoni sued the genetic counselor and the obstetrician (who was responsible for oversight of the genetic counselor) for the wrongful birth of their son, Shiva. Needless to say, Zhi denied saying that he was not a carrier!

I am, however, aware of other cases, in particular for Angelman syndrome (a severe neurodevelopmental disorder with intellectual disability and other features), where the report by a patient of a cousin with that disorder was simply ignored. There had been the opportunity yet again to demand a copy of the cousin's report. In one of those rare instances for this disorder, it was familial transmission of a defect in the chromosome 15 gene, resulting in the birth of a child with Angelman syndrome.

To make assurance doubly sure, where transmission of a genetic disorder is possible, there is the explicit burden to seek prior formal reports and to document that the request was made. The lack of documentation later allows a false claim to be brought about the caregiver's offer to test or to treat. Finally, patients who are physicians or highly educated professionals may intimidate the caregiver by their sheer force of personality or *knowledge* and override any vocalized counseling or advice. For unrelated technical reasons, this lawsuit was dismissed. In this case, once again, we have a physician patient who didn't know, he didn't know.

RUPTURE

It was a warm, balmy night, with moonbeams reflecting off a calm sea, while seemingly millions of stars

winked their beams toward earth. That evening, on this paradise island, with palms swaying gently in the

breeze, a father and his two teenage sons, Kai and Keanu, sat with an open window watching television.

The oldest son, Kai, then fifteen, had severe intellectual disability. He made most of his wishes clear by

gesticulating or signing, including wanting food or going to the toilet. Suddenly, without warning, he began

screaming, clutching himself, seeming to be in pain, but unable to explain anything. Unable to calm him

down, his father called 911, and the ambulance arrived with the paramedics five minutes after the

call. They, too, were unable to calm him down, so to protect him from self-injury, they tied him down to

the gurney and rolled him into the ambulance.

The hospital was not far away, and within thirty minutes of his sudden outburst, he was admitted to the

emergency department. The emergency-medicine physician decided to immediately obtain imaging of his

chest and abdomen, for which he needed to move the still-screaming boy onto a different trolley. He

continued to flail his arms and legs. The doctor needed his patient to stay still in order to obtain imaging,

so they placed him in a straitjacket, and he promptly died.

Shock and dismay pervaded the emergency staff, who were staggered by the sudden, unexplained death

of a fifteen-year-old.

The required autopsy revealed that Kai had an aortic aneurysm (a balloon-like bulge of his aorta), which

had burst in his chest, resulting in him bleeding to death without prior warning. The family buried him the

next day, remembering how hard they had tried to look after him, despite the sometimes-overwhelming

problems due to his severe intellectual disability. The cause of his intellectual disability had not been

determined. When he was five years old, he had a seizure. Imaging of his brain revealed a small, localized

arteriovenous malformation (a connection between tiny arteries and veins) that was not considered to be the cause of his intellectual disability but the likely cause of his seizure. Interventional treatment was not recommended because of a significant risk of death or stroke.

Two years later, the surviving son, Keanu, then age fourteen, was watching a television show when he suddenly began complaining of pain in his chest. His parents, still mourning the loss of their eldest son, did not waste a minute before calling 911. Once again, the paramedics arrived within five minutes to hear the surviving son explain that he had crushing pain in his chest. He was quickly placed on a gurney, rolled into the ambulance, and whisked off to the emergency department in the nearby hospital. Upon admission, he promptly received a morphine injection for his pain, moved to a trolley, and quickly wheeled to the radiology department for chest imaging. The radiologist was shocked to find that he too had an aortic aneurysm. He was immediately wheeled into the operating room and placed on the operating table. No sooner had they begun to anesthetize him for the surgery did he begin gasping and died. Autopsy showed that he too had ruptured an aortic aneurysm.

The family sued their primary-care physician for not referring them to a clinical geneticist who, they maintained, would have made a diagnosis of the thoracic aortic aneurysm and allowed them to save the lives of both of their sons.

Pertinent Medical Facts

An aneurysm is a localized dilatation of an artery at any site in the body. These dilatations may resemble a small or large bubble along the course of an artery, which may suddenly expand or dissect (tear) and burst. Both Kai and Keanu had an aneurysm involving the ascending aorta, which is connected directly to the heart, ascends to the arch, and then dips down through the chest into the abdomen. The aorta is the largest artery in the body. Aortic aneurysms within the chest (thoracic aortic aneurysms, or TAAs) mostly give no early warning about their presence. They quietly enlarge over time and can rupture suddenly. Not infrequently, the whole process of rupture begins in the inner layer of the aorta, and tears (called dissections) develop between layers of the now-weakened wall of the aorta. Dissections may also occur even without an aneurysm if the wall of the aorta (or other major artery) has weak, stretchable connective tissue or is damaged by fat and cholesterol deposits (atherosclerosis).

There are well-known genetic disorders that cause connective-tissue weakness due to altered structure of collagen fibers. These include Marfan syndrome, the vascular form of the Ehlers-Danlos syndrome (see chapter 17), and Loeys-Dietz syndrome. These three connective-tissue disorders may, among their many manifestations, also have aneurysms in the aorta, the brain, and elsewhere. As a matter of fact, almost 20 percent of people with TAA who do not have signs of these three disorders actually have a family history of TAA. Thus far, at least thirteen genes and their mutations are known to cause TAA. It is clear, however, that there are families with TAA whose genes are yet to be discovered. Within families with TAA, about 9 percent may have aneurysms within the brain, which may rupture or bleed. There is also an increased frequency of abnormalities of the aortic valve (bicuspid aortic valve).

Neither Kai nor his brother, Keanu, had signs of Marfan syndrome. This connective-tissue disorder primarily involves the cardiovascular system, the bones, and the eyes. Considerable variability exists in the signs an affected person might have. They may, for example, not have dislocated lenses in their eyes (a typical diagnostic feature) but rather hyperextensible joints, long arms, and a curved spine (scoliosis) with or without dilatation of the aorta. There may also be risk that the aorta might tear (dissect) or rupture, and frequently the mitral valve might stretch, prolapse, and leak. The precise diagnosis is made by analysis of the sole responsible gene (*FBN1*). Marfan syndrome is a dominantly inherited disorder, so some would have expected one of the boy's parents to have this disorder, which was clearly not the case. A new mutation occurs in 25 percent of patients. There are other less specific physical signs, and for more information please consult the Marfan Foundation. The prevalence of Marfan syndrome in the population is between one in five thousand and one in ten thousand.

The rarer Loeys-Dietz syndrome tends to be a more severe cardiovascular disorder, with some similar features to Marfan syndrome but with some additional, often unique, features that include wide-spaced eyes, a broad or bifid uvula, clubfeet, and tortuous arteries.

It is important to determine the specific culprit gene and its mutation in family members at risk in order to establish an appropriate surveillance system that could save a life. A careful family history and examination of the heart would precede gene analysis and would be followed by imaging (echocardiography). Those found to be at risk usually have their aortic diameters measured by imaging studies. Additional tests used include CT or MRI scans of the aorta.

Because TAA is transmitted mostly as an autosomal dominant disorder, an affected person has a 50 percent risk of transmitting this disorder to each of his or her offspring. Imaging is usually repeated within six months if any aortic dissection is found so as to determine the rate of aneurysmal growth. The frequency of further determinations depends upon the rate of change in the aortic diameter. There are precise measurements that dictate either watchful waiting or the need for surgical intervention. If a thoracic aneurysm has been detected, medical therapy, using either a β-blocker or the drug Losartan, is recommended to reduce the stress on the aortic wall. Additional advice includes avoidance of weight lifting, isometric exercise, and contact sports; no smoking; and attention to the cholesterol profile. Progressive enlargement of the aorta leads to the option of surgical repair well before any rupture has occurred. Major surgery involves cutting out the aneurysm and replacing that section with a graft.

Questions

- Was there any reason for the primary-care physician to refer Kai to a clinical geneticist?
- Was there any good reason to believe that, even with such a referral, a thoracic aortic aneurysm would have been detected?

Commentary

Any child with intellectual disability, even when mild, should be referred for a genetics consultation. Huge advances have been made in the identification of genes with their mutations that are causally related to intellectual disability. To date, at least seven hundred genes causally related to intellectual disability have been identified and can be accurately analyzed from a single teaspoon of blood. Notwithstanding the remarkable genetic advances, failure to determine a cause for intellectual disability is still in the 30–40 percent range. This is especially the case where there is no family history of any such intellectual limitations and when the child shows no particular unusual facial or other features (see discussion in chapter 38).

Kai, who had no outward abnormality about his features, had been seen repeatedly by his primary-care doctor. He had simply had routine childhood care, vaccinations, and so forth. A single chromosome analysis, which yielded a normal result, was the limit of the evaluation performed by the primary-care doctor. Kai also had no obvious signs of a connective-tissue disorder, such as hyperextensible joints, dislocations, or fractures. There was also no family history of any type of aneurysm and no consanguinity. The autopsy that revealed the arteriovenous malformation, with which Kai had been born, was not thought to be related to his intellectual disability but which arose as an aberration in the formation of blood vessels during early fetal development. Kai and Keanu's father was later thought to have a connective-tissue disorder, the father not having an aneurysm.

There was, in my opinion, no way that the primary-care physician or clinical geneticist would, more probably than not, have had reason to perform imaging on Kai's aorta to detect an unsuspected aneurysm. I testified in support of the primary-care doctor.

However, the jury thought otherwise and felt that a referral to a clinical geneticist had been long overdue.

OH MY LORD!

It was a spectacular spring day, and the air felt like champagne. Jill and Henry had just emerged from church after listening to an inspiring sermon from their pastor and ending the service with their favorite hymn "This Little Light of Mine." Jill could not have been happier, since she had learned that very week that she had become pregnant for the first time. An ultrasound at eight weeks of pregnancy yielded a normal result. Other than her multivitamins, including folic acid, which she had begun prior to becoming pregnant, she took no other medications. She felt simply *marvelous* throughout her pregnancy, having even more energy than usual.

Labor and delivery on a snowy night were surprisingly easy for a first timer. Labor may have been facilitated by the fact that their newborn, whom they named Calvin (after a deceased grandfather), was rather small at five and a half pounds and had a rather small head. It did not take long for their pediatrician to appear after examining Cal and to share his concern about the size of the baby's head. Due concern was expressed, and a follow-up was arranged for an office visit two weeks after Jill's two-day stay in the hospital.

At the scheduled visit, measurement of the head circumference confirmed that the head size was exquisitely small, measuring below the third percentile. During that very tearful and painful appointment, they learned that the diagnosis was microcephaly and that Cal's small brain would be associated later with very significant intellectual disability and profound limitations for his lifetime. The pediatrician initiated a series of blood tests to rule out an infectious cause and also obtained imaging of Cal's brain. Imaging confirmed a small brain without any major structural abnormality, and the other blood tests were all negative. The pediatrician next referred Jill and Henry to a clinical geneticist for further evaluation. Chromosome analysis and certain biochemical genetic tests followed, none of which revealed the cause of Cal's microcephaly.

Following guidelines, the geneticist informed Jill and Henry that the possibility was high that Cal's microcephaly was due to either an autosomal recessive disorder (where each parent would be carrying a mutation in the same gene) or a sex-linked disorder (occurring as either a new mutation or from a mutation in a gene carried by Jill). The possibility of a sex-linked disorder worried Jill, as she had a male cousin on her mother's side who had severe intellectual disability, but not microcephaly. The geneticist emphasized that if Cal's microcephaly were due to an autosomal recessive disorder, they would have a 25 percent risk of having another child with this disorder in future pregnancies. If the cause were a sex-linked gene due to a mutation carried by Jill, there would be a 50 percent risk of having an affected boy in the future, while half their girls would be carriers like Jill. Distraught by this dreadful realization, they sought comfort in prayer with their pastor and began to care for Cal as they would have with any child.

Two years later, during a routine visit to her obstetrician, Jill shared her desperate wish to have a healthy child. By that time, Cal was unable to sit unsupported and had no words or meaningful interactions. Jill's obstetrician encouraged her to have another pregnancy, promising her that he would do all the appropriate tests and reassured her that all would be well, given proper surveillance.

About three months later, Jill returned to her obstetrician's office, smiling but extremely anxious. Her obstetrician calmed her down and reassured her that all would turn out fine and that he would do the necessary tests. The ultrasound study at ten weeks yielded a normal result, and she continued the pregnancy as she had done in the past. For inexplicable reasons, she next had an ultrasound at twenty weeks of pregnancy. The fetal head was seen to be small. Jill and Henry were aghast and extremely upset. At thirty-nine weeks, one week short of her expected date of delivery, her second son, Sam, was delivered. Sam, too, had microcephaly! They then had two sons with microcephaly, who were destined to have profound intellectual disability and would need total care for the rest of their lives. Words could not fully capture the angst and anger felt and expressed by Jill and Henry. Within weeks, they sued their obstetrician for medical negligence.

Pertinent Medical Facts

Microcephaly that occurs *without* any other birth defects being present is termed "isolated or primary microcephaly." Once viral infections (such as the Zika virus or cytomegalovirus) have been excluded, the cause of recurrent microcephaly is invariably due to mutations in a single gene. The genetic cause for the overwhelming majority is autosomal recessive, with each parent carrying a mutation (not necessarily the same mutation) in the same gene. Couples who are cousins, even distantly related, are especially at risk for these types of recessive disorders, including microcephaly. (A salutary reminder that people in and from the Middle East and Asia have consanguinity rates between 50 and 70 percent!) Jill and Henry were not related but unwittingly had a 25 percent risk of having a second affected child. Sex-linked microcephaly, affecting males only, occurs much less often.

At the time this whole situation arose, none of the culprit genes and their mutations responsible for microcephaly had been identified. Today, at least seven genes have been determined to have mutations that result in autosomal recessive microcephaly. Genes that cause sex-linked microcephaly are yet to be identified. Today, prenatal diagnosis as early as eleven weeks of pregnancy can be achieved by DNA analysis. Moreover, once the gene mutations are recognized in both parents, preimplantation or prenatal genetic diagnosis is possible, enabling avoidance and prevention of this birth defect.

Questions

- Why did the obstetrician not do high-resolution ultrasound studies to determine fetal-head size early in the second trimester of pregnancy?

- Why did he reassure Jill that he would do the appropriate tests when she began to talk about a future pregnancy and then fail to do so?

Commentary

The standard of expected care at that time was for the obstetrician to perform serial ultrasound measurements from the first trimester all the way through to twenty-two weeks of pregnancy. By plotting the fetal-head circumference on a graph, it would have become painfully obvious very early that microcephaly was evident. Jill would have had the opportunity to terminate the pregnancy should she have wished to do so. The medical record showed that after the first early ultrasound at ten weeks of pregnancy, the next one was at twenty-eight weeks, too late to interrupt the pregnancy.

Sometime later, Jill encountered the obstetrician in church, which he also routinely attended. She tearfully confronted him and asked why this had all happened. He responded that he had seen her in church, decided that she would not want to abort a pregnancy, and did not want to upset her. He therefore decided to not perform earlier ultrasound tests!

Physicians should know that they cannot, and must not, visit upon their patients their own religious beliefs, racial biases, or dictates of conscience. It was unconscionable for Jill's obstetrician to assume what action she might take in the face of a recurrence. He will not have to spend the rest of his life caring for their second affected child. All he had to do was order a timely ultrasound test, placing the interests of Jill and her family first, beyond all else.

The court, in this case, not only found the obstetrician medically negligent but also levied a punitive award of $400,000 against him. (Liability insurance does not cover punitive awards.) In this case, he knew what should have been done but didn't know that certain moral imperatives demand high ethical standards from practicing physicians.

THE APPOINTMENT

Sally and the book group that she attended had just completed a lively discussion of a novel that focused on life's choices. Just before they began their discussions, Sally announced that she was pregnant for the first time. Stimulated by the thought-provoking issues about how people make choices that affect their lives, the group turned to Sally inquiring about her planned choice of an obstetrician. Instead of replying, Sally turned to the group, all but one of whom had already had children, and asked them what criteria they had considered when faced with the need to choose an obstetrician. They were not shy to offer their opinions, which were generally fairly uniform.

Some depended upon a recommendation from their primary-care physician, while others preferred a female physician. A board-certified and well-experienced physician, preferably from an Ivy League school, was a common choice. Almost all sought out a physician who was sensitive, empathetic, and gentle and had a nice personality. It was also important for them to have a thoughtful, quiet, and deliberative person who did not rush through a visit. All uniformly mentioned the importance of somebody who explained things in clear and understandable terms and who avoided jargon. One member of the group mentioned how much she appreciated her obstetrician being clean shaven and well groomed, with manicured nails and coifed hair. There were, however, vociferous responses that negatively influenced their choices or led them to leave that practice and find another doctor.

Once again, there was surprising uniformity in their individual comments.

- "He hardly looked at me, staring continuously at his computer."

- "She didn't listen to me, talked over me, and constantly interrupted."

- "Talked fast, had a difficult accent, and didn't explain anything."

- "He was insensitive and rough."

- "He rushed through a visit and said another doctor would see me next time."

- "He was too young and too inexperienced."

- "I was able to establish no relationship. I saw five different doctors in pregnancy and knew I would be delivered by any one of them. None knew me or understood my needs, nor did they display any investment in my care. I wondered if these doctors were simply technicians."

- "While taking my family history, he made unnecessary and derogatory comments about families whose members have mental illness."

Sally made her choice and relied upon the recommendation of her primary-care physician.

An ultrasound study at ten and a half weeks of pregnancy was unremarkable. At that visit, a blood sample was drawn to screen for chromosomal abnormalities, especially Down syndrome, by measuring two hormones (human chorionic gonadotropin, Papp A) and a protein (alpha-fetoprotein). The results showed that Sally had a one-in-three thousand risk for that pregnancy resulting in a child with Down syndrome. The average odds for all women are between one in seven hundred and one in eight hundred.

A month later, at her next visit, another blood sample was drawn for the same screening test, with the addition of another hormone (estriol). This time, the statistical odds that her pregnancy would end with a child with Down syndrome were 1 in 149. Her obstetrician then recommended she see a maternal-fetal-medicine specialist, without giving any details, and made that referral by having his staff send a fax with the necessary information to the specialist's office. That note, of course, indicated the stage of pregnancy as well as the reason for referral, namely increased odds for Down syndrome. The staff at the specialist's office tried multiple times to reach Sally. They simply left repeated voice-mail messages, requesting that Sally call the office to make an appointment.

Four weeks later, Sally was seen by a second physician in the same practice. There was no further discussion about the referral or the importance of the pregnancy stage. Rather, the obstetrician decided that the second screening result was probably an error. The next visit, at twenty-three weeks of gestation, was again with the same doctor, and there were no other discussions. At the twenty-seventh-week visit, her

doctor's office sent a second fax to the specialist's office. At that point, one of the nurses recognized that

the referral had been for the increased risk for Down syndrome and that the appointment had not been made.

To her horror, she discovered that the doctor's office that sent the first fax provided the incorrect contact

information for Sally. The second fax, sent from his office, again provided incorrect information. An urgent

ultrasound at this point revealed that the long bones of the fetus were unusually short and the nasal bone

was not well developed. These are typical signs of Down syndrome in the fetus. It was already too late to

have any prenatal studies that could provide an opportunity to terminate a pregnancy should

that have been Sally's wish.

At thirty-seven weeks, labor was induced, and the baby was noted to not only be small for gestational age

but also to have the features of Down syndrome. That diagnosis was quickly confirmed by chromosome

analysis.

Sally and her husband sued her doctor for medical negligence.

<u>Pertinent Medical Facts</u>

The blood test that Sally had was a routine screen for all chromosome abnormalities but especially for

Down syndrome. The biomarkers used flag pregnancies at risk, thereby signaling an indication for

prenatal genetic studies by amniocentesis sampling. The screen assists in the detection of 90–93 percent of

pregnancies in which there is an unsuspected fetal Down syndrome. There is no good explanation why the

odds for Down syndrome were so discrepant between the first and the second trimesters of her pregnancy.

One potential explanation is that she was not as far along in her pregnancy as the ten weeks suggested. In

other words, the sampling was too early. Moreover, it is not recommended to perform the screening test

both in the first and second trimesters without an algorithm (sequential or integrated screening). Statistical

data generally show that detection rates would drop by repeating the screen in the second trimester. Sally

had the automatic recommendation for an amniocentesis because of her 1 in 149 odds for Down syndrome. The most common indicator for prenatal studies in this context is when the odds are 1 in 250 or even 1 in 200.

Down syndrome, features of which were best described by John Langdon Down, was not actually discovered by him. This syndrome results from the transmission of an extra chromosome, chromosome 21, resulting in the presence of three chromosomes in the 21 group, and is hence better described as trisomy 21. This is the case for about 94 percent of cases of Down syndrome. However, 2–3 percent have a mixture of normal cells and some with trisomy 21 (called mosaicism), while 3–4 percent have a chromosomal interchange (called a translocation) that involves chromosome 21 and any other chromosome. The latter structural rearrangement conveys a serious risk of recurrence and is frequently familial. The origin of the extra chromosome is mostly maternal. Moreover, frequency of this condition escalates with maternal age, reaching a risk of at least 7 percent by the age of forty-five. However, not sufficiently well recognized is the fact that the vast majority of children born with Down syndrome are delivered by mothers who are under the age of thirty-five. This is simply because the vast majority of pregnancies occur before mothers reach the age of thirty-five.

The quintessential features of Down syndrome include the typical facial appearance, with a flat facial profile, up-slanting eyes, and folds at the inner corner of the eyes. Intellectual disability is invariable, as is short stature, loose joints, and floppy muscles. A range of minor features and other medical problems, of which there are many, I discussed elsewhere (*Your Genes, Your Health: A Critical Family Guide That Could Save Your Life*). A 2017 report in *Genetics in Medicine* estimated that in 2010, there were 206,366 people with Down syndrome living in the United States.

The provision of early intervention, including speech therapy and special education, enables those with trisomy 21 to lead meaningful lives. Considerable medical care, considering the various medical problems encountered, is necessary for a lifetime. One very important medical complication is that around 50 percent of children born with Down syndrome also have a congenital heart defect. For the most part, surgery can resolve the problem but unfortunately not always. Contrary to the past, life-spans can now be expected to exceed sixty years.

A new Down syndrome blood-screening test has largely replaced the original biomarker screens (except for neural tube defects like spina bifida). This DNA-based screen is focused on the analysis of fetal cells that circulate in a pregnant mother's bloodstream. The circulating fetal DNA from whole or broken fetal cells is separated from the mother's DNA. The analysis determines the amount of DNA specifically on the chromosome 21 pair. An extra chromosome will be detected by the presence of more chromosome-specific DNA.

The detection rate of pregnancies in which the fetus has Down syndrome approximates 95–98 percent, below 90 percent for trisomy 18, and as low as 70 percent for trisomy 13. Moreover, there is a false positive (fetus is actually normal) rate of about 2 percent. The frequency of a false negative (not true) result remains unclear, so far. In about 6 percent of pregnancy screens, no result is obtained, usually because of insufficient DNA. The same noninvasive screening test is used to simultaneously screen for two more chromosome disorders that increase in frequency with advancing maternal age—trisomy 18 and trisomy 13. Sex-chromosome abnormalities can also be detected, and some laboratories claim detection of subtler chromosome defects, as well as certain single-gene diseases.

Maternal-age risks still demand that women should be informed that direct prenatal diagnostic studies by amniocentesis or by an earlier test at eleven weeks (chorionic villus sampling) are offered from the age of thirty-five, regardless of the result of the noninvasive blood screen. It is important to remember that about 50 percent of all chromosome abnormalities will be missed by this screen!

Some of the important findings on ultrasound in the first three months of pregnancy include lack of development of the nasal bone, an increased thickness of the fold at the back of the neck, and shorter long bones seen in the ensuing weeks.

Questions

- Why did her physician not check with Sally that she had made the necessary appointment with the maternal-fetal-medicine specialist and ask for and document her reply?

- Why did the office staff of the maternal-fetal-medicine specialist not consult with him about their inability to reach a patient who clearly had an urgent referral because of her stage of pregnancy?

- Why did the other obstetrician in that same practice reinterpret the second-trimester screen as a likely error and take no further action?

Commentary

Have you ever dialed a wrong number or written down a number incorrectly? Virtually all of us have at one time or another. However, when such details can threaten a life or impair a future life, particular care has to be exercised. When a physician makes a critical referral, it is incumbent for him or her to be certain that the referral has occurred and has been properly attended to. If her doctor had taken the time, and cared sufficiently, to discover if Sally had been seen, he would have, in all likelihood, recognized that the contact information he gave for Sally and sent via his office by fax was incorrect. Moreover, the very same incorrect information was sent again, in a second fax, eight weeks later.

Despite the urgency, the staff failed to bring the physician's attention to their inability to reach Sally. The office staff were neither sufficiently well trained nor appropriately caring to have provided the correct information and to have reacted in an expected way.

The second obstetrician, who decided to reinterpret the second screening test and suggest, without proof, that it was an error, was also seriously at fault. While laboratories may well make errors, reinterpretation of a laboratory report by practicing physicians is strictly contraindicated and a hazardous exercise. It behooved that doctor to take additional steps that would have included an ultrasound that would have revealed some signs of Down syndrome and would have led automatically to the offer of an amniocentesis and prenatal chromosome studies.

So often in these legal cases, there is more than a single error. In this case again, there were multiple errors. The lawsuit was eventually settled.

THE DECIDER

The diagnostic use and accuracy of obstetrical ultrasound have evolved into a valuable tool these past fifty years. Initial use focused on the location of the placenta, with special reference to placing the amniocentesis needle in the safest position. Assessment of fetal growth followed, enabling serial measurement of the fetal-head circumference, followed by determination of the abdominal circumference and measurements of the long bones. High-resolution ultrasound made it possible to determine lack of development of the nasal bone (in Down syndrome) and to measure the translucent folds of the neck (nuchal translucency), seen especially, but not only, in Down syndrome. Remarkably precise imaging, with measurements in millimeters, enabled visualization of the ventricles of the brain and subsequently structural aspects of brain anatomy.

Recognition of fetal malformations steadily became commonplace, including heart defects, a missing limb (amelia), a partially missing limb (phocomelia), a missing digit, and missing or underdeveloped middle phalanx of the fifth finger (Down syndrome). Other abnormities that became determinable included cleft lip and other facial abnormalities, as well as even tiny bowel extrusions through the abdominal wall. Further advances included use of the Doppler effect, which enabled accurate assessment of the direction and velocity of blood flow, whether through the heart or through arteries and veins. Ultrasound studies of the ductus venosus focused on blood shunting from the left umbilical-cord vein to bypass the liver and head directly for the heart. Measurement of the blood flow through the ductus venosus and the pulsatility are also useful markers of fetal Down syndrome.

So when Irene, who was a laboratory technologist, arrived for her sixteenth-week pregnancy ultrasound, she was fully prepared. She had read about ultrasound and was looking forward to determining not only that the fetus would look good but also what the gender was. The maternal-fetal-medicine specialist was pleased to communicate that the fetus was male and everything looked fine. He did want her to return in

three weeks for an ultrasound for serial measurements. Irene had been worried, since she was an insulin-

dependent diabetic. She kept her blood sugar in tight control and was happy to hear that there were no

issues.

At nineteen weeks, the maternal-fetal-medicine specialist noticed that the umbilical cord had two blood

vessels instead of three, which he either had not seen or not documented at the sixteenth-week visit. Because

of this observation, which can be associated with an increased likelihood of a subsequent birth defect, he

recommended an amniocentesis to check the fetal chromosomes. That result, at twenty-one to twenty-two

weeks of pregnancy, yielded a normal result, and pregnancy went on with routine care. He did not share

with Irene the fact that he had noticed five midchest hemivertebrae (wedge-shaped vertebrae) and that the

spaces within the brain (lateral ventricles) in the forebrain were a little dilated. Pregnancy

continued without any problems or further studies. Labor and delivery were unremarkable.

Irene's newborn baby boy looked fine, and she was overjoyed.

At the third-month visit with Benito's pediatrician, Irene shared her observation that, compared to her

friend's newborns, he didn't hold a rattle, didn't smile when tickled, and couldn't lift his head when lying

on his stomach. The doctor agreed and recommended she see a neurologist with Benito.

The neurologist confirmed Irene's observation, noticed a normal facial appearance, except for his eyes,

which were closely spaced, and his ears, which were slightly low set. He recommended brain imaging by

MRI, which was performed some two weeks later. The results showed structural abnormality of the frontal

lobes, there being an incomplete separation between the left and right side. This disorder is termed

"holoprosencephaly."

Overcome with anger, Irene went directly to the office of the maternal-fetal-medicine specialist. She

demanded immediate access and was ushered into a side room. The obstetrician then explained that he

had noticed five thoracic hemivertebrae on the sixteenth-week ultrasound and concluded that they had little relevance, since he had seen those features in perfectly normal infants before. When he observed the two-vessel umbilical cord, he immediately recommended the chromosome studies by amniocentesis and was happy to find a normal result. The ultrasound study at twenty-one to twenty-two weeks showed slight dilation of the lateral ventricles, but he did not think it had any significance.

When Irene angrily asked him why he did not share these observations with her, he responded that "he will decide when and what to tell a patient," upon which she clutched Benito, grabbed her pocketbook, and stormed out of his office. Shortly thereafter, she sued that doctor for depriving her of the opportunity to decide whether she would continue a pregnancy in the face of three significant structural anomalies of the fetus, despite having no definitive-named diagnosis at that time of pregnancy.

Pertinent Medical Facts

Holoprosencephaly is surprisingly not rare, occurring in about 1 in 250 miscarried embryos. About 1 in 10,000 live-born infants have this structural abnormality of the forebrain. Strangely, infants of diabetic mothers have about a 1 percent risk (which represents a 200× increase) of having holoprosencephaly. Women with uncontrolled insulin-dependent diabetes have about a threefold increased risk of bearing a child with a major birth defect, intellectual disability, or a genetic disorder. This increased risk approximates 10 percent. However, in very well-controlled insulin-dependent diabetes, there is not an increased frequency of birth defects. There are also suspicions that cholesterol-lowering drugs (e.g., statins) causing low cholesterol values may result in fetal holoprosencephaly.

Between 25 and 50 percent of those with holoprosencephaly have a chromosome abnormality. The amniocentesis study Benito had excluded that particular cause. DNA studies have revealed that 10–20 percent of offspring with holoprosencephaly have a tiny deletion or duplication in the genome (see chapter 38). Up to 25 percent of those with holoprosencephaly have a mutation in a single gene, at least fourteen of which are known. The mutation may occur out of the blue or may be transmitted as a dominant disorder by a carrier parent (who may show nothing more than closely spaced eyes and a single central incisor tooth). Transmission may also be via a recessive mode of inheritance where each parent carries a mutation in the same culprit gene or as an X-linked trait where 50 percent of males would be affected from a carrier mother.

The precise cause for Benito's holoprosencephaly was not established. His development was severely delayed, and seizures made their appearance before he was one year old. He was floppy, held his bottle poorly, had difficulties feeding, and often had reflux with choking and gagging. He slept poorly and woke his parents multiple times every night. Taking him out was more easily accomplished using a wheelchair. Eventually, they had to insert a G-tube through the abdominal wall and into this stomach to provide adequate calories, since he was failing to thrive.

The umbilical cord normally contains two arteries and one vein. In about 1 percent of newborns, one artery is missing, and yet the infant is normal. However, when there is only a single umbilical artery present, there are increased obstetrical and newborn risks. These risks approximate 2.6 percent for there being a fetal abnormality, including complex heart defects. In addition, reported associations include lower birth weights, intrauterine growth restriction, fetal loss during pregnancy, stillbirth, death of the newborn, and an increased likelihood of preterm delivery. In 1.5–9.8 percent of twins, a single umbilical artery is missing. In this group, regardless of whether they are identical or fraternal twins, somewhere between 27 and 50 percent are found to have fetal abnormalities, most being complex and severe.

Questions

- Was it required for the maternal-fetal-specialist to share his ultrasound observations with Irene?

Commentary

Physicians are accustomed to issuing therapeutic directives upon which their patients depend in order to remedy their health issues. However, when it comes to decisions related to the continuation of a pregnancy with or without fetal abnormality, nondirective counseling is the order of the day. Guidelines issued by the American College of Obstetrics and Gynecology and the American College of Medical Genetics and Genomics emphasize patient autonomy in reproductive decision making. The maternal-fetal-medicine specialist had a duty to Irene to share the observations he had made. He should have explained that he was unable to make a definitive diagnosis of a named disorder but that the combination of hemivertebrae, a two (instead of a three) vessel umbilical cord, and dilated lateral ventricles implies a significant risk of future intellectual disability. No real comfort could have been obtained by seeing the normal chromosome report. By not providing Irene with information about these anomalies, he deprived her of the opportunity to terminate the pregnancy and spare her and her partner a lifetime of grief.

All decisions concerning pregnancy termination in the face of abnormalities are parental and do not hinge on medical *recommendations*. The quintessential qualities a physician needs in these circumstances include maturity, experience, warmth and empathy, sensitivity, knowledge, communication skills, and insight into the psychology of human relationships, pregnancy, and grieving. This physician failed miserably by taking the remarkable position that he would decide what and when he would tell a patient, even about fetal abnormality. Ignorance and arrogance make good bedfellows.

The case was settled.

DUTY TO WARN

In 1998, Kimberly Molloy and her second husband, Glenn, had a son with the Fragile X syndrome. This is a genetic disorder with multiple symptoms and signs, the most challenging being at least moderate intellectual disability. Soon after discovering that their son, MM, had this disorder, Kimberly learned that her daughter, SF, from her first marriage, also had Fragile X syndrome and that she herself was a carrier of the disorder. SF had been born about ten years earlier, and Kimberly had two other daughters from her first marriage. Kimberly and her first husband divorced when SF was approximately one and a half years old. Her ex-husband was awarded custody of all three children. Subsequently, Kimberly married Glenn and had two children, KM and MM, who were born in 1993 and 1998, respectively.

Kimberly went to see Dr. Diane Meyer when SF was four to determine the cause of her developmental delay. At that time, she told Dr. Meyer about her brother with intellectual disability and her wish to determine if SF's problems were genetic. Dr. Meyer wrote in her notes at that time "? chromosomes + Fragile X" and ordered chromosome testing of SF. At that time, Dr. Meyer also referred SF to Dr. Reno Backus at the Minneapolis Clinic of Neurology.

About one month later, SF was seen by Dr. Backus and was also told about Kimberly's brother. Dr. Backus concluded that SF had developmental delay and autistic signs of unknown cause. Kimberly told Dr. Backus that she had remarried and enquired about her risk of having another child with similar problems as those suffered by SF. He told Kimberly that risks were extremely remote, especially with a father other than her ex-husband. In addition, Dr. Backus told Kimberly that SF's problems were not genetic but were "just one of those things that happen." This doctor later claimed that he was not involved with SF's care and that he was only asked to evaluate her from a neurological point of view and was simply acting as an advisor to the referring physician, Dr. Meyer.

A month later, SF was brought to the North Memorial Medical Center for chromosome testing that had been ordered by Dr. Meyer. Later, Dr. Meyer admitted that it was her intention to order Fragile X testing, but, for unknown reasons, this test was not performed. Needless to say, the chromosome studies were normal and were reported as such. Kimberly believed that the normal results included Fragile X testing.

About six months later, in a consultation for SF with Dr. Meyer, she still did not determine whether SF had been tested for Fragile X.

SF was referred to another pediatric neurologist, Dr. Kathryn Green, who examined SF and reviewed the family history, noting a maternal half-uncle with intellectual disability. Dr. Green also did not order or recommend Fragile X testing. She testified that she had not been asked to make a diagnosis but rather to provide an opinion on how to manage SF's hyperactivity.

After MM began showing signs of developmental delay, but before he or SF were diagnosed with Fragile X, Kimberly underwent surgical sterilization because of her concern that she was a carrier of genetic defects. At two years of age, MM was diagnosed with the Fragile X syndrome, and subsequent testing confirmed that SF was similarly affected. Kimberly was then shown to be a carrier of Fragile X syndrome.

The lawsuit, initiated by Kimberly in 2001, claimed that Drs. Meyer, Backus, and Green, and their employers, were negligent in the diagnosis and treatment rendered to SF, Kimberly, and MM. Furthermore, they failed to order Fragile X testing of SF, failed to read and interpret the laboratory results from the test that SF underwent, negligently reported to SF's parents that SF had been tested for Fragile X and that she did not have that condition, and failed to counsel them about their risks of having affected children in future. They further claimed, and this is important, that had they known about SF's condition, they would not have conceived MM and that, as a result of all of these doctors' negligence, they incurred and would continue to incur medical, educational, and other expenses relating to MM for a lifetime.

An effort was made by the doctors' attorneys to get rid of this lawsuit by seeking summary judgment. This was subsequently denied by the district court, and they moved on to the appeals court of Minnesota.

The facts of this case have been taken from the opinion of the appeals court judge, G. Barry Anderson, addressing doctors' claims challenging the district court's denial of their summary-judgment motions. Judge Anderson wrote affirming the district court's conclusions and addressed three specific issues. First, he wrote that a physician-patient relationship existed between doctors and Kimberly Molloy because they had the duty to inform her of the existence of a genetic disorder. Second, Kimberly Molloy's cause of action accrued at the point of conception of MM and thus was not time-barred from Minnesota law. Finally, Minnesota law did not bar Kimberly Molloy's cause of action because it was not a suit alleging that had the doctor's negligence not occurred, an abortion would have been sought. This, then, was a case of wrongful conception and not prohibited in Minnesota.

Pertinent Medical Facts

The primary manifestation of the Fragile X syndrome is intellectual disability. Early development is characterized by delayed sitting and walking as well as speech, which might only begin around twenty months of age. Throughout childhood, speech is especially problematic but is compounded by an abnormal temperament that includes tantrums, hyperactivity, and autistic behaviors. Affected boys are recognizable by their features that include a rather large head, a prominent forehead, large protuberant ears, a prominent jaw, and a long face. The severity of intellectual disability in boys is reflected in their IQs, which range between thirty and fifty. After puberty, autistic behavior often remains and requires attention, together with a certain shyness and unwillingness to look the examiner in the eye. Common features include strabismus (cross-eyes) and lax and loose joints, including flat feet. The stretchable connective tissue may also be reflected in the heart's mitral valve, which may prolapse and leak. On occasion, there may be dilatation of the aorta. The skin is usually soft and smooth or velvety, and curiously, after puberty the testes are found to be large.

The cause of this disorder is a complex alteration resulting in disruption and alteration of a gene that is located near the tip of one arm of the X chromosome. Since boys have only one female (X) chromosome, serious interruption of a gene will almost invariably lead to serious clinical consequences. Girls who have two X chromosomes will have at least one that is normal and will *balance* the other X with the abnormality, thereby modifying and mollifying clinical consequences.

This disorder is transmitted as an X-linked condition, in which a carrier female has a 50 percent risk of transmitting the disorder to each of her male offspring and 50 percent of her female offspring would be carriers. The actual interruption in the gene (*FMR1*) leads to a repetitive series of so-called triplet repeats or runs of three of individual blocks (nucleotide bases) that make up our gene structures. These blocks, abbreviated by the letters ACTG, reveal runs of CGG triplets, which, if they exceed fifty-four, become a potential problem. Triplet repeats between fifty-five and two hundred are termed "premutations" and for the most part are not associated with significant signs. However, if there are greater than two hundred triplet repeats, the full spectrum of intellectual disability and other signs becomes obvious. For the reasons mentioned, girls are less seriously affected, but some have intellectual disability that may require extra educational attention.

Not well enough recognized is the fact that about 21 percent of premutation female carriers develop premature ovarian insufficiency and hence difficulty in achieving a pregnancy. Women who experience *infertility* should routinely be tested for their Fragile X carrier status. In fact testing for Fragile X in infertile women is a common way carriers are discovered.

Given the X-linked mode of inheritance described above, women who are carriers may choose to have either preimplantation or prenatal diagnosis.

One not-sufficiently well-recognized long-term consequence for both males and females with a premutation (less than two hundred triplet repeats) is the increased risk for neurological disorders. Often after the age of fifty, progressive balance issues and a tremor may make their appearance. This risk is about 17 percent by the age of fifty-nine, 28 percent by the age of sixty-nine, and 47 percent by the age of

seventy-nine. After eighty, that risk approximates 75 percent. Those risks pertain to males. Female

estimates range up to 16.5 percent total. Quite often, balance and tremor issues are not recognized as

manifestations of the Fragile X syndrome but are mistakenly thought to be due to aging or some other

degenerative neurological disorder. On occasion, as I have seen, detection of this balance and tremor

disorder (called Fragile X tremor ataxia associated syndrome) in a male after the age of fifty may lead to a

diagnosis of the Fragile X syndrome in his grandson, transmitted via his unaffected carrier daughter.

Very often, family history on the mother's side reflects some male brothers, nephews, and uncles with

intellectual disability, typical of an X-linked disorder.

Autistic behavior occurs in as many as 25 percent of affected boys. In some families with affected grand

and great-grandchildren, the signs and severity of the Fragile X syndrome tend to be more severe over

generations (a process called anticipation). The prevalence of females who are unaffected but are

premutation carriers ranges between 1 in 77 and 1 in 259.

Questions

These are the three questions posed to the appeals court after a district judge had already ruled in favor of

Kim Molloy. The physicians sought a summary judgment to get rid of this case, and the questions that the

appeals court had to address were as follows:

- Does a physician who fails to test for and diagnose a genetic disorder in a child owe a legal duty

  to that child's parents who have a subsequent child who also has that disorder?

- When does a cause of action accrue in a medical-malpractice case, alleging failure to test for and

  diagnose a genetic disorder in a child, when a subsequent child is born with the same disorder?

- Does the state statute (in Minnesota) prohibit parents from bringing an action alleging they would

  not have conceived the subsequent child described in the second question?

Commentary

Judge Anderson systematically analyzed the issues and position taken by the doctors in their appeal to reverse the district court's decision against allowing summary judgment. In his analysis, the judge explored each issue and contention. First, he established that the doctors had a duty to SF, who was their patient. Earlier, the district court had concluded that the duty might also extend to Kimberly Molloy because a "doctor performing genetic tests on a minor child owes a duty to the biological parents of the child."

Judge Anderson drew attention to other cases in which a duty had been found between a physician and a minor patient's parents. In that case, the Supreme Court held that the physician was liable for negligently advising the parents. Emphasis was given in Kimberly Molloy's case that the record showed that she had received and relied upon direct advice from her doctors and that they were fully informed about the family history. In addressing whether physicians owe a legal duty to parents in these circumstances, previous cases recognized a physician's duty, based on reasonable foreseeability, to act as a matter of law. Kimberly Molloy's doctors should have foreseen that negligently rendering care to SF or erroneously reporting genetic tests to SF's parents could result in the birth of another child with Fragile X. They could also have reasonably foreseen that a parent of childbearing years, in the absence of the knowledge that SF suffered a genetically transferable condition, would conceive another child.

Clearly Dr. Backus had no idea about the mode of inheritance of Fragile X and erroneously believed that Dr. Meyer's testing had included analysis for Fragile X. The judge concluded in his opinion that Dr. Backus, after entering into a relationship in which a duty existed to Kimberly Molloy to render correct and appropriate medical advice, should have known that Dr. Meyer had failed to properly complete chromosomal testing. Furthermore, the judge opined, he had negligently assumed that the Fragile X test had been completed and that he owed Kimberly Molloy a duty to render medical advice pursuant to the appropriate standard of care when he advised her regarding the risks of conceiving another child with the same problems as SF.

Dr. Green was seen to be negligent even though she had been asked to provide an opinion regarding the management of SF's hyperactivity. As a treating physician, she also failed to order Fragile X testing and was seen to have a physician-patient relationship with SF.

All three doctors conceded that physicians are expected to notify family members when a genetic abnormality is detected so that those family members may obtain testing as well, if desired. If the patient is an adult, the duty to diagnose a genetic disease ends with the notification of the patient. However, for a minor child, the physician must notify a biological parent. These doctors would have fulfilled their duty if they had rendered appropriate medical services to SF and correctly communicated the resulting information to SF's parents. This, they did not do.

The appeals court denied the doctor's efforts to reverse the district-court ruling against a summary judgment.

The description given above is a truncated version of the appeals-court decision, which has been published. The case focuses on an extremely common set of circumstances seen continuously by clinical geneticists and genetic counselors. Our duty to inform is a constant, as is the requirement to document information transfer. Our usual practice, which we initiated many decades ago, is to provide a summary letter following a genetic evaluation or counseling that ends with a postscript, advising patients to remain in touch if further reproduction is planned given continued and major advances in genetics.

Given the remarkable progress in genetics, another issue concerning duty had arisen. A correctly performed and reported gene test may conclude that the result is a variation and *probably benign* or that the finding is of *uncertain significance* (not uncommon since we have twenty-one thousand to twenty-two thousand genes). Some years later, new advances reveal that the variation was not benign and then recognized as disease causing. Similarly, the gene change deemed of uncertain significance may no longer be uncertain.

Who has the duty to recontact and inform the individual and family about the vitally important new realization? The laboratory? The geneticist? The primary-care doctor? Is it the patient's responsibility to remain in touch with the geneticist or laboratory? We receive samples from all over the United States and from forty-five countries. Moreover, over forty million change their addresses each year in the United States.

At best, those who have been tested need to know the importance of knowing their laboratory result so that they can check with any geneticist if a reinterpretation is needed in the face of possible advances and changing family circumstances (births, deaths, new diagnoses, divorce, remarriage, etc.).

Huge advances in human genetics have left a majority of physicians out-of-date about the *new genetics*. Thus far, about forty-five hundred genes and their disease-causing mutations have been identified. About one in twelve people are affected, knowingly or not. Prenatal genetic diagnosis or preimplantation genetic diagnosis has to be offered (and documented) to all couples in whom disease-causing mutations can be identified.

This means that doctors first need to recognize that a disorder is genetic and second, that the causal gene is known. For a busy practitioner, any requirement that demands time and expertise to search the massive gene databases for this information would be absurd. Being alert to the possibility of a genetic disorder should simply have the doctor confer with or refer to a specialist.

Sadly, a lack of basic knowledge about the mode of inheritance displayed by the doctors in question reflected an even more pervasive lack of caring or attention. None of these three doctors recognized that they didn't know, they didn't know.

The case was eventually settled.

DAD, DAUGHTER, AND DUTY

Robert Batkin, complaining of pain in his back and abdomen, was diagnosed as having a tumor in his abdomen by his physician, Dr. George Pack. During surgery, in addition to the tumor, a huge number of colon polyps were seen. His entire colon and a portion of the small bowel were resected. This left Mr. Batkin with an ileostomy pouch. The pathology report confirmed that cancer had begun in at least one of the polyps. Incidentally, the surgeon also treated Mr. Batkin's wife for a different but benign disorder.

Two years later, Dr. Pack discovered that Mr. Batkin's cancer had spread to his liver, after he reappeared with a yellow color in his eyes (jaundice) and complaints of pain radiating down his leg. Within a month, and at forty-five years of age, Robert Batkin died. At that time, his daughter, Donna, was ten and her sister was seventeen.

About twenty-six years later, when Donna Safer was thirty-six years of age, she began to complain of abdominal pain. She was found to have polyps that had already developed into cancer. She too underwent surgery with a total colectomy and a portion of the small bowel being removed. She was also treated with chemotherapy. Only at that point did they discover that Donna's father had had the genetic cancer called familial adenomatous polyposis (FAP), upon which they filed a lawsuit against Dr. Pack. They claimed in their suit that the hereditary nature of FAP was well known and that Dr. Pack, according to the expected standard of care, should have warned immediate family members of their risk so that they would have the opportunity of surveillance and early diagnosis, thereby enabling timely treatment.

An effort was made by Dr. Pack's attorneys to seek a summary judgment aiming to dismiss the case, especially given the fact that records were scant and Dr. Pack had already died over twenty years earlier! Remarkably, Robert Batkin's widow testified that neither her husband nor Dr. Pack had ever even told her about the cancer and moreover that he was simply treating her husband for an intestinal blockage or an unspecified *infection*. Apparently, upon inquiry about any risk to her children, she was told by Dr. Pack not to worry.

Remarkably, the trial court held that a physician had no "legal duty to warn a child of a patient of a genetic risk." Among the reasons advanced was the opinion that there was no physician-patient relationship between Dr. Pack and Donna Safer and that the transmission of germs versus genes was not the same in respect of the duty to warn since "the harm is already present within the non-patient child, as opposed to being introduced by a patient who was not warned to stay away. The patient is taking no action in which to cause the child harm."

In denying Dr. Pack's estate from getting rid of the lawsuit through a summary judgment, the superior court opined that early monitoring of those at risk could effectively avert some of the more serious consequences of FAP. The court went on to state that "the duty to warn of avertable risk through genetic causes, by definition, was a matter of familial concern and sufficiently narrow to serve the interests of justice." The court went on to state that the duty to warn, especially with respect to young children who may be at risk, was required and that reasonable steps had to be taken to ensure that the necessary information reaches those likely to be affected. In passing, it is interesting to note that no statute of limitations was breached, which hence allowed Donna Safer to pursue her claim.

Pertinent Medical Facts

Familial adenomatous polyposis (FAP) is a distressingly grim genetic disorder. In an affected person, polyps begin to appear in the teens or twenties, the average age being about sixteen. By thirty-five years of age, some 95 percent of affected individuals have polyps. This is not a disorder with a few polyps but rather, once polyps have appeared, they rapidly increase in number to reach hundreds, if not thousands, resembling a nobly carpet. Risk of cancer is effectively 100 percent. If not diagnosed, 7 percent of untreated individuals develop colon cancer by the age of twenty-one, 87 percent by the age of forty-five, and 93 percent by the age of fifty.

To make things worse, if that was possible, there are risks for cancers in other organs that include the intestine closer to the stomach and thyroid cancer, as well as very infrequent cancers of the pancreas, brain, liver, bile ducts, and stomach.

The mutated gene (*APC*) is transmitted as an autosomal dominant, in which an affected person has a 50 percent risk of transmitting this culprit gene and its mutations to each of his or her offspring. However, between 20 and 25 percent of affected individuals have a brand-new gene mutation in the *APC* gene. For Robert Batkin, there was the 50 percent risk of transmitting this mutation to his children, including his daughter Donna Safer. She was only ten years of age when he was initially diagnosed.

There is an attenuated form of FAP with somewhat later onset, later development of cancer, and slightly better prognosis.

Thankfully, FAP is not common, ranging somewhere between 1 in 6,850 and 1 in 31,250 live births. It is shared equally between the sexes and fairly constant worldwide.

Anyone diagnosed with FAP should inform his or her immediate and extended families, since early diagnosis can be lifesaving. Surgery to remove the entire colon (colectomy) is available for treatment or as a preventative option. Curiously, benign tumors of bone and skin may also appear and require excision.

For many years, colonoscopy was recommended from the age of ten. Today, analysis of the *APC* gene will release at least those without a gene mutation from further invasive procedures. However, those found to harbor a gene mutation will enter a surveillance program of colonoscopy at least annually and examination of the esophagus, stomach, and duodenum via the mouth, beginning between twenty and twenty-five years of age, at intervals ranging between six months and four years. In addition, screening of the thyroid gland by ultrasound is recommended annually.

An affected person, with a 50 percent risk of transmitting the gene mutation to each of his or her offspring, has the option of preimplantation or prenatal genetic diagnosis in future pregnancies.

There are a number of other colon cancers that are also hereditary. Almost all are diagnosable via colonoscopy but, even more important, can be anticipated by gene analysis. For one such colon cancer, termed "hereditary nonpolyposis colon cancer" (HNPCC or Lynch syndrome), susceptibility can be detected by sequencing five genes. Fortunately, this cancer accounts for only 1–3 percent of all colon cancers. Unfortunately, however, mutations in any one of these five genes are associated with an increased lifetime risk for cancer in other organs: 52–82 percent for colorectal cancer (HNPCC), 35–60 percent for cancer of the internal lining of the uterus (endometrial cancer), 6–13 percent for stomach cancer, and 4–12 percent for ovarian cancer. One very important realization is that, even in families with a single mutation in one gene, different cancers may appear and may not be recognized as being due to the same single-gene mutation. For virtually all of these different types of colon cancer, an autosomal dominant mode of inheritance applies. Once again, there is a 50 percent risk of transmission to offspring of affected individuals.

Commentary

The roots of the duty to warn lie directly in the decision reached in the *Tarasoff v. Regents of the University of California* case in which the parents of Tatiana Tarasoff, a young student murdered by a psychiatric patient, sued the university-employed psychotherapists who had been treating that patient. Tatiana's parents claimed that the therapist failed to warn their daughter or the authorities of the imminent danger posed by the assailant and failing to have him confined as required under a statutory provision.
The court stated, in rejecting any claim of confidentiality by the therapist, that "protective privilege ends where the public peril begins." The court concluded that the therapist knew or should have known how serious a risk of violence the patient posed, that the threat of violence was foreseeable to a third party, and that the therapist had a duty of reasonable care to protect that party from harm by their patient.

Subsequently, courts have extended the duty to warn to fields beyond psychiatry. The duty to warn concerning contagious or communicable diseases has been followed by lawsuits brought by car-accident victims whose physicians failed to warn their impaired patients not to drive. The expansion of the duty to warn about genetically transmissible disease was simple, rational, and expected.

A third case (*Pate v. Threlkel*) further informs the discussion about a physician's duty to warn.

Heidi Pate was the adult daughter of her mother who had been diagnosed with medullary thyroid cancer. Three years after her mother's diagnosis of this serious malignancy, Heidi was found to also have this same cancer. This dominantly inherited cancer is caused by a mutation in a single gene (*RET*). However, in about 70 percent of cases, the mutation is brand new but transmissible to 50 percent of that person's offspring. At least in the adult, presenting symptoms include pain in the neck, an enlarged thyroid gland, and persistent diarrhea. Metastatic spread is early and potentially fatal. The concern is so great that even in infancy the recommendation is to remove the thyroid gland surgically before one year of age! If a mutation is detected, the parents of the affected should be tested immediately, and, if positive, their siblings should be tested in turn.

Heidi had no idea, until her mother was diagnosed, that this was an autosomal dominant disorder and that her risks had been 50 percent. Heidi claimed in her suit that as the direct and proximate cause of the doctor's negligence, she suffered from advanced medullary thyroid cancer. In her lawsuit against her mother's physician, she claimed that he owed her mother a duty to warn her about testing her children for this malignancy. This would have enabled Heidi to establish careful surveillance, enabling an early diagnosis and made a surgical cure more probable than not.

Initially, the trial court dismissed Heidi's suit, holding that the requirement of privacy and confidentiality between the doctor and the patient governed any requirement for communication. The appellate court agreed with the trial court's dismissal of Heidi's complaint. The court did add, however, that the doctor's duty may in fact apply to a third party when a "foreseeable zone of risk to the third party" exists. Incredibly, however, the court reasoned that Heidi was not within this foreseeable zone of risk and that there was therefore no duty to warn her (see chapter 18 for discussion about judges and science).

Fortunately, the Florida Supreme Court reversed both of these lower courts, concluding that the doctor had a duty to warn Heidi's mother of the cancer's genetically transferrable nature. Incredibly, the Court went on to opine that patients are responsible for warning their children, maintaining that if a doctor were to warn a party directly, he or she would breach his or her duty of confidentiality. The Court also claimed that the duty to warn a third party was impractical and burdensome.

Physicians have much to worry about, given the circumstances of these cases. At the time of the trial on the FAP case, medical records were scant and Dr. Pack had died over twenty years earlier. Therefore, his estate, and hence his widow and children, became the defendants. The trial court did not appear to consider the possibility that Robert Batkin may not have wanted to inform his family about his cancer. It is also conceivable that Dr. Pack was unaware of the hereditary nature of FAP and its extremely high risks of transmission. Nevertheless, the appellate division of the superior court of New Jersey refused to dismiss Donna Safer's complaint and confirmed that there was potential liability. The case was eventually settled.

The trial court dismissed Heidi's complaint, holding that she was not in a physician-patient relationship with Dr. Threlkel, which was necessary for her to bring a medical-malpractice action. The district court affirmed the trial court's dismissal. That court rejected the argument that Heidi's case was no different to previous decisions that recognized a doctor's duty to inform third parties of a patient's infectious disease. The court also rejected Heidi's position that pointed to the parents of a four-year-old child whose suit alleged that the child's pediatrician failed to diagnose cystic fibrosis early enough to prevent the parents from having a second child with that disorder. That court, however, did recognize that a physician's duty may extend beyond a patient to the members of that patient's family.

The Supreme Court of Florida focused on the prevailing standard of expected care that included both Heidi and her mother. The Supreme Court concluded that "when the prevailing standard of care creates a duty that is obviously for the benefit of certain identified third parties and that the physician knows of the existence of those third parties, then the physician's duty runs to those third parties." The Court recognized that a patient's children fall within the zone of foreseeable risk. The Court went on to recognize that it was difficult or impractical to require a physician to seek out and warn *various members* of a patient's family about a specific risk. The court held that, in any circumstances in which the doctor has a duty to warn about a genetically transferrable disease, the duty would be satisfied by warning the patient.

Three other published cases further inform this discussion. The first was a thirty-six-year-old man who was diagnosed with the long QT syndrome (see chapter 47) following repeated episodes of fainting. He was found to harbor a mutation in a specific dominant gene that causes this potentially fatal disorder due to the cardiac arrhythmia that occurs in this condition. Since his father had died sometime in his forties, this gentleman was left with the potential burden of informing his three siblings who were all at 50 percent risk of having the same disorder. There were also nine nephews and nieces who also would have been at risk.

In this case, there were both ethical and legal issues if he decided not to communicate this vital information, especially if a relative died as a consequence of not having had the available lifesaving treatment, which included medications as well as an implantable cardiac defibrillator.

The second case was of a Connecticut woman who had an extensive family history of breast cancer. Her physician failed to warn her of her increased risk for ovarian cancer, which she later developed. The Connecticut Supreme Court upheld the jury verdict (*Downs v. Trias*, 2012).

In the third published case, a patient was seen by a geneticist because of her concern about a family history of breast cancer. She was unaware that a family member with whom she did not speak had consulted that same geneticist. Gene studies for a specific analysis of the two common breast-cancer genes (*BRCA1* and *BRCA2*) had been performed on the relative, and a precise mutation was found. The ethical, and ultimately legal, question was if the geneticist should inform this woman that it was possible to simply check her DNA for the precisely known familial mutation breaking the privacy of the family member. Once again, the issue of confidentiality was in potential conflict with the demands of privacy. Of course, simply testing the two culprit genes, cost issues aside, would simply resolve all questions.

If you were witness to a big Mac truck heading directly at an innocent bystander, would you hesitate while considering the legal precedents about the duty to warn? Or would you react reflexively to warn that person at risk? Duty to protect should require no legal demand.

TOO MUCH AIR

Her pregnancy was plagued by anxiety and depression. Erica had, however, begun to feel much better when she learned that she was pregnant for the first time. Although not married, Erica, at twenty-three, had a good job and was "looking forward to raising her child" but did admit that she had thoughts of harming her baby.

Pregnancy was largely uneventful, and serial ultrasound examinations confirmed normal fetal growth. One week overdue and with no sign of spontaneous labor, the decision was made to induce her to get the delivery moving. After a few hours, her membranes ruptured spontaneously, and clear amniotic fluid was noted. Her physicians decided to let her rest overnight and in the morning began to augment her labor and provided her with an epidural anesthetic to control pain. Labor progressed and her cervix dilated, and she began a period of pushing for some two hours. However, it soon became clear, despite the fact that the electronic fetal monitor revealed no abnormality of the fetal heart rate, that an arrest of descent was the problem. Through Cesarean section, they extracted her son, who weighed in at eight pounds seven ounces. She named him Lenny.

Lenny was limp, had a slow heart rate, and was not breathing. Immediate chest compressions and two minutes of positive pressure ventilation served as sufficient resuscitation for him to begin breathing on his own, not requiring a ventilator. Measurement of the blood gases in his umbilical cord raised no special concern (pH 7.24, base excess −7). His Apgar scores were three, six, and seven at one, five, and ten minutes, respectively. These scores reflect the child's status of the heart rate, respiratory effort, muscle tone, reflex response, and color. At delivery, Lenny was covered all over with meconium (first stool).

A family-medicine resident was present at the delivery, and direct visualization of Lenny's larynx (laryngoscopy) was not done, nor was he intubated in order to remove by suction any of the meconium that may have reached beyond his vocal cords.

Respiratory distress continued. He had an elevated respiratory rate and a heart rate of 160 per minute. Measurement of his oxygen level revealed a 92 mmHg level of saturation.

Because of the concern about his breathing, Lenny was transferred to another hospital that had a higher level of neonatal care. On departure from his delivery hospital, Lenny's oxygen saturation was 123 mmHg.

It took about thirty-five minutes to reach the hospital. On admission, his oxygen saturation was measured at 322 mmHg (normally 75–100 mmHg). A small leak from his lung (called a pneumothorax) occurred while continued supplemental oxygen was used. His oxygen saturation reached values as high as 378 mmHg for more than fourteen hours.

Initial imaging of his brain by ultrasound and by MRI was reported as normal. By three days of age, however, they noticed that his normal head circumference had suddenly increased, and further imaging was consistent with brain swelling (cerebral edema) (similar to a burn, fluid pours out when the cell membranes become permeable, due to, for example, a lack of oxygen). It was then that Lenny had a number of seizures, which were quickly controlled. Lenny slowly improved and was discharged from the hospital three weeks after his birth.

By two months of age, Lenny was seizure free, but his head had become small, and his anterior fontanel (soft spot) was not palpable. At three months of age, he was tremulous and his legs spastic. A CT scan of his brain at six months of age revealed extensive damage to his brain (cystic encephalomalacia).

By four years of age, Lenny could not sit, crawl, stand, walk, or talk. He also could not eat and had to be fed through a tube to his stomach via his abdominal wall (G-tube). His head was tiny (microcephaly), and his limbs had developed contractures due to his spasticity.

Erica sued the physicians and hospitals who cared for Lenny, holding them responsible for his severe brain damage.

Pertinent Medical Facts

It has been known for a long time that administration of supplemental oxygen, while critical for survival, has the potential to cause long-term damage to the back of the eye (retina), lungs, and the brain. Excessive oxygen (hyperoxia) initiates a series of events within and between cells that involve about one thousand genes, which function like a sensor to oxygen levels and control the necessary adaptations. These genes, via their proteins, act "like a thermostat," except they do not *measure* temperature but rather react to elevated oxygen concentration. Elevated levels of oxygen trigger enzyme systems within cells that then self-destruct (called "apoptosis"). The cascade of events set in motion by hyperoxia interferes with the cell biochemistry, altering the brain's continued development. If oxygen concentrations reach the astronomical levels Lenny was subject to, profound irreversible brain damage occurs, as brain cells "commit suicide"!

Lenny was also clearly exposed to low levels of oxygen during labor and delivery before his Cesarean section. However, immediate resuscitation, including chest compressions, quickly revived him, only for him to be felled by hyperoxia in the ensuing twenty-four hours.

Questions

- What did the standard of expected care require for Lenny's resuscitation at birth?
- Why did Lenny have prolonged exposure to hyperoxia?
- Did Erica's two hours of pushing limit the oxygen supply to Lenny's brain?

Commentary

Guidelines issued by the American College of Obstetricians and Gynecologists recommend that when there is neonatal depression, meconium staining of the amniotic fluid, and the need for resuscitation, intubation and tracheal suctioning should be performed. The family-medicine resident in this case did not do what was required and thereby violated the expected standard of care. Oversight of that resident was also lacking. It is highly likely that the subsequent development of respiratory distress that Lenny suffered was caused by his aspiration of meconium into his lungs and the subsequent development of the pneumothorax. However, there was also a failure to measure Lenny's oxygen saturation during his resuscitation. The standard of expected care was to use a pulse oximeter to record the skin-oxygen saturation. This simple step would have helped monitor his oxygen concentration, thereby avoiding hyperoxia.

It is almost a reflex for nurses to reach for oxygen when their patients in labor are noted on the monitor to have concerning or nonreassuring changes in the fetal heart-rate tracing. The intention is to increase oxygen supply to the fetus via the umbilical-cord vein. Caution, however, is needed in light of a 2017 study from the Washington University School of Medicine. From an analysis of 7,789 newborns, they concluded that there was a small but significant increased risk of complications for those newborns who during delivery had some oxygen deprivation. This was almost certainly the situation with Lenny.

It is likely that the two hours of pushing by Erica in her second stage of labor deprived Lenny of a noncritical level of oxygen to his brain. Born limp, not breathing, and with a very slow heart rate clearly indicated that oxygen deprivation had indeed occurred during that two-hour period. In all likelihood, Lenny's brain cells were already susceptible to the greater damage caused by excessive oxygen levels.

The American Academy of Pediatrics now recommends that room air rather than oxygen be used to initiate resuscitation of a newborn because of the danger of hyperoxia.

Lenny's caregivers, including the nurses who were also expected to monitor his oxygen as well as the hospitals, were held accountable. It seems they didn't know, they didn't know, that too much oxygen can permanently damage the infant brain.

The case was settled.

DEATH BY TELEPHONE

Shauna's pregnancy was far from smooth. She developed diabetes during pregnancy and was obese, and her hypertension needed increased medication for control. While she accomplished a vaginal delivery after a prolonged labor, heavy bleeding followed, rendering her anemic. Her son, Louis, was hardly breathing at birth and required oxygen for the first five minutes using a bag and mask, in addition to suction. After that initial scare, he did well. His weight was 7 pounds 15.5 ounces, and pregnancy was at full term. He had a normal-duration stay in the nursery and went home with his mother. His blood sugar initially was a little low, but this was not surprising for the infant of a diabetic mother. Because of the initial scare, a series of chemical and biochemical tests were done, all of which yielded normal results. Prior to his discharge from the hospital, he was feeding well, voiding, and stooling normally. His chest was clear, his heart rate and rhythm were regular, and his limbs were normal and well perfused. Examination of his limbs, including his hips, fingers, toes, and spine, was all normal. Shauna was asked to bring him back for a two-week well baby visit.

At that visit, Shauna reported that Louis was spitting up at least once or twice a day, as well as having some loose nonmucous stools. He apparently seemed well hydrated, and no physical abnormality was evident. His doctor noted that his vomiting or spitting up was neither forceful nor projectile, and the conclusion he reached was that Louis had gastroesophageal reflux or lactose intolerance. It was noted that Louis had not only failed to gain his birth weight in two weeks, but that he had actually lost weight. Changes were made to his diet, his feed was thickened, and advice was provided for antireflux positioning. Shauna was instructed to call back in three days if he was not better.

Three days later, Shauna's husband, Eric, called Louis's doctor when he returned from work. He communicated clearly that Louis continued to spit up, passed urine, did not appear lethargic, did not feel hot to the touch, and that he would mostly spit up when lying down for a diaper change.

On the telephone, the doctor opined that Louis's symptoms were most consistent with reflux but did suggest a change in the liquid that Louis was being fed, as well as initiating a milk-free soy formula.

The very next day, Eric, called again, this time speaking to the doctor on call who had never seen Louis and was not fully aware of his history. Once again, the father emphasized that Louis continued to spit up. The covering doctor instructed him to simply carry on and continue with the course of treatment he was on. Later that same day, on a second call, Eric was frantic and called the covering doctor to report that Louis was limp, less responsive, and seemed to be breathing fast. The doctor instructed them to call 911 and take him immediately to the emergency department in the nearby hospital.

Upon admission to the emergency department, it was obvious that Louis was critically ill. He was immediately intubated and ventilated. Examination of a blood sample revealed a very high level of acid in his blood (called "metabolic acidosis") as well as an extremely high white-blood-cell count and cell types that indicated a bacterial infection. Despite heroic efforts, Louis died the next day.

At autopsy, bleeding into his lungs and his nose was noted, and infection was considered to be the most likely cause of his death. He had been given intravenous antibiotics the day before he died, so it was not unexpected that blood cultures yielded no detectable bacteria.

The family sued both doctors for their failure to both diagnose and treat their son, resulting in his death.

Pertinent Medical Facts

Evaluation of the full-term newborn for early-onset infection is both common and important. The risk of infection is higher in the newborn than at any other time of life. Even though the mortality rate for full-term newborns with serious infection is less than 2 percent, brain damage can result in up to 50 percent.

The American Academy of Pediatrics and the Centers for Disease Control have published national guidelines addressing this subject.

The premature infant, the newborn, and the elderly have weak defenses against both infection and dehydration. The immune system that protects us from infection is still developing in the premature and newborn infant, while in the elderly, that system is weakened and less effective. Signs of infection in the newborn are often subtle and nonspecific. Symptoms include not feeding well; spitting up; irritability; a weak cry; a below-normal, normal, or elevated temperature; and unexpected drowsiness. The penalty for missing the diagnosis of infection in the newborn can be a quick and unexpected death. Even when benefiting from direct face-to-face physical examination of the newborn, diagnosis of infection can often be based more on caution than from an observation of any physical signs, white-blood-cell count, or the nonspecific C-reactive protein test. This realization leads pediatricians to quickly obtain blood samples and, if necessary, a sample of cerebrospinal fluid by lumbar puncture for bacterial cultures and to initiate treatment with antibiotics immediately, even without a definitive diagnosis. If test results return as normal, antibiotic treatment is discontinued.

Questions

- Why did Louis's doctor not recognize that, at two weeks of age, he was below his birth weight, symptomatic, and not doing well? Why did he not hospitalize him immediately?

- Why did the covering doctor choose to guess what was wrong, without having even seen the patient, despite the obvious worry and anxiety expressed by his father?

Commentary

In recent years, an increasing awareness of medical negligence by primary-care doctors has become apparent with more available data. In Massachusetts, during a recent five-year period in which there were 7,224 malpractice claims, 551 (7.7 percent) were focused on primary care doctors. The real problem was diagnostic failure, as noted in 397 (72.1 percent) cases, while medication issues occurred in 12.3 percent, communication problems in 2.7 percent, and other medical treatment issues in 2.4 percent. Failure to diagnosis infections was on the list of conditions of diagnoses that were missed. Other conditions included cancer, heart disease, blood-vessel diseases, and stroke.

An earlier national study with 239,756 closed malpractice-liability claims showed that 11.5 percent (27,556) involved family doctors. Once again, the most common allegation against family doctors was diagnostic failure.

The first warning sign, missed by Louis's doctor, was his loss of weight that registered below his birth weight at two weeks of life. This occurred against a background that his mother provided about his persistent spitting up and feeding difficulties. That was the point at which hospitalization was necessary and almost certainly would have saved his life.

The second grievous error in the care and treatment of Louis was rendered by the covering doctor. His flawed thought process failed to properly consider that he did not know the patient, had never seen the child, was treating a sick newborn, was making a diagnosis of lactose intolerance intuitively, and not insisting that he see the child. Clearly, this was death by telephone.

As physicians, we all face concerned and worried parents and patients. Calls come in at any time of the day or night. Knowing the family, the patient and his or her illness, the treatment in place, and the potential seriousness of the illness enables appropriate responses. If there is any doubt in the mind of the caring physician, a newborn should be seen or sent directly to the emergency department in a hospital. Certainly, with newborns, there is no room for delay. Here, clinical judgments are paramount, since these kinds of telephone calls are common in pediatrics.

Louis's health deteriorated rapidly, with his overwhelming infection, reflected by his very high white-blood-cell count and the type of cells circulating in his blood, compounded by dehydration and metabolic acidosis. Sometimes the white-blood-cell count, even in the face of infection in the newborn or the elderly, might actually drop below normal. The metabolic disturbance in body chemistry occurs when too much acid is produced or when the kidneys fail to remove enough acid from the body. Because of the compounding effect of sick cells, infection, dehydration, and diminished levels of oxygen, hydrogen ions pour out of the cells into the bloodstream, causing the acidity. Metabolic acidosis is especially dangerous, having neurological effects that can cause drowsiness, seizures, stupor, coma, and death. Effects on the heart may lead to potential rhythm disturbances and death. One or both of these effects led to Louis's death.

The American Academy of Pediatrics guidelines emphasize the fact that infections in the newborn are a major cause of morbidity and mortality.

Once again, we see errors compounded. Failure to recognize the ominous indicator of a weight below birth weight in a neonate having loose stools and vomiting was regarded as negligence. Advising a parent about a newborn with these symptoms who the covering physician had never seen invited disaster.
Neither physician recognized the obvious risks that led to Louis's death.

The case was settled.

TALIA...*OH, TALIA*

If you prefer not to cry, do not read on.

Talia was a vigorous, smart, creative artist and a resourceful twenty-three-year-old who had struggled and coped with a lifelong connective-tissue disorder (called Ehlers-Danlos syndrome). Her joint hypermobility and associated joint aches and pains were constant reminders of this genetic disorder. She had bilaterally subluxing shoulders, wrists, and one thumb. She had five ACL ligament reconstructions on her right knee. It was only in her teens that involvement of multiple organ systems became increasingly problematic. The symptoms and signs she experienced and lived with daily were typical of this disorder.* Standing up suddenly from a recumbent position would make her light-headed and even close to fainting. She recognized this feature, so when she played soccer, she remained standing whenever she came off the playing field during half time, because if she sat down and then stood up, it would take her over ten minutes to regain her balance and overcome her dizziness. Due to her orthostatic symptoms, Talia experienced brain "fog." She would find it harder to think and felt she needed to clear the cobwebs away. This symptom would manifest, for example, when entering a room and not remembering the original purpose. Intestinal symptoms, including abdominal pain and distention, with bouts of diarrhea, were diagnosed as "irritable bowel syndrome." She had an extremely irritable bladder. Talia had Raynaud's phenomenon (fingers [mostly] and toes turn white and then blue, numb, and painful). She had mild scoliosis. When she was seventeen, Talia had surgical correction of an underdeveloped jaw and bilaterally subluxing temporomandibular joints. She had blue sclera, and her skin was soft and velvety and extremely sensitive, and she would sometimes feel a burning sensation, especially in her arms and

---

*I am grateful and appreciative to have Talia's mother provide all the details of Talia's symptoms and signs and suffering at the end of her life. Retelling and reliving Talia's terrible last days evoke a profound deep sadness and sorrow.

legs. Because of the autonomic nervous system dysfunction, she would have intermittent bouts of flushing. As she got older, Talia's sleep became disturbed, and fatigue became more and more of an issue.

In her later teens, however, the headaches became more severe, and sudden movement of her head and neck sometimes resulted in blackouts. Increasingly, she developed severe pains in her neck and the back of her head and eventually sought the opinions of several neurosurgeons who were familiar with EDS to determine if a cervical spinal fusion would help.

She duly underwent neurosurgery to correct a small Chiari I malformation (see below) and a spinal fusion of the vertebrae in her neck. The surgery was performed at Swedish Cherry Hill Hospital in Seattle by a prominent neurosurgeon.

Many of the following details were reported by Mike Baker of the *Seattle Times*, some of which was derived from court records.

When Talia woke from the anesthesia, she could hardly speak or open her mouth enough to squeeze in a finger. Her lower jaw was ajar, jutting forward, as Mike Baker reported, "like a bulldog." With her voice a harsh rasp, she complained to the nurse that she was having difficulty breathing and promptly vomited twice in the bed. The nurse paged Dr. Delashaw, the neurosurgeon, and he did not respond. Then the nurse paged the neurosurgical resident. As the family became more alarmed and more insistent, a rapid response team was called. Talia's father, a primary-care physician who was present, explained that Talia's jaw was locked and her neck immobile from the rods affixed to her vertebrae and that she might need an emergency cricothyrotomy if her airway occluded. After some resistance, that discussion resulted in Talia being moved to the intensive-care unit. Her breathing difficulty, however, continued even in the ICU and through the night.

The next morning, Dr. Delashaw and his team made a brief visit to Talia in the intensive-care unit. Talia explained her trouble breathing and that her jaw would not open. The neurosurgeon's response was that there was nothing he did that would have put her jaw out of place, and he suggested that she see a specialist after leaving the hospital. The doctor's note described Talia as having "mild difficulty breathing," which they thought was due to her being intubated during surgery. They thought she was ready to transfer out of intensive care. Later that morning, Talia texted her friend, reporting that "my throat is nearly swollen closed." To her cousin, she texted that she couldn't even talk or swallow.

All this time, her father, gravely concerned, repeatedly expressed to the ICU staff his concerns that Talia's airway was not being managed and that they needed to evaluate her and deal with her airway before she occluded, which would result in her requiring an emergency tracheostomy. Talia's breathing got no better, and the ICU staff continued to ignore Talia and her parents, in spite of an evaluation by a speech pathologist indicating that Talia had stridor, could not breathe when on her back, could not open her mouth wider than a centimeter, and that she was having trouble swallowing. As Talia's parents became more insistent that Talia was having more difficulty breathing, the doctor's plans were to transfer her out of the ICU and onto the regular ward, and they gave her intravenous Valium to calm and sedate her.

Early in the afternoon, about eighteen hours after Talia's father had first expressed his concern about Talia's airway and raised the possibility that Talia would need an emergency tracheostomy, Talia suddenly gave a harsh cough and called for a suction tube to try to clear her throat. A sudden terror crossed her face, and she croaked urgently, "I can't breathe! Help me! I can't breathe!" Talia's blue eyes bulged; she struggled to breathe but was unable to get any air. Her mother ran to call for help. A respiratory therapist and nurse practitioner placed an oxygen mask over her nose and mouth while Talia thrashed momentarily in her bed, but unable to draw in any air, she went still very quickly. Her father cried out that Talia needed an immediate tracheostomy while the respiratory therapist and nurse practitioner tried to force an oral airway into her mouth. They frantically tried different sizes, which they couldn't pass through her clenched teeth, while her father screamed that they could not use an oral airway because her jaw was locked and her mouth would not open—she needed an tracheostomy *now*! But the two staff members continued to try in vain to pull Talia's jaw open anyway.

The code team entered the room ten minutes after Talia's cry for help. The respiratory therapist remained at Talia's head, where he tried unsuccessfully to use a bag and mask, while other members of the code team began to establish additional intravenous access. Talia's father again called for a tracheostomy, but his pleas fell on deaf ears. Talia's oxygen saturation dropped precipitously; she remained still, and her skin turned dusky. Over fifteen minutes after Talia stopped breathing, an anesthesiologist entered the room and, upon observing Talia's condition, decided immediately that she needed a tracheostomy. There was no tracheostomy kit at the bedside. Talia went into cardiac arrest, and the anesthesiologist was eventually able to complete the tracheostomy while the staff were performing CPR on Talia.

Shortly after that, about twenty minutes after Talia occluded, her heartbeat and blood pressure stabilized, but she was left comatose. Over the next nine days, brain imaging and electro diagnostic studies confirmed that Talia had sustained massive brain destruction due to the lack of oxygen and that she would remain in a permanent vegetative state. The physicians then left it to Talia's parents to decide when to take her off life support.

Talia had a large and loving extended family, and they came from as far away as Toronto to say good-bye before life support was terminated. Her parents and her sister remained at her bedside for thirty-seven painful hours, watching her die from lack of oxygen for the second time in ten days. They still haven't recovered from the experience of losing their beloved daughter, Talia, after helplessly witnessing the series of events that led so unnecessarily to her death.

The required autopsy did not reveal the precise cause of Talia's inability to breathe, which was obviously due to swelling of the throat, mucus, or vomitus, given no physical obstruction.

A week after Talia's death, a letter addressed to her arrived in the mail from Swedish Cherry Hill Hospital, asking Talia to complete a survey that described her stay in hospital. "By sharing your thoughts and feelings, you can help us improve the care we provide," the letter stated.

Talia's parents sued the hospital for medical negligence. The hospital, hoping to avoid further public

embarrassment, settled the case. Three years later, in conjunction with a series of articles about Talia and

Swedish Cherry Hill that appeared in the *Seattle Times*, the hospital extended their "deepest sympathies to

any family who is grieving the loss of a loved one." But one wonders if there was ever any direct apology

to the family.

Pertinent Medical Facts

There are about sixteen different clinical types of the Ehlers-Danlos syndrome. Talia certainly had a

classical type with joint hypermobility, the gene for which was not determined. These types and subtypes

are almost invariably transmitted as autosomal dominant disorders, with an affected person having a 50

percent risk of transmitting the disorder to his or her offspring.

Talia, throughout her teens, suffered from multiple aches and pains in multiple joints as well as extremely

hyperextensible joints. Despite all of that pain, she was an avid skier, soccer player, and pole vaulter. Other

manifestations include joint dislocations and, frequently, subluxations (bones popping in and out of joints).

Chronic and disabling pain is common and frequently psychologically disabling. Disorders similar to

irritable bowel syndrome are often unrecognized. An almost constant feature is orthostatic intolerance (e.g.,

dizziness or feeling faint when standing up suddenly from a recumbent position), which can be associated

with a sudden increase in the heart rate with or without palpitations (typically called POTS— postural

orthostatic tachycardia syndrome).

Another feature of this orthostatic intolerance is the excessive fatigue that people with this disorder

experience. It can be so disabling that those affected have difficulty getting out of bed and going off to

school or work. In addition, another manifestation is brain "fog." This is an extremely common feature,

and patients relate that they often enter a room and do not know why they did or what they came for.

They could be driving somewhere and forget where they are. They often make notes of things that they

need to do in order to avoid forgetting. Both the excess fatigue and the brain "fog" may have their origins not only in the commonly associated low blood pressure but also in involvement of the autonomic nervous system. The latter may also be at the root of complaints of painful, blue, or cold fingers and toes (called Raynaud's phenomenon). Mitral valve prolapse is not uncommon, due to a floppy mitral valve, and often the source of palpitations.

The skin is often soft and velvety, and easy bruising is common. It is also often translucent, thin, or hyperelastic. Degenerative joint disease is common and a source of neck and back pain. Muscle spasms are common, frequently involving the legs and back. Malalignment of the vertebral column shows up as scoliosis. Well recognized is a tiny part of the posterior brain poking through the skull into the spinal canal (called Chiari I). This may be a source of aggravating and frequent headaches and pain at the back of the head and other aggravating symptoms. When the brain extrusion into the spinal canal reaches a certain length (e.g., 0.6 cm), neurosurgery may be recommended. Headaches and migraines are common, often debilitating, and may be triggered by pain in the temporomandibular joints of the jaw.

Disturbance in the autonomic nervous system results in sudden episodes of flushing and sweating of the face; sweating all over the body for a few minutes; and episodes of sudden burning sensations in the limbs, fingers, or toes, due to neuropathic pain. This is thought to be likely due to the involvement of the small nerve fibers in the limbs. Following surgery, wounds may not hold together well (wound dehiscence), and hernias may occur at the sight of surgical scars.

Talia suffered disabling joint instability of her neck, which became the source of debilitating pain. The neurosurgery Talia chose was to have rods and screws inserted into the vertebrae of her neck to stabilize the spine in that region and to free her from the disabling pain.

Given the chronic pain and multisystem difficulties, psychological dysfunction and emotional problems are common and may include anxiety, depression, affective disorders, and a feeling of hopelessness or desperation. Chronic pain inevitably disturbs sleep, which then interferes with the ability to cope with all of the other manifestations. Everything is made worse by the fact that physicians often miss the diagnosis of Ehlers-Danlos syndrome. Those who are affected feel misunderstood, disbelieved, often wrongly

diagnosed as having mental health problems, or accused of malingering. Some are diagnosed as having

chronic fatigue syndrome.

There are many other features and details of treatment that are not pertinent to this discussion but can be

examined through the Ehlers-Danlos Syndrome Society.

Questions

- How was it possible for Talia to die in the intensive-care unit, simply not being able to breathe?

- Was Talia's jaw, anchored by loose ligaments, dislocated by the anesthesiologist, who needed to

  have her chin thrust upward to open her airway even though she was placed on her stomach for

  surgery?

- Why did anesthesiology not do a routine check on Talia after she was out of recovery, and why

  was an anesthesiologist not called in for a consult, given her difficulty breathing in the presence

  of a fused neck and a locked jaw that would not open?

- Since direct physical examination of Talia's throat could not be done, why was imaging not

  performed to determine the reason for the difficulty in breathing that she experienced?

- Why were Talia and her parents' requests systematically ignored, even with Talia's father being a

  physician?

- What was wrong with the working atmosphere of Swedish Hospital?

Commentary

It is essentially incomprehensible to consider the incompetence of the Swedish Hospital intensive-care

unit staff, who allowed a patient to die because of an inability to breathe through a physiological

obstruction that they were unable to diagnose. Where were the senior attending surgeon, physician,

anesthesiologist, or intensivist who should have made the decision for a tracheostomy in order to avoid a disastrous outcome? Worse still, why was there no tracheostomy kit available at the bedside when it was needed? Was the idea of anticipatory medicine a foreign subject to those who work in the intensive-care unit at Swedish Hospital? Why were a respiratory therapist and nursing staff with experienced physicians messing with efforts at intubation via her mouth when a tracheostomy was overdue? Again, why was Talia's father's request for a tracheostomy ignored?

The response by the neurosurgeon, Dr. Delashaw, was that "there was nothing that he did that would have put her jaw out of place." Apparently, he suggested that she see a specialist after leaving the hospital. One can question why Dr. Delashaw didn't simply call for another specialist opinion. Long gone are the days when a surgeon should be considered simply a technician, but rather somebody who cared for a patient, requiring a mind-set that went beyond manual dexterity.

The failure to diagnose the reason for her obstructed breathing again reflected pathetic clinical skills evident in the intensive-care unit. Imaging by ultrasound or x-ray certainly would have assisted in determining the cause of her obstructed breathing. If indeed she aspirated on mucous or vomitus, the tracheostomy would have saved her life.

How important was the pervasive culture, the hubris, and the arrogance that compromised patient welfare at Swedish Hospital? The published comments on Facebook by a Swedish Hospital physician addressed this issue as follows:

> I am a Swedish clinician with many years of experience at the institution. The events happening in the Neuroscience Institute are not unique. They are indicative of the current culture of the organization and are reflected in departments across it. The key problems plaguing Neuroscience, greed that compromises patient care and staff well-being, dismissal of staff reports of serious patient care issues by management and administration, and resultant retaliation, both tacit and blatant, are all prevalent in my area of practice. The so-called culture of safety is a culture of fear. In my area of practice for the past five years or so my colleagues and I have reported issues of

unethical and substandard practice, harm and potential harm to patients, and various forms of abuse of staff members, repeatedly. We have reported these to managers, up through various levels of administration, and to the anonymous Culture of Safety reporting hotline, to have them routinely dismissed. Those speaking up have been recipients of a range of retaliatory actions, from consequent slaps on the hand, to termination. The level of moral distress, (a phenomenon in which one knows the right action to take, but is restrained from taking it), my colleagues and I endure on a daily basis borders on unmanageable. Thank you for this investigation. I hope it is only the beginning of an inquiry into Swedish's current culture and practices, and will force changes that are desperately needed to protect patients and staff.

The report by Mike Baker and Justin Mayo in the *Seattle Times* on February 10, 2017, detailed their investigation of clinical neurosurgical practice at the Swedish Cherry Hill Hospital in Seattle. They focused on the Swedish Neuroscience Institute in this hospital acquired by Providence Health and Services. Their outstanding investigative journalism uncovered disturbing findings that are summarized here directly from their reports.

They found that physicians in the neuroscience unit were incentivized to pursue high-volume patient numbers, especially those needing complicated surgical techniques. In 2015, the neurosurgeons generated half-a-billion-dollars net, of operating revenue, which represents a 39 percent increase compared to three years before. The neurosurgeons' focus was on invasive brain and spine procedures. They noted that neurosurgeons were running two or three operating rooms concurrently, appearing for less than fifteen minutes for any one operation, and using less experienced surgeons-in-training in order to achieve a high volume of patients. Also noted was the fact that more invasive techniques were being used at Swedish Cherry Hill Hospital, such as opening the skull instead of using less invasive procedures.

One result of this high-volume approach was to overload the intensive-care unit, leading to decreased attention by intensive-care unit nurses to individual patients. Some of the nurses ended up working some twenty hours per day. Also noted was increased numbers of blood clots, collapsed lungs, and serious surgery complications, including strokes.

Current and former staff of the Neuroscience Institute reported an array of concerns that included inadequate patient care, inappropriate surgery, poor documentation, lack of accountability for postoperative complications, and poor decision making that resulted in patient harm and death. One staff neurosurgeon talked to Dr. Tony Armada, the CEO of Swedish Hospital, about the "toxic, repressive environment" that impacted patient care.

Providence Health and Services recruited Dr. Johnny Delashaw, the neurosurgeon who operated on Talia. In his first sixteen months, he treated 661 patients, billing more than $86 million! During that period alone, Dr. Delashaw faced forty-nine internal complaints, mainly about the quality of his patient care, his performing unnecessary surgical procedures, and having allegations about unprofessional behavior. He had been recruited from Oregon Health Sciences University, where, in fourteen years, he was sued in twelve different cases, including surgery on the wrong part of the spinal cord. He had also worked at the University of California at Irvine. In 2013, the American Association of Neurological Surgeons censured Dr. Delashaw for questionable testimony he gave as an expert witness in a medical-malpractice case.

You the reader must be thinking who on earth was responsible for the disaster. The real facts are outlined above, but the accountability is much more far-reaching. Why did it take an expose from the *Seattle Times* to get the attention of those in authority? Why did the board of directors of Providence Health and Services, the board of governors of Swedish Cherry Hill Hospital, and the CEO of that hospital not take any timely action? Were any of the board of trustees of Swedish Hospital held accountable? How was it possible they didn't know about the toxic atmosphere in the hospital? And if not, why not? Did they all abdicate their responsibilities? Why was the state Board of Registration and Medicine normally responsible for disciplinary actions not overtly involved? It is now clearer how a dollar-splitting, greed-obsessed, egotistical, but expert technical neurosurgeon accomplished surgery that nevertheless resulted in the terrifying death of a young, creative woman. What a terrible shame and disgrace!

Litigation arising as a consequence of negligent care in intensive-care units (ICUs) is unfortunately not rare. An analysis of 313 claims in England made between 1995 and 2012, and reported in the *British Journal of Anesthesiology*, concluded that sixty-three (20 percent) were due to respiratory/airway problems. Of the claims made because of death in the ICU, 30 percent were for respiratory/airway issues.

Talia came from an extremely kind and caring family. When Talia was still young, her parents became foster parents to two young girls whose mother had been murdered. They also had two other girls, friends of Talia and her sister, join them in their home after their mother committed suicide. These girls remained part of their family. Consequently, when all the girls went off to college, Talia's parents adopted two children from Ethiopia. These two children, who grew up hungry and the victims of abuse by their father (who later died from AIDS), were both adored by Talia.

Her parents named her Talia, which means morning dew, a divine blessing, a tender nourishment of life. Talia...*oh, Talia*!

GENES OR HYPOXIA

Pregnancy with a maternal weight that reached 350 pounds at the time of delivery is a recipe for disaster. Such was the situation for Kimberly, who had struggled for a lifetime with her obesity. To make a bad situation worse, Kimberly had gained 90 pounds during her pregnancy. Morbidly obese women, as Kimberly would be described, have a clear risk of delivering a very large (macrosomic) baby. Diabetes during pregnancy is common in this situation. Kimberly's glucose-tolerance test yielded a borderline normal result. She only had one early pregnancy glucose-tolerance test and should have had another later in pregnancy. She was almost certainly a gestational diabetic, explaining her baby's large size. The infants of diabetic mothers have excessive fat deposition, especially around their shoulders and trunk, which leads directly to difficulties in traversing the birth canal during labor and delivery. Pregnancies with macrosomic babies frequently require a Cesarean section because of the disproportion between their size and the outlet from the pelvis. Ultrasound is often used to track and estimate fetal weight, especially in the last three months of pregnancy, particularly when the baby is large, and to determine amniotic fluid volume, which Kimberly had in excess (called polyhydramnios).

The decision was made to induce labor using the drug Pitocin to stimulate uterine contractions. Kimberly reached a stage where she was pushing for some two hours before delivery was achieved. Worrying heart-rate decelerations were noted on the electronic fetal monitor. That delivery, unfortunately, was traumatic. Her daughter, Markell, weighed ten pounds five ounces at birth. In trying to extract Markell, her collarbone was broken, and there was bruising of her head, her left arm, left nipple, and right forearm. She was briefly depressed at birth and had mild respiratory distress. Imaging of her brain showed a tiny amount of blood near the back, but on the surface, of her brain (subarachnoid hemorrhage).

Though battered and bruised, and with a broken collarbone, Markell's heart rate, tone, and level of consciousness were all within normal limits, and her color was good. Moreover, a blood-gas evaluation of her cord blood revealed no increased acid output (metabolic acidosis), usually due to a lack of oxygen, despite having come through two hours of second-stage labor. Her head circumference was also close to the ninetieth percentile, in sync with her large size.

In the months following birth, it became clear that Markell was slowly becoming spastic, and her developmental milestones were delayed. Moreover, her brain was not growing according to expectations, resulting over time to a progressively small head (brain) size (microcephaly). Neurological evaluation led to brain imaging that revealed abnormalities concerning a genetic disorder or possibly the effects and consequences of damage due to lack of oxygen. These consultations also led to questions of a specific genetic disorder, primarily because of the typical brain-imaging observations of the hind brain (cerebellum) that strongly suggested a genetic disorder.

In due course, DNA studies enabled a definitive diagnosis of the autosomal recessive disorder called pontocerebellar hypoplasia. Markell's neurological signs were typical for this disorder.

Pertinent Medical Facts

Pontocerebellar hypoplasia is an autosomal recessive disorder characterized by spasticity, incoordination of sucking and swallowing, major delays in motor and cognitive development, visual impairment, and seizures. Some newborns may also have multiple joint contractures, impaired control of breathing, and possible early death. Despite being born with a normal head size, the brain's failure to grow results in microcephaly (small head) by the end of the first year of life. During that period, development of severe involuntary movement is characteristic and is accompanied by developing spasticity. Death often occurs before the age of ten, but survival can be prolonged by the insertion of a G-tube into the abdomen for nutrition and prompt treatment of recurrent infections.

Two of the types of pontocerebellar hypoplasia are extremely severe and are mostly preceded by excess amniotic fluid (polyhydramnios) and joint contractures while still in the womb, which are associated with severe spasticity soon after birth. Polyhydramnios occurs due to impaired fetal swallowing, and lack of fetal movement (fetal akinesia) could result in congenital contractures of the limbs. Difficulty with breathing and dependency on ventilation may often lead to death in the newborn period.

Brain imaging typically shows atrophy of the posterior part of the brain (the cerebellum) with particular diagnostic signs and patterns. Involvement of the cerebral cortex and other areas of the brain may also occur.

While typical clinical features and characteristic findings point directly to the diagnosis, precise and specific diagnosis is made by analysis of the culprit gene (*TSEN54*). Once the mutations have been determined, parents of an affected child, who are facing a future 25 percent risk of recurrence, have the option of future preimplantation or prenatal genetic diagnosis.

Difficulties in achieving a prompt diagnosis are experienced when, as in this case, problems arise during labor and delivery, where an alleged lack of oxygen may have a critical role in causing additional brain damage. Confusion may well arise when the images of the brain following prolonged or partial prolonged lack of oxygen (hypoxia) are compared with abnormalities in pontocerebellar hypoplasia. Teasing apart the relative contributions of the gene defect from the hypoxic exposure on the brain can be challenging.

Not unexpectedly, pontocerebellar hypoplasia, being an autosomal recessive disorder, may well result as a consequence of consanguinity. Related parents may well be carrying the same inherited mutation from a common ancestor.

Notwithstanding the genetic diagnosis, Kimberly sued the hospital and her doctor.

Questions

- Why was it not clear that Kimberly was carrying a very large baby?
- Why was Kimberly induced with Pitocin when the baby was so large, and why was the Pitocin continued even when some irregularities (decelerations) were seen on the electronic fetal monitor?

- Despite the baby's size and traumatic delivery, was the baby's genetic disorder the root cause of her subsequent global delay in development?

Commentary

Kimberly was morbidly obese, a condition that is accompanied by a distressing number of maternal and newborn complications. Maternal morbid obesity is associated with double the risk of an adverse outcome to pregnancy and the need for interventions. Mothers like Kimberly have an increased rate of diabetes developing in pregnancy, increased risk of hypertension either before or during pregnancy with preeclampsia, a higher rate of Cesarean section, and a greater likelihood of wound complications. During labor, there is an increased likelihood that the baby would get stuck in the birth canal (shoulder dystocia) and that vaginal and anal tears, with the possibility of subsequent urine and fecal incontinence, may occur. Postpartum, they have an increased frequency of deep vein thrombosis and later an increased mortality rate from coronary-artery disease.

The newborns of morbidly obese women, compared with those of normal weight, are also more likely to have been stillborn. There is an increased rate of preterm (less than thirty-seven weeks) births and an increased rate of birth defects, cerebral palsy, seizures, birth injury to both brains and bones (fractured skull, arm, or collarbone), and other problems including respiratory distress, low blood sugar, bacterial infection, and death.

Given that Kimberly was morbidly obese, a macrosomic infant should have been anticipated. Moreover, estimates of fetal weight should have been followed serially by ultrasound, providing a much better assessment of the likelihood of passage of the baby through the pelvis. Clinical assessment in the face of such massive obesity is extremely difficult if not impossible, insofar as determining fetal size by palpation. An ultrasound performed in the twenty-four hours prior to delivery might have helped, except for the fact that the films got mixed up with another patient's and were never seen!

The decision to use Pitocin to induce labor when the baby was so large was debatable, according to testifying experts. The occurrence of some irregularities (decelerations) during administration of Pitocin raises the question of why it was not discontinued. Pitocin has a risk of causing hyperstimulation of the uterus, with frequent contractions that have the potential of seriously interfering with blood flow (oxygen) to the fetus during contractions. Notwithstanding the potential issues with Pitocin, the baby's state at birth, despite being battered, was surprisingly good, and, more important, no metabolic acidosis, the telltale sign of oxygen lack, was evident.

The genesis of errors in clinical reasoning, especially in complex situations where uncertainty coupled with pressure of time coexist, has multifactorial origins. Fatal failures may occur when full information is neither obtained nor analyzed. This would include past medical and pregnancy history, ultrasound reports, and genetic or chemistry results. Adverse events frequently occur as a consequence of errors of execution, reasoning, and decision making.

I have had the privilege of reviewing the medical records of well over fifteen hundred cases, for which claims of medical negligence that led to brain-damaged babies were made. At the same time, working as an expert witness equally for the plaintiff and defense, I carefully read the opinions of experts in obstetrics. From this disheartening experience, I recognized recurring patterns of care prior to, during pregnancy, and through labor and delivery, as well as in the newborn.

Preconception care remains abysmal. We have yet to educate all women (in school) that pregnancy care begins *before* conception. By the time the vast majority of women attend for obstetrical care, they have missed at least one, often two, menstrual periods, placing the fetal age at six to ten weeks at the first visit. By that time, it is too late to prevent spina bifida (see chapter 4) or the effects of medications that cause birth defects (teratogens).

Standards of expected care now in place require all women to be offered appropriate genetic-carrier tests preferably preconception (chapter 20) or at least at the first obstetric visit at six to ten weeks of pregnancy. Failure to offer, document, and communicate carrier-test results has invited litigation, since indicated prenatal diagnostic tests, for example by amniocentesis, would otherwise not have been offered.

Information during pregnancy that pertains to subsequent labor and delivery is surprisingly often ignored. Worse still, the rotating attending obstetrician may not know key details about the patient's history when called to render care in a developing crisis. In addition to the lack of awareness about the patient's medical records, I have noted recurring breaches of the expected standards of care. These failures have included the following: failure to serially graph fetal growth measured by ultrasound (including the critical head-circumference measurements), failure to recognize relative growth discrepancies between the head and abdominal circumferences, failure to recognize the implications of trouble ahead when the maternal-serum screen for chromosomal abnormalities and neural tube defects is abnormal (in the face of a normal amniotic fluid alpha-fetoprotein), failure to heed a mother reporting decreased fetal movements, and failure to properly assess fetal size relative to the maternal pelvis (cephalopelvic disproportion). All these (and other) factors should be (and often are not) in the minds of obstetricians when making critical decisions about the need for Cesarean section.

Allegations of failure to provide an expected standard of obstetrical care are universal and similar, almost regardless of country. Analyses of claims made for brain damage or death in Sweden (472 cases) and Norway (315 cases) are instructive. The Norwegian report on 161 paid claims emphasized that human error was the common reason, including inadequate fetal monitoring (50 percent), lack of clinical knowledge and skills (14 percent), noncompliance with clinical guidelines (11 percent), failure to obtain Department of Medicine assistance (10 percent), errors in drug administration (4 percent), and system errors.

The Swedish report was similar, albeit with slightly different categorization, which included choice of a "non-optimal mode of delivery" (52 percent).

A similar report in the United States of 189 closed perinatal claims concluded that 70 percent were due to substandard obstetrical care.

Decisions made in the face of uncertainty and potential crisis (to pursue vaginal delivery or do an immediate Cesarean section) provide the invariable sharp focus of attention in litigation. All the foregoing facts and information bear on these decisions and remarkably are often ignored in the heat of crisis.

Christopher Chabris and Daniel Simons in their book, *The Invisible Gorilla*, recount a striking demonstration of the consequences of intense focusing (not unlike the fixation on the electronic fetal monitor and the frequency and efficiency of contractions in labor).

These psychologists made a short video of two teams, one wearing white and one wearing black, passing basketballs. Viewers of the video were instructed to count the number of passes made by those wearing white, ignoring those wearing black. Halfway through the video, a woman appeared wearing a gorilla suit and crossed the court, thumped her chest, and disappeared. The "gorilla" is in view for only nine seconds. Of the many who have seen this video, half failed to notice the gorilla. The instruction to focus intensely on only one team vividly demonstrated how we can be blind to the obvious.

Urgent decision making under pressure of time and in the face of uncertainty introduces an entire array of factors that can initiate the action and color the consequences. The challenge of managing labor and delivery is compounded by the reality that at least two (or more) lives are at risk. Experiences loom large in that decision arena. I noticed the recurring factor grounded in experience but manifesting as intuitive action. Unfortunately, errors of intuitive thought are difficult to prevent. Imagine the young trainee listening to the attending obstetrician who "has seen this before," countering with objective evidence.

Intuition may be valuable to the experienced physician, as long as clinical judgment is based on clear evidence. Every now and again, testimony exposes physicians who believe that they can do what others cannot. Some physicians are remarkably confident, even when they are wrong, occasionally resulting in profound errors in judgment.

Some decision makers seem to have been guided by emotion rather than by reason and even swayed by trivial details, resulting in an inability to distinguish the degree of risk. While risk perception varies among us all, encountering a risk-taker who is an attending obstetrician can lead to disaster.

Famous psychologists Amos Twersky and Daniel Kahneman concluded that many decisions are based on beliefs concerning the likelihood of uncertain events. The endless cases of brain-damaged-baby claims I have reviewed have been populated by examples of inexperience, poor judgment, fatigue, hubris, arrogance, failure to listen to an experienced midwife, failure to communicate, failure to establish rapport, failure to appear in time, failure to follow standard guidelines, ignorance, and patient anger.

In his outstanding book, *Thinking, Fast and Slow*, Nobel Laureate (in economics) Professor Daniel Kahneman explores judgment and decision making and how the mind works. He points to two systems of thought: intuitive (fast thinking) and a slower, more deliberate, effortful form (slow thinking). The intuitive form incorporates "the entirely automatic mental activities of perception and memory." The intuitive form, he maintains, is responsible for many of the choices and judgments made. Clearly, in the heat of labor, anticipatory forethought primed by factual knowledge of that pregnancy should preferably precede unprocessed intuitive thoughts.

Professor Kahneman quotes Nobel Laureate Herb Simon (economist and psychologist), who concluded from a study of chess masters that "intuition is nothing more and nothing less than recognition." I believe that intuition (perhaps translated into prior experience) is insufficient alone and must have the company of deliberate thought and knowledge, if labor and delivery are to be successful. There is also the absolute requirement needed to fully comprehend the role and importance of genetic disorders that contribute, confound, and complicate labor and delivery.

In my view, the trial court's comprehension of the genetic issues and implications in this case fell far short of reasonable and rational expectations. This has been my experience in trials in which I have testified in the past. Mine is not a lone opinion. A distinguished professor of law, David L. Faigman, at the University of California Hastings College of Law wrote about judges as "amateur scientists":

> While the importance of science to society is likely to expand geometrically in the century ahead, judges, on the whole, have little training in, knowledge of, or inclination to learn science. Scientifically illiterate judges pose a grave threat to the judiciary's power and legitimacy. Like all ignorance, scientific illiteracy casts knowledge into the shadows, where only forms can be made out and detail is impossible to discern. Scientifically illiterate judges abdicate power and shun responsibility. In the twenty-first century, no judge will deserve the title if he or she does not know science, according to professor D. Faigman*.

Very similar sentiments were expressed by Judge Posner in the US Court of Appeals for the Seventh Circuit in *Jackson v. Pollion*. This entirely "meritless case" (of mild hypertension in a prison inmate untreated for three weeks without significant consequences) meandered through the lower courts for four years. The appeals court opinion indicated "widespread and increasingly troublesome discomfort among lawyers and judges confronted by a scientific or other technological issue."

***

The trial court in this case decided in favor of Kimberly. The case was appealed by the hospital and the doctor all the way to the Michigan Supreme Court. After a heated argument, the plaintiff emerged victorious, regardless of the fact that the child had a precisely defined genetic disorder.

*Faigman DL, 2006. "Judges as 'Amateur Scientists'. Boston University Law Review 86: 1207-1211

THE ROTATION

Carol's labor and delivery were difficult and prolonged. She was barely five feet tall but had an uneventful pregnancy up to the time she delivered. She was a single mother, whose job was a cashier in a supermarket. She had a longtime relationship with a coworker. Upon their son Jimmy's birth, they married and were excited to become parents for the first time.

Jimmy weighed seven pounds fifteen ounces and came out bruised but otherwise deemed healthy. He was discharged from the hospital, together with his mother, on day three of life. A physical examination before leaving the hospital confirmed that, other than some bruising, he was well. As with all newborns, he had his heel pricked in order to get a tiny drop of blood on a special filter paper for a newborn screen, which the resident had ordered as is routinely done.

The newborn screen is primarily for the early detection of biochemical genetic disorders and is especially focused on early diagnosis in order to initiate immediate treatment when required. The resident who ordered the test rotated off the newborn service, and the discharge note indicated that Jimmy would be seen by his family doctor two weeks later. That visit was Jimmy's first well baby appointment, and Carol left reassured that all was well. Jimmy was gaining weight, feeding, and stooling well. Carol had insufficient milk, so she had discontinued breastfeeding, but Jimmy took well to his bottle.

Subsequent visits to the family doctor were not particularly noteworthy, except for the observation that Jimmy had eczema. The doctor thought that the eczema had allergic origins and treated him with a cortisone cream.

Sitting in the park one Sunday afternoon with friends, all of whom had baby carriages and their joyful bundles, one mentioned that she thought Jimmy was "doing much less" than the other babies of similar age. This observation upset Carol, since she too had begun to notice that Jimmy did not seem to be as responsive as other babies. In particular, he did not seem to bring his hands together or play with his hands. He also did not appear to recognize his bottle and did not roll from side to side. Getting him to laugh was difficult.

Carol revisited the family doctor, who confirmed her observations and ordered a chromosome analysis. The result was normal, and he tried to reassure her that Jimmy would catch up. However, Jimmy's development clearly lagged well behind babies of his age. Consultation with a neurologist was arranged, and the conclusion was reached that, because Jimmy was rather stiff, he had cerebral palsy, together with intellectual disability.

Years went by, and even when special education was provided, it made no difference. When he was eighteen, his mother, then divorced, decided that he should see an internist and switch from his family doctor, who mainly saw children. The internist inquired about Jimmy's development and sought the notes and records of his past care and tests. He said that he would start from scratch to try and precisely determine the cause of Jimmy's intellectual disability. He ordered a few other genetic tests but immediately requested a copy of the newborn-screen result from the primary-care doctor, who responded that he had no copy. Since the newborn screening is performed in the state laboratories, he sought the report directly. He was staggered to receive the report, which clearly indicated that Jimmy had phenylketonuria (PKU). Neither the hospital file nor the family doctor's file contained a copy of this report.

Carol was devastated to hear from the internist that Jimmy had a biochemical disorder that is usually diagnosed by the newborn screen and requires immediate treatment to avert the development of intellectual disability. Carol sued the hospital and her Jimmy's family physician.

Pertinent Medical Facts

Phenylketonuria (PKU) is an autosomal recessive disorder due to a liver-enzyme deficiency that inevitably results in severe intellectual disability if untreated. Carol and her ex-husband were each carriers of a mutation in the same culprit gene but had no idea they were carriers with a 25 percent risk of having an affected child. The immediate treatment required is a specific, very low-protein diet. That alone enables development to proceed normally. A low-protein diet together with a phenylalanine-free formula was the treatment that should have been initiated soon after Jimmy's birth.

In retrospect, Jimmy had been noticed to have light skin and hair pigmentation, typical eczema, and a small head. His internist ordered brain imaging, which revealed abnormalities in his white matter, which is typical in PKU. The effects of Jimmy's PKU were irreversible.

Today, it is possible to determine the carrier state for PKU by analysis of the gene (*PAH*). While it was no longer important to Carol, since she had no wish to have more children, it was important for her to inform her siblings and her nieces and nephews that they should be tested to determine their carrier status for PKU. Couples who are found to both be carriers but plan to have children have the options of prenatal genetic diagnosis and preimplantation genetic diagnosis. Among people who are of Irish descent, the approximate carrier rate is one in thirty-three. For those of northern European or East Asian origin, the rate is one in fifty. For most of the Western world, the prevalence of PKU is between one in forty-five hundred and one in ten thousand births.

Questions

- Who was responsible for seeing the laboratory result of newborn screening when the ordering resident rotated off the service and for communicating the result to both parents and the family physician?

- Was the state laboratory responsible for immediately communicating the abnormal result of the newborn screen to a physician on the newborn service and to document the date and the name of the caregiver?

Commentary

Once again, we bear witness to an abysmal failure by more than a single party. The handoff point by a resident to a colleague is a known period of hazard. One exhausted resident trying to exit the service may forget a detail or two about a patient, especially if the matter is routine and not urgent. The attending physician had the duty to ensure that the laboratory results were obtained, seen, and communicated to Jimmy's mother and doctor. (On one occasion, when I was unable to reach a family with a critically important result, I sought the help of the local police, who quickly reached the family).

The failure of a hospital system to ensure receipt of critical important results that have life-threatening or life-changing implications reminds us once again of common systemwide administrative incompetence often seen in hospitals (also discussed in chapter 2). The state laboratory that performed the newborn-screening test bears the brunt of responsibility. It was required of them to be sure that the critical result reached a responsible caregiver who was able to communicate the extremely important result (see chapter 24). Some eighteen years later, the state laboratories could find no record of the documentation and neither could the hospital.

Not unexpectedly, trainees (interns, residents, and fellows) are especially vulnerable to commit errors. As a group, they are inexperienced, often fatigued, have limited knowledge, and frequently poorly supervised at night and on weekends or public holidays. One major study of errors made by trainees in 240 cases, revealed errors in judgment in 72 percent of cases, breakdown in teamwork in 70 percent of cases, and technical incompetence in 58 percent of cases. Teamwork problems reflected a lack of supervision and failures when residents hand off at the end of a shift or when they rotate off a service. Failures of technical competence involved decision making for diagnosis and monitoring of patients, as well as a lack of surgical skill. Data from one large malpractice insurer of eight thousand physicians showed that residents were named in 22 percent of claims.

The Accreditation Council for Graduate Medical Education whose required core competencies aim to advance patient safety places supervisory responsibilities squarely on the attending physician.

The need for medicolegal education of medical students has been recognized for many years. For the most part, only lip service has been paid to this obvious need. More than fifteen years ago at Boston University School of Medicine, I proposed that a few hours in the curriculum be spent on this subject. The curriculum committee heard me out, but my plea fell on deaf ears.

Medicolegal education of interns and residents is also inadequate. I estimate that the overwhelming number of doctors in practice today never had any medicolegal education in medical school or during training.

Timely treatment in the weeks after birth would have prevented the development of Jimmy's intellectual disability. The case was settled, but Jimmy was left with severe irreversible intellectual disability for life and his mother with the burden of caring for her disabled son.

ANCESTRY

Nellie and William could hardly contain their excitement when Nellie's menstrual period, which always appeared like clockwork, didn't arrive on time. They had been hoping and planning for a pregnancy and attempting to time it so that she would deliver in the summer, when she would not be teaching. At her first doctor's visit, pregnancy was confirmed. At the same visit, her obstetrician suggested a general carrier-screening test that covered more than 160 genetic disorders. She was happy to submit to that blood test as well, even while the doctor was saying that she knew little about more than half of the disorders that were being tested. She returned for a second visit at eleven weeks of pregnancy to have a blood-screening test for chromosome abnormalities, such as Down syndrome. The test result showed no increased risk for Down syndrome or two other important chromosome abnormalities (trisomies 13 and 18). At sixteen weeks, she had yet another blood test screening for alpha-fetoprotein for detection of open defects like spina bifida. That test, too, was negative.

When she returned for her sixteenth-week visit, the doctor shared the result of the extensive carrier-test screen. It showed that Nellie was a carrier of a mutation in the Tay-Sachs disease gene (*HEXA*). The report indicated that her partner, William, should be tested, and he materialized the next day for that purpose. In less than a week, he learned that he was not a carrier of a mutation in the *HEXA* gene for Tay-Sachs disease.

Pregnancy continued uneventfully, and labor and delivery "was a breeze." Baby Diane weighed six pounds fifteen ounces and went home with Nellie and William on the morning of day three of life. Diane met all of her milestones for the first six months and was sitting unsupported, was alert, was interactive, stretched out her arms to be picked up, played peekaboo, and was able to roll from her back to stomach. During the following two months, she was pulling herself to stand and to hold on to furniture. She was able to wave bye-bye, babble, and crawl. At ten months, however, it seemed that she was losing some of the developmental milestones she had already accomplished. The doctors were puzzled and concerned. They reviewed the pregnancy records, including the test results from Nellie and William, but were at a loss to explain the mild regression that had occurred.

During the ensuing few months, Diane became floppy, losing her ability to stand and to sit unsupported. Extensive genetic testing revealed that Diane had inherited Nellie's mutation for Tay-Sachs disease as well as a previously unidentified mutation also in the *HEXA* gene, which must have come from her father, William. Diane had inherited two mutations in the *HEXA* gene, resulting in a diagnosis of Tay-Sachs disease.

Nellie and William sued their obstetrician and the laboratory that performed the tests on Nellie and William's blood samples.

<u>Pertinent Medical Facts</u>

Warren Tay was a British ophthalmologist who, in 1881, described the cherry-red spot in the retina of the eye that is uniformly seen in infants with Tay-Sachs disease. Bernard Sachs was a Jewish American neurologist who graduated from Harvard in 1887. His contribution was to provide a comprehensive description of the disease and for noting its increased frequency among Ashkenazi Jews from eastern Europe.

Tay-Sachs disease is a fatal neurodegenerative genetic disease caused by a deficiency of a certain enzyme (*hexosaminidase* A) within all cells, especially affecting the brain. It is an autosomal recessive disorder, with each parent being a carrier of a mutation in the *HEXA* gene. When both parents are carriers, they have a 25 percent risk of having an affected child. Children born with this disorder appear perfectly normal and healthy. In fact, they most often have beautiful complexions, much like porcelain dolls, due to the accumulation of a particular chemical (ganglioside) within their cells because of the enzyme deficiency.

Development and accomplishment of the typical milestones appear normal for the first three to six months, after which parents begin to notice a marked startle response to a sudden noise, diminished attentiveness, and steadily progressive weakness and loss of the ability to sit unsupported or to even roll over. Slow but steady deterioration follows, with seizures making their appearance while the child becomes spastic and blind. The head typically begins to enlarge by the age of eighteen months, but this is not due to hydrocephalus. Examination of the eyes always reveals a cherry-red spot on the retina. Continued deterioration throughout the second year of life results in intermittent arching of the back, difficulties in swallowing, increasing number of seizures, and eventually the child lapsing into a vegetative state.

Death most often due to bronchopneumonia ensues for all between the ages of two and six years.

There are other forms of Tay-Sachs disease, even in adults, that are not the subject of this discussion.

Tay-Sachs disease used to be a disorder largely confined to the Ashkenazi Jewish population. However, with systematic testing of Jewish couples, the original prevalence of one in thirty-six hundred Jewish births has changed dramatically. Today, the incidence of Tay-Sachs disease in the Ashkenazi Jewish population has been reduced by more than 90 percent. Between one in twenty-seven and one in thirty Ashkenazi Jews are carriers of a mutation in the *HEXA* gene. Analysis of that gene in the Ashkenazi Jewish population revealed three common mutations that account for some 98 percent of all carriers.

Among Sephardic Jews or non-Jews, Tay-Sachs has been seen with a frequency of one hundred times less than that of the Ashkenazi Jewish population. Carrier frequency in the Sephardic and non-Jewish population is between 1 in 250 and 1 in 300.

Once a mutation has been detected, as it was in Nellie, William would have needed to be tested. However, even though a mutation in one of the common Ashkenazi Jewish mutations was found in Nellie, William, being non-Jewish, needed to have his serum tested for the enzyme (*hexosaminidase* A). That test would have enabled determination of a non-Jewish carrier in almost all cases and is indeed the required test for

that group.

Determination of a mutation in both Nellie and William would have enabled them to have prenatal genetic

diagnosis or, in a subsequent pregnancy, preimplantation genetic diagnosis. Furthermore, once a mutation

is discovered, the parents of the couple, and also their uncles and aunts, should be offered carrier testing.

All of us have the potential of being carriers of certain genetic disorders that may have an increased

frequency due to our ethnic or ancestral origins. Interestingly, the frequency of Tay-Sachs disease carriers

in the French Canadian and Cajun populations is similar to Ashkenazi Jews. A large study of Ashkenazi

Jewish individuals was reported from the Icahn School of Medicine at Mount Sinai in New York. The

aim was to determine the likelihood of being a carrier of at least one of eighteen relatively common

genetic disorders in this ethnic group. The study revealed that one in six were carriers of at least one of

those eighteen disorders (also see table 1).

In table 1, the specific disorders found especially in particular ethnic groups are shown together with the

frequency of carriers. Previous lawsuits have been adjudicated when physicians have not known or

remembered these ethnic burdens. Consequently, cases of infants with Tay-Sachs disease or sickle-cell

disease have been adjudicated and physicians found liable for not ordering carrier testing and not

documenting their recommendations.

Today, because of carrier testing (especially preconception), it is rare for a Jewish couple to have a child

with Tay-Sachs disease. Almost all infants born affected are now mostly delivered by non-Jews.

Unfortunately, there is no known effective treatment for Tay-Sachs disease.

Commercial companies have introduced carrier screening for 160 or more genetic disorders performed

simultaneously on a single blood sample. This extensive carrier screen has not been endorsed by either

the American College of Medical Genetics and Genomics (ACMG) or the American College of Obstetrics and Gynecology. Both have published extensive guidelines and recommendations. The vast majority of disorders tested include a few selected mutations in the gene being examined. The provided result is a statistical expression of residual risk after a negative (no mutation) result. It invariably *does not mean the tested person is not a carrier*. Moreover, many of the disorders tested are rare, and most practicing physicians know little about most of them or have not even heard or read about them.

Based upon the criteria published by the ACMG, a reported analysis of carrier tests for recessive disorders offered by commercial laboratories showed that only 27 percent fulfilled necessary criteria for screening. The most common reasons were the low frequency (less than one in one hundred) of carriers or a detection rate of less than 70 percent. Remember, for recessive disorders, the partner must also be a carrier of a mutation in the same gene for the couple to have a 25 percent risk of having an affected child with the tested disorder.

As a basic tenet for preconception population-carrier screening, certain guidelines are universally accepted. Fourteen of the most important are the following:

1. The carrier frequency should be one in one hundred or greater for screening to be offered, according to guidelines from the American College of Obstetrics and Gynecology.

2. The patient's ethnicity and family history should be known prior to screening.

3. Carrier screening and counseling should ideally be done before pregnancy.

4. The disorder being screened for is of such severity as to prompt couples to consider prenatal diagnosis and possible pregnancy termination.

5. Genetic counseling should be offered routinely to those with a detected mutation.

6. The disorder should have well-known disease-causing mutations such that a positive or negative result reliably predicts that an individual is or is not a carrier.

7. The laboratory test is accurate, reliable, reproducible, and cost-effective.

8. The clinical manifestations of the disorder do not vary from almost any signs to significant impairment without any ability to determine severity.

9. The disorder is routinely detected at birth, for which an established effective treatment is available.

10. Methods that employ nontargeted specific mutations will inevitably encounter possible mutations (variants) of unknown significance. It is accepted that informed consent and genetic counseling prior to such testing be obtained in anticipation of such potentially problematic results.

11. Many direct-to-consumer genetic tests fail to provide a clear statement about whether an individual will develop a specific disorder. Instead, the information provided only conveys the risk or probability of developing a particular condition.

12. Reports from direct-to-consumer screening should make it clear that their results can neither confirm nor exclude the possibility of a genetic disorder or that unexplained and unrelated results may emerge and which could have implications for their family members.

13. Prior to screening, consumers must be informed as to who will have access to their test results, how privacy will be assured, whether results may have personal or family-related implications for health, life, long-term care, and disability insurance.

14. For direct-to-consumer testing, assurance is required that the consumer's DNA will not be shared with third parties and will not be sold.

Guidelines promulgated by professional colleges improve and safeguard clinical practice. Practitioners who choose to ignore guidelines open the door for litigation should an adverse event occur. In the inadvisable circumstances that a physician chooses to ignore or reinterpret a specific guideline, very detailed and documented reasoning will be needed for defense. Even then, any egregious practice is likely to fall foul of the jury.

Questions

There was only one question: How could the very extensive tests for carriers have failed to detect that William was a Tay-Sachs disease carrier?

Commentary

Examination of the medical records revealed a cascade of errors.

The initial blood sample taken from Nellie that yielded a report of her being a Tay-Sachs disease carrier came with the written recommendation for genetic counseling as well as the recommendation to test her partner. The obstetrician felt that she could deal with this rather straightforward issue and did not refer Nellie and William for genetic counseling. When William came in for his blood sample, she instructed the phlebotomist to be sure that she wrote on the requisition form that his partner was a Tay-Sachs disease carrier. The phlebotomist, after drawing the blood sample, completed the requisition form, filling in the space that said "Race," with the word "Caucasian," and filling in the space that said "Ethnicity," with the word "Caucasian." The phlebotomist was an employee of the laboratory.

William's report indicating that he was not a carrier came on a form with the heading "Ashkenazi Jewish Mutation Analysis"! As just stated, the phlebotomist had not identified William's ethnicity. Both he and Nellie were of Irish descent!

The Ashkenazi Jewish mutation analysis in that laboratory incorporated eighteen genetic mutations in the *HEXA* gene. (At least 182 mutations are known for this gene.) For someone of Ashkenazi Jewish ancestry, that analysis provides a high degree of exclusion, exceeding 98 percent. However, for a non- Jewish person, the detection rate by mutation analysis is poor and possibly in the 50 percent range. In fact, the standard recommendation by the American College of Obstetrics and Gynecology as well as the American College of Medical Genetics and Genomics is to initially test the non-Jewish patient's *serum* for the *hexosaminidase* A enzyme. In a male, this provides an almost 100 percent detection rate and is indeed the standard of expected care for detection in a non-Jewish person.

The laboratory also had a genetic counselor who had initially called the obstetrician's office about the test result. However, she left no message and never did get a callback. She never bothered to call again, nor did she notice the absence of a stated ethnicity on the requisition form. If the laboratory had been alert to the information about ethnicity, they would have been expected to make an immediate inquiry and, upon notification, recommended by telephone and in writing that the enzyme-based test for William was critically important.

Once again, we witness the compounding of errors, beginning with the obstetrician and continuing with the phlebotomist, the laboratory director, and the genetic counselor. Collectively, they didn't know, they didn't know, and left Nellie and William to care for a slowly dying and suffering child.

Table 1: Likelihood of Being a Carrier for Various Ethnic Groups[1]

If You Are	The Chance Is About	That You Carry a Gene Mutation for
Afrikaner (white South African)	1 in 400	Porphyria[2]
Armenian, Jewish (Sephardic) Turks, Arabs	1 in 3 or 1 in 8	Familial Mediterranean fever[2]
Black	1 in 8 to 1 in 10	Sickle cell anemia[2]
	7 in 10	Milk intolerance as an adult
Black and male or	1 in 10	Hereditary predisposition to develop
Black and female	1 in 50	Hemolytic anemia after taking sulfa or
	1 in 4	Other drugs[3]
		High blood pressure[3]
Finns	1 in 36	Aspartylglucosaminuria[2]
French Canadian	1 in 49–90	Aspartylglucosaminuria[2]
Italian American or Greek American	1 in 10	Beta-thalassemia[2]
Jewish (Ashkenazi)	1 in 111	Bloom syndrome

	1 in 40 (women)	Breast/Ovary cancer gene mutation
	1 in 40	Canavan disease
	1 in 26	Deafness (nonsyndromic)
	1 in 96	Dihydrolipoamide dehydrogenase deficiency
	1 in 127	Galactosemia
	1 in 18	Gaucher's disease
	1 in 32	Dysautonomia
	1 in 8	Factor XI deficiency
	1 in 5 to 1 in 7	Familial Mediterranean fever
	1 in 66	Familial hyperinsulinism
	1 in 92	Fanconi anemia
	1 in 71	Glycogen Storage disease type 1A (Von Gierke disease)
	1 in 92	Joubert syndrome
	1 in 122	Maple syrup urine disease type IB (MSUD)
	1 in 81	Mucolipidosis type IV
	1 in 90	Niemann-Pick disease type A
	1 in 25–30	Tay-Sachs disease
Asian	1 in 1	Milk intolerance as an adult[3]
White	1 in 25 to 1 in 29	Cystic fibrosis[2]
	1 in 31	Deafness[2] (nonsyndromic)
	1 in 10	Hemochromatosis[2]
	1 in 40 to 1 in 60	Spinal muscular atrophy[2]

[1]These disorders can occur in any ethnic group but are more rare.
[2]DNA carrier and prenatal diagnosis test available
[3]No DNA test available
From Aubrey Milunsky. *Your Genes, Your Health: A Family Guide That Could Save Your Life.* Oxford University Press, 2012.

NEVER EVENTS

"Never events" actually occur! This term was originally introduced in 2001 by Ken Kizer, MD, who was the former CEO of the National Quality Forum. He aimed to reference devastating medical errors that were meant to never occur. However, by September 20, 2009, the Joint Commission (an independent, nonprofit organization that accredits and certifies nearly twenty-one thousand health-care organizations and programs in the United States) reported a total of 6,428 so-called sentinel events, that is, events that are beyond complications that should never have occurred. That accumulated total included 867 cases of wrong-site surgery, 710 operative or postoperative complications, delays in treatment in 536 cases, medication errors in 526 cases, suicide while under care in 770 cases, and patient falls in 406 cases. In all of these case reports, death or significant disability eventuated and were invariably preventable. Subsequently the National Quality Forum in 2011 constructed a list of 29 events that were grouped into categories and which I will briefly summarize. Disturbing as it should be, there are actual cases (frequently multiple) in *all* the examples given.

Surgical Events

This category includes surgery or other invasive procedures performed on the *wrong body part*, the *wrong patient*, or the *wrong procedure* used. Also included are deaths during surgery or immediately after surgery or a procedure, as well as the unintended *retention of a foreign object* inside a patient after surgery or another procedure.

Product or Device Events

This category includes patient death or serious injury associated with the use of *contaminated drugs*, *devices*, or *biologics* provided by health-care personnel or as a consequence of the use or function of the device for purposes other than intended. Also included are patient deaths or serious injury associated with *intravascular air embolism* that occurred while under care.

Patient-Protection Events

This category includes the *discharge or release* of a patient who is unable to make decisions or to someone other than an authorized person. Included in this category is patient death or serious disability associated with the *patient's disappearance* or the patient's actual or attempted *suicide* resulting in serious disability while under care.

Care-Management Events

This category includes patient death or serious injury associated with a *medication error* (*wrong drug, wrong dose, wrong patient, wrong rate of administration, wrong time, wrong preparation*, or *wrong route of administration*). Additional inclusions are patient death or serious injury due to *unsafe administration* of blood products, maternal death or serious *injury associated with labor* in a low-risk pregnancy while under care, death or serious *injury of a neonate* associated with labor or delivery in a low-risk pregnancy, artificial insemination with a *wrong donor sperm or egg*, patient death or serious injury associated with *a fall* while under care, serious *pressure ulcers* while under care, patient death or serious disability resulting from irretrievable *loss of an irreplaceable biological specimen*, patient death or serious injury resulting from a *failure to follow up* or *failure to communicate* laboratory, pathology, or radiology test results.

Environmental Events

This category includes patient or staff death or serious disability associated with *electric shock or burns* in the course of patient care in the health-care setting and any incident in which a line designated for oxygen or other gases to be delivered to a patient contains *no gas*, the *wrong gas*, or is *contaminated by toxic substances* (see chapter 7 for disconnected oxygen supply). In addition, this category includes patient or staff deaths or serious injury associated with a *burn* incurred from any source in the course of patient care or as a consequence of the use or lack of use of *restraints or bed rails* while under care.

Radiologic Events

This includes death or serious injury of a patient or staff associated with introduction of a *metallic object into the MRI area* or radiation of the *wrong patient*.

Criminal Events

This includes *impersonation* of a physician, nurse, pharmacist, or other licensed health-care provider; *abduction* of a patient; *abuse or assault* while under care; *drug use* by a care provider; and death or significant injury of a patient or a staff member resulting from assault or assault with a deadly weapon that occurs within a health-care setting.

While "never events" were regarded as rare, a Johns Hopkins study in 2013 estimated that four thousand surgical "never events" occur yearly in the United States. These events are recognized as being devastating, with some 71 percent of cases reported to the Joint Commission in a twelve-year period proving fatal.

The Joint Commission strongly recommended that hospitals report "sentinel events," defining them as an "unexpected occurrence involving death or serious physiological or psychological injury or the risk thereof." The Leapfrog group (an independent, national nonprofit organization focused on patient safety, care quality, and availability of care) urged that organizations should disclose errors and apologize to patients as well as reporting the "never event" and waiving all costs associated with that incident. Moreover, the Centers for Medicare and Medicaid Services took the position that they would no longer pay for additional costs associated with many preventable errors, including "never events." Unfortunately, many states have not mandated reporting of "never events." In some states, such as Minnesota, recognizing hospital systems' problems mandate not only reporting incidents but also performing a root-cause analysis.

Two widely publicized "never event" mastectomy cases among a surprising number in the United States, Canada, England, and elsewhere serve as yet another wake-up call about surgical mistakes:

In 2003, Linda McDougal publicized the fact that she had had a double mastectomy after she was told she had an aggressive form of breast cancer. Her doctors had recommended bilateral mastectomy, and forty-eight hours after her surgery, she was told that she did not have cancer. Apparently, her file had been switched with another patient's. The mistake occurred when two physicians failed to check the names, identification numbers, and birth dates of the two patients when they inadvertently switched the name on the slides with the pathology paperwork. Apparently two patients' sets of slides were on a single tray. Two patients' sets of paperwork were available to the pathologist who picked up the wrong sheets with the slides and failed to validate the name and identification number on the slide with the name and identification number on the paperwork. There was no safeguarding color-coding of the slides and the paperwork. What should have happened was that only a single patient's set of slides should have been placed on the tray and a second pathologist should have reviewed all aspects of the case.

Linda McDougal required special attention since her wound became infected, and subsequently, of course, she needed reconstructive surgery. At the time of her going public, she noted that only the surgeon had apologized, but not the pathologist or the hospital. Nor did the insurance company step up immediately either!

In 2013, a woman in Halifax, Nova Scotia was told that she had breast cancer and opted for mastectomy. She was subsequently told that the tissue samples had been switched and entered incorrectly on the patient's charts. It took over six weeks for the Capital District Health Authority to notify this patient of this egregious error. No one lost jobs because of this error.

There are a disturbing number of patients who have had surgery on the wrong side of their body or on the wrong organ. The Johns Hopkins study mentioned earlier concluded that physicians perform wrong procedures on patients twenty times a week and that surgeons operate on the wrong body part twenty times per week as well.

Once again, these cases have been well publicized:

> At St. Vincent Hospital in Worcester, Massachusetts, a surgeon mistakenly removed a normal kidney from the wrong patient. He had relied on the CT scan of another patient with the same name but a different birth date but who had a large kidney tumor. A similar case occurred at the Mount Sinai Medical Center in New York, where a surgeon removed the wrong kidney.

> Also in Worcester, at the University of Massachusetts Memorial Medical Center, Nelson Gonzales received a liver transplant from a donor with an awful brain tumor (glioblastoma). He was only told after that cancer had spread in the donor, about the origin of his donated liver. Needless to say, cancer developed in his donated liver. Nelson Gonzales died exactly one year after his transplant.

> At the Massachusetts General Hospital, a tragic mix-up occurred that resulted from an overdose (thirty times too high) of an anticoagulant given by a nurse. This mother had previously broken her shoulder and was being treated for an infection. She bled internally to death over twelve hours while in the hospital.

> Some years earlier, the chief of neurosurgery at the Staten Island University Hospital operated on the wrong side of the brain in two patients. Previously, that neurosurgeon had been fired from Memorial Sloan Kettering Hospital for operating on the wrong site of a patient's brain after confusing two patients. That doctor eventually surrendered his license to practice medicine. One of the errors perpetrated was the failure to bring the patient's CT scans into the operating room

prior to an incision being made into his brain. That hospital was also cited for failing to make timely reports of these incidents.

For the third time in one year, surgeons at the Rhode Island Hospital operated on the wrong side of a patient's head. In one case, surgery was required to stop the bleeding between the brain and the patient's skull. Once they realized the error, they switched to operating on the correct side of her brain to remove a dangerous clot. In remediation of errors, the hospital put in place rules that included greater continuity in the transmission of patient information between departments, availability of patient records during surgery, requirement of a second physician to review the site and side of all surgical cases before surgery, and the presence of monitors to eliminate potential sources of medical error.

A patient at the Halifax Hospital Medical Center in Florida was admitted for the vascular disease she had that was causing pain in her left leg. She agreed to have vascular surgery on her left leg, and the day before the surgeon marked that leg with a pen. Nevertheless, the surgeon operated on the wrong leg and then, in an attempt to justify his action, stated that it was also necessary on the other side. Apparently, in the first six months of 2013, thirty-five patients in Florida had operations on the wrong site, six had wrong surgery performed, and in a single case, surgery was performed on the wrong patient. The surgeon involved is apparently no longer on that hospital's staff, and the hospital suspended the operating-room team. The federal Centers for Medicare and Medicaid terminated their provider agreement with that hospital. That meant that no payments would be made to that hospital for patients who were the victims of wrong-side or wrong-organ surgery.

Multiple cases are known of the wrong patients undergoing biopsy, having endoscopies (such as colonoscopies), or having a catheter inserted into the bladder. A patient was also given radiation treatment for cancer he did not have. All of these instances occurred due to a failure to properly identify and confirm the patient's identity. Cases of amputation of the wrong leg are also well known.

I would like to believe that the following can be categorized as an exception in the grim arena of "never events." The *Boston Globe* Spotlight team reported in July 2017 about the Manchester, New Hampshire, Veterans Hospital. Because of flies in the operating room, it had to be abandoned. Exterminators were unable to get rid of the flies. Surgery in an adjacent operating room had to be cancelled after surgeons found either rust or blood on two sets of surgical instruments, supposedly sterilized.

Neurosurgeons elsewhere to whom veterans had been referred found that some had suffered permanent spinal damage due to lack of proper care. One surgeon wrote that such disabled patients lacking care would be seen in a third-world country.

Do we have a government that asks soldiers to lay down their lives in an operating room under their care?

Three senior leaders, including the medical and nursing directors, were dismissed following the Spotlight report. How much will that change if the poor climate of care remains so cloudy?

A multicenter study, using the National Practitioner Data Bank, identified a total of 9,744 paid malpractice settlement and judgments for surgical "never events" between 1990 and 2010 and a total of $1.3 billion paid. Death occurred in 6.6 percent of patients, 52.9 percent sustained permanent injury, while all others had a temporary injury. Surgeons who were named in a "never event" claim were again named in at least one more "never event" claim 12.4 percent of the time.

Included among the many risk factors for "never events," specifically for wrong-site operations, were the presence of several surgeons involved in the same operation, multiple procedures, the pressure of time, emergency surgery, abnormal patient anatomy, and morbid obesity.

Selected additional disturbing cases or events to partially add to a dishonor role that provide salutary lessons include a few more examples:

Death of a six-year-old boy at the Penn State Hershey Medical Center who was placed under a heating blanket and whose temperature exceeded 107°F. His temperature had not been taken for ten hours, as reported by Associated Press.

An eighteen-year-old largely recovered from acute lymphoblastic leukemia mistakenly given a toxic drug (Vincristine) into his spinal canal causing his death some three weeks later.

A nurse incorrectly recalibrated a syringe pump delivering a morphine injection into a patient with stomach cancer, resulting in a fatal overdose.

A UK trainee who aimed to remove an infected appendix from a pregnant patient inadvertently removed an ovary. Days later the infection spread; she delivered a stillborn child and died on the operating table.

The body of a stillborn premature twin was lost at the University of Cincinnati Medical Center, discovered only when the family was making funeral arrangements that included the other twin who had survived for one hour.

A surgeon, chief of vascular and thoracic surgery at Hoboken University Medical Center in New Jersey, removed a portion of a healthy lung when the opposite side had the malignant tumor. He lied to the patient, stating that the removed lung tissue contained a life-threatening tumor. The patient died about three years later when the tumor he had, ruptured.

Operating-room fire during anesthesia has caused patient burns. A review of closed malpractice claims (1985–2012) in the American Society of Anesthesiologists Closed Claims Database revealed 103 operating-room fires, 90 percent with electrocautery as the cause, with open oxygen delivery close by. Alcohol-containing solutions or volatile compounds were present in 15 percent of cases. Most electrocautery fires occurred during head, neck, or upper-chest procedures.

In 2003, in a nationally known case, Jesica Santillan, a Mexican seventeen-year-old received a heart and lungs transplant at Duke University Medical Center in North Carolina. Despite the very experienced surgeon and team, there was a failure to check that the donor's organ matched Jesica's blood type. They didn't! This incredible snafu, discovered near the end of the complex surgery, resulted in a second operation with organs from another donor. Sadly, however, antibodies in Jesica's blood had rapidly begun attacking her mismatched organs. By the time of the second surgery, she was near death. She had in fact suffered irreversible brain damage. The machine keeping her alive was turned off.

Her anguished mother accused the Duke Hospital of trying to murder her daughter!

This desperately sad case resulted from a series of failed communications, even though a dozen physicians were involved. The surgeon took responsibility for this awful but simple error. The Carolina Donor Services and the New England Donor Bank had policies that required blood types of donors and recipients be matched before organs are released for transplantation. They didn't!

In 2012, in yet another transplantation case, a brother donated a kidney to his twenty-four-year-old sister who had end-stage kidney disease. The brother's kidney was removed first and placed in a special container, while his sister was undergoing her preparative surgery. A part-time nurse, at the University of Toledo Medical Center in Ohio, returning from lunch, began cleaning up and threw his kidney away!

The sister returned for surgery two months later and received a kidney that was a poorer match and of poorer quality than her brother's.

The Joint Commission on the Accreditation of Healthcare Organizations published *National Patient Safety Goals* in 2017 and outlined three categorical steps to prevent wrong-site, wrong-side, and wrong-patient operations. The categorical recommendations were preoperative verification, site marking, and time-out. The first verification step aims to gather all the necessary information with access to the patient's medical records, consent for the procedure, laboratory and pathological reports, radiological results, and review of pertinent medical information if necessary. The next step is marking the exact or correct site. Site marks include the surgeon's initials or "yes." The surgical site needs to be marked before entering the operating room and done when the patient is still awake and who can then confirm the appropriate operative site. The responsible surgeon or an assistant surgeon who is directly involved should mark the site. The third step, or time-out, requires a pause before any incision is made and is primarily a communication tool between the surgeon, nurses, and anesthesiologist. This includes verification of the patient's name, medical record number (or Social Security number), date of birth, procedure to be done, site and laterality, patient position, and implants or any special equipment necessary for the surgery.

We have known long before the Institute of Medicine report in 1999 that to err is human. Unfortunately, mistakes happen, and the point has been repeatedly made that anticipation of our fallibility must be met with organized and ready backup to anticipate the rare and not so rare, but inevitable, potential error.

Professor Peter Pronovost, a pioneer in patient safety, has written about nine patient harms that pose risks for most patients, besides their loss of dignity. These harms include:

- Adverse drug events
- Catheter-associated urinary-tract infections
- Intravenous central line–associated infections
- Fall injuries
- Pressure ulcers (with infection)

- o   Surgical-site infections

- o   Blood clots (e.g., deep vein thrombosis leading to pulmonary embolism)

- o   Ventilator-associated pneumonia

- o   Obstetrical adverse events

Professor Pronovost has emphasized that inpatients often experience multiple harms. Moreover, each type of harm requires its own set of preventative steps. He has made an impassioned plea for the development and implementation of a systems approach to managing patient care. This will require, he maintains, an engineering mind-set by clinicians and a melding of professional cultures. Viewing the carnage of deaths and harms, progress thus far is hard to perceive.

Why, other than litigation, are there no strictures or penalties for surgeons or other physicians found culpable for causing "never events," with 12.5 percent being recidivists?

According to a Leapfrog Group Hospital survey in 2016, more than twenty-five states and the District of Columbia have mandatory reporting of "never events." Why have so many states not made reporting a requirement? Who is being protected?

Moreover, only a few of the states report publicly! Why are legislators not acting in the interest of patients? That is, for all of us who will become patients! Minnesota has had a reporting program since 2005, with 100–150 "never events" each year.

As future patients, we need to know which hospitals have zero to low rates of "never events" when we need care.

CRIMINAL

Neurosurgeon Christopher Duntsch was born in Montana from where his family moved to Memphis, where he grew up. His story, and the catastrophes that follow, were reported in detail in *D Magazine*, by Matt Goodman in November 2016. Details are derived from his reports.

His father was a missionary and physical therapist, while his mother was a teacher. He graduated from the University of Memphis and subsequently from the medical school at the University of Tennessee Health Science Center. His résumé apparently indicated that he had earned a doctorate in microbiology from St. Jude's Children's Research Hospital, graduating summa cum laude. However, St. Jude's maintained that there was no such program in their hospital at that time. He did well in medical school and was among the 12 percent of medical-school graduates in his class named to the elite Alpha Omega Alpha medical honors society. He remained at the University of Tennessee for his surgical training, where he also became involved in research, serving both as a principal and coprincipal investigator. During that period, Dr. Duntsch's behavior had become noticeably erratic. A woman with whom he had a relationship reported him eating a paper blotter of LSD and taking prescription painkillers as well as snorting cocaine.

After seeing two of Dr. Duntsch's patients for corrective surgery, a spine surgeon in Dallas faxed a photograph of Duntsch to the University of Tennessee to determine if the surgeon was an imposter. He was told that Duntsch had been sent to an impaired-physician program for refusing to take a drug test after someone had reported him using cocaine. Nevertheless, he had been allowed to return to finish his residency in surgery. The Dallas neurosurgeon also heard, upon his inquiry, that Duntsch was not allowed to operate independently. The university refused access to his personnel file.

Duntsch had also filed two patents for discoveries related to stem-cell work performed by two other scientists. By 2011, he had started two companies based on those discoveries. A lawsuit was brought by a high-school friend who joined one of the two companies, because he had reneged on payments that were promised. Duntsch subsequently filed for bankruptcy and was removed as a board member and chief scientific officer.

Pursuing further clinical work, he was hired by the Minimally Invasive Spine Institute in North Dallas. He also sought privileges at the Baylor Plano Hospital, which received a letter of recommendation, from his previous chief simply verifying Dr. Duntsch's training. That letter apparently contained the statement that "his work ethic, character, and ability to get along with others were beyond reproach." Immediately following his first and only surgery at the Spine Institute, Dr. Duntsch just flew off to Las Vegas without arranging any cover for his patient. The hospital, needing his attention, called the institute director. Dr. Duntsch was fired when he returned. From court documents, apparently, people had expressed concern at the institute about the possibility that he was impaired due to drugs, alcohol, or mental illness.

A series of botched surgeries followed, including patients with severe residual pain, quadriplegia, as well as death in a number of patients. At one point at Baylor Plano Hospital, Duntsch was not allowed to operate. Moreover, multiple lawsuits alleged that Baylor did not report Duntsch to the National Practitioner Data Bank, which was created by Congress to be a private clearinghouse of physicians who have been suspended or have had their privileges revoked. According to court filings, he was supposed to be overseen by an attending physician in the operating room, which apparently did not occur.

Dr. Duntsch left Baylor with a letter that stated "there have been no summary or administrative restrictions or suspensions of Dr. Duntsch's medical staff membership or clinical privileges during the time he has practiced at Baylor Regional Medical Center Plano." Armed with that reference statement, he began work at the Dallas Medical Center in July 2012. During that time, he performed three procedures. One patient died, and another was partially paralyzed during surgery. One surgeon at that institution reported that he had direct knowledge of seven patients whom "Dr. Duntsch had maimed or killed." That surgeon described Dr. Duntsch as the most careless, clueless, and dangerous spine surgeon he had ever seen.

In yet another patient who was to have two vertebrae fused and linked by a metal plate, a grim outcome was recorded. She awoke with severe pain and could not stand, and the spinal fusion plate was located in the soft tissue of her back. One nerve root had been amputated, and multiple screw holes were nowhere near where they were supposed to be, while another screw had been placed in another nerve root at the bottom of her spine. This case resulted in the revocation of Dr. Duntsch's privileges. Baylor, when questioned, responded that they did not file their own complaint to the Texas Medical Board because they were aware that someone else already had! Baylor stated that they had "references from multiple sources who worked with him in his residency and fellowship training programs."

In yet another case at a different surgery center, Duntsch operated with another grim outcome. The patient's vocal cord was paralyzed, and her esophagus and trachea became connected, which was regarded as an "unheard of complication."

Throughout 2013, Dr. Duntsch was apparently snorting cocaine.

Dr. Duntsch then went into private practice in Dallas, where he thought he would be well protected due to Texas's tort reform laws that capped the amount that patients can sue physicians for malpractice at $250,000. And more important, to successfully sue a hospital in Texas, patients must prove that the facility acted with malice and that, in granting a physician privileges, it intended to harm the patient. This, of course, was an incredibly difficult thing to prove. With privileges at University General Hospital, Dr. Duntsch operated yet again with another disastrous outcome. The hospital, desperate with this case, granted Dr. Randall Kirby emergency privileges to reoperate on a patient Dr. Duntsch had treated. He found not only a significant esophageal injury that interfered with the patient's breathing but also a sponge that had been left in the soft tissue of his neck. The patient also had an injury to his left vertebral artery, and the incision, which was far from where it should have been, had begun to leak pus. Dr. Kirby then, together with the patient's family, brought the case to prosecutors and asked to press charges. He said, "I am beginning to think the police are the only ones intellectually and physically capable of getting to the bottom of this matter." During the ensuing months, Dr. Duntsch was struggling financially and was stopped for driving under the influence, with an arrest report stating that he had been driving on two tires, one of which was completely gone and was on the rim. He was also arrested for stealing sunglasses, watches, shoes, ties, briefcases, a wallet, cologne, necklaces, and a walkie-talkie from Walmart. He again filed for bankruptcy while staying with his parents.

In July 2015, the Dallas County District Attorney Office returned five indictments of aggravated assault and one of harming an elderly person. Duntsch pleaded not guilty and was jailed pending trial. In 2017, a Texas jury addressed the allegations against Duntsch of numerous cases of malpractice, including crippling four patients and killing two others between July 2012 and June 2013. He was convicted of felony injury to an elderly person and was sentenced to life in prison.

D Magazine reported that prosecutors had proclaimed that Duntsch was the first physician in the nation to be sentenced to life imprisonment for what he did in the hospital operating room. The grand jury had indicted him on five counts of aggravated assault with a deadly weapon (a scalpel) as well as a single count of harming an elderly patient. As the magazine reported, Duntsch's surgery resulted in a patient bleeding to death during surgery, his best friend being left quadriplegic, one patient dead from a stroke, and at least thirty patients at four hospitals who were seriously harmed.

Pertinent Medical Facts

Neurosurgeons have among the highest risk of malpractice lawsuits of all specialties. Failures in spinal surgery rank as the most common cause of claims. In one study, the most common causes of claims were faulty surgical technique in 33 percent of cases, delayed diagnosis/missed diagnosis in 17 percent, and delayed treatment in 12 percent. Operating on the spinal vertebrae, one would think, is reasonably straightforward with reference to selecting the correct vertebra. In a study in which 169 spine surgeons responded, almost 50 percent reported having performed wrong-level lumbar-spine surgery at least once! About 10 percent admitted to having performed wrong-site lumbar surgery at least once. Almost 20 percent of the responding surgeons admitted to having been sued at least once in relation to these errors. All of this occurred despite superb imaging availability.

Neurosurgeons in the United States are not alone with these risks. A study in England of 6,017 closed claims, reported between 1997 and 2011, concluded that the leading causes of damages paid for cranial surgical errors were delayed diagnosis in 29 percent and delayed treatment in 24 percent. Leading causes of damages paid in spinal surgery were delayed diagnosis in 32 percent and surgical negligence in 29 percent.

There are reports of physicians begin charged with manslaughter in other countries. The reader will also recall the sentencing of Dr. Conrad Murray to four years in prison after being convicted of the involuntary manslaughter of Michael Jackson. His actions were regarded as an example of an extreme departure from the standard of care. Apparently, he inappropriately treated insomnia with a surgical anesthetic (propofol), did not obtain informed consent, administered the propofol without the necessary monitoring equipment, delayed contacting the emergency services, and, finally, made ineffective resuscitation efforts.

Questions

- How was it possible for a neurosurgeon to cause death and so much harm to so many patients in multiple institutions without being stopped?

- Why were good references or simple factual statements made that enabled him to repeatedly obtain hospital privileges in different institutions?

- Why did the Texas Medical Board wait until June 2013 to revoke his medical license?

Commentary

The cascade of catastrophes that occurred in this case is not only appalling but also an absolute disgrace. The unimpeded killing and maiming of so many patients without those in authority in multiple institutions taking preventative steps to protect patients is a damning indictment of our senior leaders in the named Texas hospitals, the Tennessee Medical School, the Texas Medical Board, and the Texas legislature.

I have previously served on a promotions committee within a medical school and find it incomprehensible that there were no issues raised relative to the behavior or performance of Dr. Duntsch through his years at the University of Tennessee Medical School. That school, abiding by the strict laws relating to privacy and confidentiality, refused access to his personnel file. Do the tenets that hold privacy and confidentiality statutes as sacrosanct need to be maintained in the face of murder and mayhem? Can the Tennessee legislature not amend their laws to accommodate their primary requirement to safeguard the public in the face of such atrocities? Was it not the responsibility of the medical school to prevent the emergence of someone who became a grave danger to the patients he treated?

What prime factor led the Baylor Plano Hospital, the Minimally Invasive Spine Institute, and the Dallas Medical Center to provide hospital privileges to Dr. Duntsch? The devastating realization is that the answer is greed! Neurosurgeons are the first or occasionally second most important revenue earners in a hospital. Turning a blind eye to repeated catastrophes doesn't interfere with the bottom line! Why else would they have hired Dr. Duntsch, who in fact was not a board-certified neurosurgeon? According to the Board of Neurological Surgery, he never sat for the oral examination and was never board certified as a neurosurgeon. He had been reported to the American Board of Neurological Surgery, but since he was not a diplomate, they had no power over his disastrous surgical performance.

Even more problematic are the series of letters of recommendation or simply *factual* letters or statements that enabled him to obtain sequential hospital appointments. The cowardly and dangerous actions of his previous chiefs enabled his sequential hospital appointments by virtue of their letters. Refusal to provide a letter of recommendation does not introduce the threat of a lawsuit. I have, however, seen instances where inferior candidates have received letters of recommendation in order to rid an institution of that individual. Dr. Duntsch left Baylor Plano Hospital with a letter making no reference to his series of botched surgeries. They apparently also did not report him, as required, to the National Practitioner Data Bank.

Texas state laws that were promulgated to protect any prominent public institution undoubtedly were not meant to also protect an individual against manslaughter in that hospital. Surely leaders in such hospitals should be vulnerable and liable.

The steep descent of this impaired, addicted physician would have continued to wreak havoc on unsuspecting patients had it not been for the courageous stand taken by a general surgeon, not a neurosurgeon, to seek the help of a prosecutor, who eventually stopped the carnage.

Remarkably, the Texas Medical Board, to whom a report about Dr. Duntsch had been made, also took far too long to revoke his medical license. Their tardiness to act contributed to Dr. Duntsch's opportunity to maim and kill more patients. Their slow reaction time almost certainly reflects an endemic problem throughout the United States, where Boards of Registration in Medicine are seriously underfunded and, as a consequence, are understaffed. Once again, legislatures, whose attention is focused elsewhere, fail to see the dangerous consequences of an inadequately funded Board of Registration.

Multiple factors, as always, were at the root of the grievous harm that was visited upon so many patients. Among these, the most important included blind adherence to confidentiality and privacy laws, greed, wishes to avoid being a victim of a lawsuit, abysmal leadership, legislative impotence, and a general failure to care. Almost no one with institutional authority recognized that they didn't know, they didn't know, about the consequences of their inaction.

If the havoc wreaked on the patients of Dr. Duntsch were an example of a rare case, some reassurance might be possible. However, recent history provides no reassurance whatsoever. The *Houston Chronicle*, some years ago, and again in Texas, drew attention to yet another surgeon. The *Chronicle* reported that under Dr. Eric Sheffey, four of his patients died, two others committed suicide while pursuing malpractice claims, and many others suffered either botched surgeries or unnecessary operations. Dr. Sheffey acknowledged that he and his insurers had paid out more than $10 million to settle claims. Apparently, two administrative-law judges examined some thirty operations performed by Dr. Sheffey and found that twenty-nine of them were partially or completely unnecessary, as they reported to the Texas State Board of Medical Examiners. Some patients apparently had multiple operations that were unjustified, some being left worse than they were before. Dr. Sheffey was given warnings, and apparently there were other disciplinary actions. Nevertheless, he was eventually arrested while driving a car containing cocaine and admitted that he was a user. Incredibly, the board placed him on probation rather than to remove his license to practice medicine.

We are not alone in the United States in our misery with these issues. Between 2006 and 2013, eleven doctors in England were charged with manslaughter due to gross negligence. Some other claims have been made elsewhere, including France, Taiwan, and other countries.

Neurosurgery maintains its position as the highest malpractice risk specialty in all Western countries. An analysis of 617 closed malpractice claims between 1997 and 2011 were recorded by the UK National Health Service Litigation Authority. Considering both brain and spine surgeries, the leading causes that resulted in payment for damages were delayed diagnosis, delayed treatment, and surgical negligence.

We all eventually become patients and trust that our care providers act in a way that will protect us from harm. The expectation we all have is that anyone at all who witnesses situations that may or will cause harm will speak up, alerting team members or those in authority. The principles of medical ethics are well recognized. The Physician Charter on Professionalism was developed through collaboration with the American Board of Internal Medicine Foundation, the American College of Physicians Foundation, and the European Federation of Internal Medicine. That charter highlights three key fundamental principles: privacy of patient welfare, patient autonomy, and social justice. These three principles are similar to the well-known principles of medical ethics that are beneficence (the duty to promote patient welfare), nonmaleficence (the duty to prevent or do no harm), patient autonomy (the duty to respect patients and their rights), and justice (the duty to treat patients fairly). The physicians in authority in the institutions noted above simply disregarded these fundamental principles.

The jury took only four hours of deliberation to reach a guilty verdict that resulted in a life sentence for Dr. Duntsch.

THE DONOR

Paul and Lorraine Hawks were a happily married couple who, according to the *Boston Globe*, were planning to build a new wheelchair-accessible home in Tampa. Paul was fifty-six and in his own business as an electrician. They had planned to start a small Christian ministry in Tampa, Florida. He was known as a kind man with a generous spirit who had driven elderly worshipers to and from church for the past nine years.

The remarkable beneficence that living organ donors have is likely to be akin to the thoughts and character of those who, in action, lay down their lives to save others. Such must have been the thoughts of the generous and self-sacrificing Paul Hawks, when he consented to donating a portion of his liver to his brother-in-law. That operation occurred at the Lahey Clinic in Burlington, Massachusetts. The quintessential points that are summarized here are taken from the *Boston Globe* report of this troublesome incident.

The recipient, Tim Wilson, had a diagnosis of end-stage liver disease and liver cancer. After a full evaluation of both Tim Wilson and Paul Hawks, and after obtaining consent, the surgery began.

After about 60 percent of Paul Hawks's liver had been removed by the surgeon, Dr. Elizabeth Pomfret, uncontrollable bleeding occurred. This was some four hours after surgery began. A subsequent report from government investigators, obtained by the *Boston Globe* through a freedom of information request, revealed that a vein tore partially away from the large inferior vena cava, a major blood vessel attached to the liver. Apparently, they tried to clamp the smaller vein, but it ripped away entirely from the vena cava, the largest vein in the body, and the bleeding was catastrophic. The surgeons could hardly see through the blood while they stitched the hole in the vena cava. Further complicating their attempt to stem the bleed was their use of three small incisions for the operation, instead of one long incision. Then, further bleeding began at another site in the vena cava. In trying to locate the precise bleeding spot, the surgeons removed the section of Paul's liver, which had already been almost completely detached, and rushed the organ to the adjacent operation room, where Tim was on the operating table ready for the transplant. Despite about seventy pints of blood (about the amount of blood in seven people), Paul Hawks's heart stopped. The surgeon cracked open his chest and massaged his heart with her hands but in vain. Paul Hawks, the donor, was dead.

Lorraine Hawks sued the doctors and Lahey Clinic.

Pertinent Medical Facts

Liver cancer, more accurately called hepatocellular carcinoma (HCC), is the sixth-most common cancer worldwide and the leading cause of death among patients with cirrhosis of the liver. This cancer is the third-most common cause of death related to all malignancies. There are an estimated twenty thousand new cases each year in the United States. Hepatitis C and alcohol are among the key causes leading to cirrhosis of the liver, which becomes the root cause of liver cancer. The five-year survival rate appears to be less than 12 percent. Men are about three times more likely than women to develop HCC, while Asians and Hispanics are at significantly higher risk than whites.

Because 80–90 percent of patients with HCC have cirrhosis of the liver, the American Association for the Study of Liver Diseases recommends that patients with cirrhosis be screened for HCC using ultrasound every six months. Treatment options for HCC include cutting out the tumor, mainly applicable to patients without cirrhosis. Otherwise, the options are (1) inserting a catheter through the arterial system to the artery serving that region of the liver and administering chemotherapy followed by an effort to block the blood supply to the tumor (called chemoembolization), (2) attempting to destroy the tumor with radioembolization/radiofrequency, and (3) liver transplantation. Great surgical skill and a multidisciplinary team are necessary to achieve effective treatment and possible cure for this devastating cancer.

The real cure is achievable by liver transplantation from a deceased or living donor. Five-year survival rates for transplantation are in the 68–75 percent range. However, case selection is critical if sense is to be made of survival statistics. In addition to the patient's general health, the presence of one or more tumors within the liver and their size impact the survival rate. While efforts are made to determine the spread of the cancer to the lymph nodes and elsewhere, guarantees of no spread cannot be provided. Strict patient selection, using either the Milan criteria or the Barcelona criteria, has been valuable in determining which patients could be recommended for transplantation. These criteria have been widely accepted, for example, by the United Network for Organ Sharing. Additional guidelines have been created by the Organ Procurement and Transplantation Network in classifying liver cancer within cirrhotic livers. Liver transplantation has a much better survival rate compared to all other treatments.

Organ allocation in the United States is based on a scoring system called the Model for End-Stage Liver Disease. This system employs various biochemical measurements of the recipient's blood and allows prioritization of patients on the transplant waiting list.

Not unexpectedly, the layout of the arteries supplying the liver may not be the same in each person. Available data indicate that some 10–15 percent of the population may have an anomalous arterial architecture, which may have been the case with Paul Hawks.

Questions

- Was the evaluation of the donor beyond reproach?
- Were the rules to protect living donors properly followed?
- Was the recipient's prognosis sufficiently favorable to merit a transplant, which had risks for the donor?

Commentary

Thousands of lives have been saved by organ donation. Nevertheless, the stringent requirements are necessarily burdensome and go far beyond the expected surgical skill, which the Lahey surgeons clearly had. Critical consideration is the health evaluation of the donor. In this case, Paul Hawks was known (by the Lahey team, but not Lorraine) to have some type of minor electrocardiographic abnormality in his heart, but more important, the surgeons were aware that he had additional possibly anomalous blood vessels serving his liver. He was also fifty-six years of age, which is regarded as near the upper limit for a living donor. Of further importance was the knowledge that Tim Wilson had two different tumors in his liver that would clearly impact his prognosis.

Reasonable questions can be asked about the wisdom of performing liver-transplant surgery when serious issues of prognosis for the recipient are known. The decision to proceed with the transplant in the face of a worrying prognosis for the recipient suggests seriously flawed thinking. As it was, Tim Wilson's tumors did not allow him to get priority on the New England Transplantation waiting list for a deceased-donor liver. Priority is given to patients with liver cancer who are most likely to live for years after surgery. That was not the case for Tim Wilson. Over a year later, Tim Wilson died.

Mortality figures vary for *donor* deaths for liver transplantation. Some say the risk of death is one in one thousand, while others say the risk of death is one in two thousand. Fortunately, in the United States, over one hundred million adults have registered as donors. Nevertheless there is a severe shortage of livers for transplantation and a high mortality rate for those on the waiting list.

The *Boston Globe* reported that, in the three years before Tim Wilson's death, the Network for Organ Sharing (the nonprofit organization that oversees transplants under government contract) failed to adopt rules to protect living donors that satisfy federal officials. The aims of these policies were to have hospitals provide donors with their own advocates independent from the transplant program, with directions that all medical information about recipients should be provided. Paul did not have an independent advocate, which was out of compliance with the federal Centers for Medicare and Medicaid

Services rules. Some have argued that there is the need to balance the donor's right to know with the recipient's right to privacy. My view, however, is clear. If someone is willing to risk his or her life, he or she needs to know everything about the recipient's state of health.

In this case, inevitable legal argument will encompass issues of informed consent that is focused on a patient's right to self-determination. A 2015 case in England (*Montgomery v. Lanarkshire Health Board*) before their Supreme Court brought the matter into sharp relief. A woman with insulin-dependent diabetes (often associated with a big baby) had difficulty in labor (called shoulder dystocia) and delivery of the large infant, who sustained brain damage due to severe oxygen lack (anoxia). She claimed that had she been fully informed about the risks, she would have opted for a Cesarean section.

The Court's final decision made it clear that what physicians tell patients about risks, benefits, and options will no longer be determined by what physicians deem important but rather by what a reasonable patient regards as important.

In the United States, about half of the states use the reasonable-patient standard.

Paul Hawks's wife, Lorraine, stated after Paul's death that transplant programs should be required to disclose everything that is known about donor deaths as well as the recipient's health. Furthermore, she stated that donors can only be truly protected if they are evaluated at a separate hospital. In recognition of the huge monetary rewards received by hospitals performing transplantation, this is a position that requires careful attention.

Lorraine Wilson has suffered depression since her husband died, and she continues to struggle with increasing symptoms of multiple sclerosis. Paul died on Lorraine's fifty-seventh birthday. It didn't help her mental state to learn that Tim Wilson had never been on the waiting list for a deceased-donor organ.

INCIDENTALOMAS

Soon after Marjorie's fiftieth birthday, she began experiencing some nonspecific chest pain. These symptoms created not-unexpected anxiety, given that her father had died suddenly at the age of fifty from what was thought to be a heart attack. He had been known to have an elevated level of cholesterol. She quickly sought an appointment with a cardiologist, who immediately performed an electrocardiogram, which yielded a normal result. He followed that immediately with an echocardiogram, images from which revealed that Marjorie had a bicuspid aortic valve. There was some dilatation of her aorta as that major blood vessel left the heart. This was seriously concerning and was followed by the recommendation that she have a CT angiogram of her aorta. This test involved injecting contrast medium that could be seen as it flowed through the aorta.

This study aimed to determine the integrity of her aorta, the largest artery in the body. Imaging of her aorta revealed an ascending thoracic aortic aneurysm (ballooning of an artery that can burst). In the CT angiogram radiographic images, her lung was clearly visible. That view, on retrospective examination many months later, showed a spiculated mass measuring 1.4 × 1.3 cm in the left-lower lung field. This mass was neither seen nor reported by the radiologist.

About five months after the aneurysm was discovered, Marjorie began complaining of a chronic cough, headaches, dizziness, and losing her balance. Her doctor ordered a CT scan of her chest, abdomen, and pelvis. An obvious cancerous lesion of 4 × 1.7 cm was observed in her left lung. This mass was precisely at the same location in her lung as the then-smaller mass that was seen five months earlier. Imaging studies of her head revealed that the cancer had spread to three areas of her brain. She received chemotherapy and radiation treatment and was alive one year later.

Marjorie sued the radiologist for having missed an operable lesion in her lung that had metastasized to her brain and threatened her life.

Pertinent Medical Facts

Aneurysms are bulges along the course of arteries, which may burst with catastrophic consequences. Even without bulging and bursting, a weak spot in the wall of the artery may tear and burst (called dissection), causing a fatal hemorrhage. Aneurysms with or without dissections share causes in common. Most often, multiple different factors collude leading to weakness in the arterial wall. These include various interacting genes as well as conditions such as atherosclerosis with fat and cholesterol deposits in the arterial wall. These multiple factors that interact include not only the various genes but also inflammation, hypertension, and disturbances of cell growth and multiplication, as well as fat biochemistry that results in plaques in the inside lining of arteries.

There are, however, some very well-recognized familial aneurysm genes, especially involving the aorta. These familial connective-tissue disorders are due to mutations in single genes, the more common of which is Marfan syndrome (see chapter 9). In addition to that disorder, there are a number of other named syndromes, including Ehlers-Danlos syndrome (see chapter 17) and the Loeys-Dietz syndrome, that could result in thoracic and abdominal aneurysms. For each of these, analysis of specific genes is available for precise diagnosis. At least another thirteen single genes are known, together with their mutations, that cause these aneurysms.

Anyone with a family history of an aneurysm should seek an evaluation by a clinical geneticist. That evaluation, in addition to imaging of the aorta or other arteries (e.g., in the brain), would include analysis of the specific genes that are known to be associated with aortic aneurysms. About 20 percent of individuals with thoracic or aortic aneurysms or dissections, but who do not have one of these named syndromes, do have a family history of these vascular defects. About 30 percent of families with familial thoracic aortic aneurysms or dissections who do not have one of the named syndromes have a mutation in one of the other thirteen genes.

Once a gene mutation is determined, there is a 50 percent likelihood of that gene being transmitted to each of the individual's offspring. Various surgical approaches are used to remedy these very high-risk situations. For reasons that are unclear, abdominal aortic aneurysms occur more than six times more frequently in males than in females.

Questions

- How was it possible to have missed the lung lesion that was in plain sight on the radiographic images?

Commentary

The laser-like focus of a radiologist charged with describing the state of the aorta, as was the situation with Marjorie, may easily result in a failure to see an abnormality visible within the same radiographic field. A superb example of the consequences of mental absorption, concentration with intense focusing, was provided by Christopher Chabris and Daniel Simons in their book *The Invisible Gorilla* (chapter 18). Experienced radiologists know that they simply have to systematically look at the entire exposed field so as not to miss a potentially important anatomical abnormality. Failure to do due diligence will very occasionally result in a disastrous miss, which was the case with Marjorie's lung cancer. It didn't help to know after the fact that the radiologist was not board certified. A strict discipline is necessary to ensure a systematic examination of an entire radiographic field, even though the radiologist may be examining thousands of images per year.

Radiologists rank eighth among those likely to be sued for medical malpractice among all specialties. A 2016 report based on the Comparative Benchmarking System Database, a repository of more than three hundred thousand medical-malpractice cases in the United States, was used to examine closed claims over a five-year period (2008–2012). Not unexpectedly, in that report radiology malpractice claims most commonly involved diagnosis-related allegations, with special reference to missed cancer diagnoses. Among all failures to make any specific diagnosis, there was a striking 44 percent that pertained to cancer diagnoses.

In another study of 8,401 radiologists in forty-seven states, the researchers noted that 31 percent reported they had been sued at least once in their career. By far the most common cause for litigation was the failure to diagnose breast cancer. Additional reasons for radiologists being sued include failures to communicate and failures to recommend additional testing. The American College of Radiology has Practice Guidelines for Communication of Diagnostic Imaging Findings. In essence, radiologists are required to expedite reports that indicate significant or unexpected observations and to communicate with the referring physician in a timely manner.

The occurrence that is far more common than a missed diagnosis is the detection of a lesion that is noted incidentally while focused on an organ or tissue that is being examined. The secondary or incidental findings have been termed "incidentalomas." Along with the remarkable advances in radiographic resolution, using both the CT and MRI scanning with next-generation equipment, more and more incidental findings are being noted and reported. Professor Leonard Berlin, a distinguished professor of radiology from Skokie Hospital in Illinois, has summarized the frequency of incidentalomas reported during specific procedures as follows.

Incidentalomas in various organs have been reported in

- 70 percent of those CT screens of the colon;

- 34 percent of individuals suffering from blunt trauma;

- 35 percent of patients having thoracolumbar CTs for blunt trauma;

- 25 percent of patients having a chest CT;

- 40 percent of those having abdominal and pelvic CT examinations simply for research purposes;

- 49 percent of patients undergoing aortic CT angiograms;

- 50 percent of patients having chest CT examinations;

- 15 percent of those having CT of their kidneys and liver during abdominal examinations; and

- 67 percent of patients having ultrasound studies of their neck to examine the thyroid gland.

Others have pointed out that the likelihood that an incidentaloma represents a lethal cancer is less than 1 percent. This, however, was only from a single report. Guidelines have evolved to assist in the management of incidentalomas with special reference to their size in specific organs. The larger the incidental lesion, the more likely further examination will be recommended, despite increasing radiation risks.

A report by M. Niel in the *Chicago Daily Law Bulletin* recounted the sad experience of Sandra Hogan. She had a routine set of x-rays prior to planned surgery on her back. A few years before, a radiologist reported the presence of an abnormality in her lung and made recommendations for follow-up. A number of Sandra Hogan's physicians saw that report, but none followed the recommendations. Moreover, she was not notified of that abnormal shadow. Some two years later, the diagnosis of lung cancer was made, and her chance of recovery was considered to be less than 5 percent. The jury awarded Sandra Hogan $14 million damages for lost wages, medical expenses, and pain and suffering.

There has been considerable discussion about whether or not incidentalomas should be reported, if they appear benign. Once reported, findings cannot be ignored and inevitably spawn a combination of anxiety and the initiation of an additional sequence of tests to determine the nature of the incidentally discovered lesion. In some of these cases, a precise diagnosis or determination of the nature of the lesion may never be achieved, leaving the patient worrying about potential inconsequential findings for years on end. Practice in all specialties, including radiology, is governed by the American Medical Association Code of Ethics, which requires a physician to present all of the known medical facts accurately to the patient.

The Quality and Safety Division of the Massachusetts Board of Registration in Medicine also weighed in on this subject in 2016. The division made it clear that incidental findings must be communicated to physicians who must inform patients in a timely and appropriate manner.

The frequency of incidentalomas is increasing because of the incredible escalation in the number of CT examinations, notwithstanding the risks of radiation. Professor Berlin has pointed out that the frequency has increased geometrically from three million CT examinations a year in 1980 to close to eighty million by 2012! Clearly, the closer one looks, the more one sees and finds. The practice guidelines for communication of diagnostic information from the American College of Radiology clearly advise expedited reporting of significant or unexpected findings. The European Association of Radiologists and the United Kingdom's Royal College of Radiologists have both adopted similar guidelines.

Once an error has been discovered and acknowledged, the question of apology needs to be addressed. Doctors are generally good ethical beings, and intuitively most, I believe, would want to apologize. Their lawyers, however, will often instruct them not to apologize for fear that sentiment might trigger a lawsuit. Absent any apology, all may remain quiet until the patient discovers that his or her physician either had not been honest and forthright or had purposefully misled them. Anger is then the steam that drives the ensuing lawsuit and inflates the demands.

Not only lawyers discourage or instruct physicians to resist apologizing. Insurance companies who carry the liability may impose a duty of cooperation and may demand silence as they defend a claim of negligence.

Apology is best made in person and as soon as the error has been recognized when humility, sensitivity, and sincerity are most effectively communicated. A written apology (constructed or edited by a lawyer) may be effective but will invariably lack the emotional tone of personal expressed and admitted fault, regret, remorse, and sympathy.

Professor Berlin has also pointed out the remarkable fact that thirty-five states have passed laws that do not allow admission of an error and apology to be revealed in the courtroom! He goes on to emphasize that ethical and moral considerations enjoin physicians to disclose errors and offer apologies.

As in the case of the high-resolution advances in imaging in radiology, technological advances in human genetics have also enabled incredibly detailed examination of our genomes. Not unexpectedly, the closer we have looked, the more we have found, including incidental observations of changes that were not being looked for. For example, an analysis aimed at the examination of all our coding genes in a single test (called whole exome sequencing) may reveal a gene with a mutation that may cause colon or breast cancer or a fatal neurological disease. Because of the real and not rare experiences in this context, the American College of Medical Genetics and Genomics (ACMG) has published specific guidelines about the management of incidental observations made during gene analysis for a different disorder that has potential serious health implications. The ACMG has listed fifty-nine genetic disorders for which treatment, surveillance, or interventions are available. We are required to communicate the finding of any disorder on this actionable list to patients, even though this observation was incidental. Patients having whole exome or whole genome sequencing can opt out of being informed of results about diseases for which no remedy is known but will be told about an actionable disorder.

As patients, we need to choose our primary-care doctors and specialists carefully. Recommendations from friends are best checked with the state Board of Registration in Medicine for a doctor's malpractice record.

THE NOVICE

At birth, Kenneth was a healthy, good-looking baby with normal weight, length, and head circumference. His milestones through the first two years of his life were achieved well within the normal range. However, when he began to walk, marked instability of his hips and knees was noted. By three years of age, his instability was considered by his orthopedic surgeon to be due to lax ligaments, confirmed by his hypermobility in other joints. Kenneth soon found that even in elementary school, he could not keep up with his friends. As he advanced to elementary school, he began to experience progressive problems with his hips and with his thighbones popping out of his hip joints regularly (subluxations). Also, particularly bothersome was his progressively worsening knock-knees. Not only did this cause him knee pain, but it also made him look odd while walking. Sure enough, classmates soon began to tease him that he walked like a duck.

By the age of six, x-rays had revealed that he had abnormal developing bones (a skeletal dysplasia), which was characterized as a biochemical genetic storage disorder called Morquio disease. He also began to develop a curved spine (scoliosis), hunching of his shoulders (kyphosis), and beaking of his sternum (pectus carinatum).

At puberty, Kenneth was dramatically short, which, together with his gait and knock-knees, made him acutely aware of how different he was from his classmates, especially with his deformed back. Fortunately, being unable to participate in any type of sports, Kenneth spent a great deal of time with his books. Consequently, he was well read and doing well in class. Unfortunately, however, anxiety and depression became chronic problems.

At sixteen years of age, he convinced his parents that he wanted to drive his own car with the necessary handicap arrangements that would allow manual control. But before pursuing this plan, he urged his parents to arrange for surgery to remedy his severe knock-knees, which would enable him to drive. This they did, and Kenneth entered the hospital to have that surgery. He walked into the hospital, clambered onto the bed in his room, and happily contemplated having straight legs. Because his rib cage had become progressively deformed due to his generalized bone disorder posing a risk of lung infection, the decision was made to do the surgery under epidural anesthesia. Kenneth was even more delighted that he would be able to be awake during the surgery. He was pleased to see a relatively young female anesthesiologist who came to administer the epidural anesthesia. They bent him over with some difficulty and introduced the spinal needle into his malaligned spine and spinal canal, through which the epidural anesthesia was injected. His legs went numb almost immediately, and he settled down in the operating room, thinking about the car his parents promised him after he obtained his license.

The surgery went off without a hitch, and his knock-knees were largely repaired. It took only a few hours after surgery for the physicians to notice that his sensation had not returned. Moreover, they also observed that he could not move his legs. An MRI of his spine was duly ordered, and the devastating observation was made that the anesthetic had been injected directly into his spinal cord, which had been destroyed at that location in his lower back. It became clear that Kenneth had been rendered totally paraplegic, lacking sensation and movement in his legs and had no control of his bladder or bowel.

His parents sued the anesthesiologist and the hospital for causing such a devastating injury and especially for allowing an inexperienced anesthesiologist who had never performed epidural anesthesia on any patient with a deformed spine to administer the epidural anesthesia.

Pertinent Medical Facts

Morquio disease belongs to a group of biochemical genetic disorders that result from the absence or malfunction of certain enzymes (lysosomal) that our cells use to break down long, complex chains of carbohydrates (called glycosaminoglycans). These particular carbohydrates within our cells construct and maintain the integrity of our bone, cartilage, tendons, ligaments, skin, and even corneas. When there is a deficiency of particular lysosomal enzymes, these complex carbohydrates accumulate in our cells, causing

progressive damage, especially to our bones and connective tissues. Given that all of our cells accumulate

these carbohydrates, many organ systems may seriously malfunction, including our brain cells, and

intellectual disability may occur as a consequence. There are a group of biochemical genetic disorders in

which these carbohydrates accumulate in our cells (called mucopolysaccharidoses), most of which are

associated with intellectual disability and involvement of our bones, among other organs. Morquio

disease, fortunately, is not usually associated with intellectual disability. Unfortunately, however, the

enzyme deficiency in this disorder leads to profound abnormalities in the formation, structure, and

function of bones.

Early signs in the more severe form become evident usually by one to two years of age and progress

variably. Kenneth had a moderately progressive form.

There was no family history for this disorder, typical for an autosomal recessive disorder, with both of his

parents being unaffected carriers of a specific gene mutation. They unwittingly had a 25 percent risk of

having a child with Morquio disease.

For the first one to three years of life, children with Morquio disease may show few, if any, abnormalities in

physical development. Their intellectual development remains intact. However, instability of their hips and

knees due to lax ligaments and developing bone abnormalities leads to an evaluation that ultimately results

in this diagnosis. Progress throughout childhood is marked by disproportionate growth, resulting in very

short stature and a very short trunk but normal-length limbs. Some deviation of the wrists is typical, as is the

development of beaking of the breastbone (called pectus carinatum) and flaring of the lower rib cage.

Progressive deformity of the chest and spine causes marked disfigurement, including scoliosis, and marked

curvature (kyphosis) that may be further complicated by a prominent jutting out of some

vertebrae along the back. Severe knock-knee often develops, resulting in a waddling gait.

Deformity of the chest often leads to respiratory difficulties, and obstructive sleep apnea is common.

Other problems that can occur include leaking heart valves, hearing impairment, clouding of the corneas,

dental abnormalities, and an enlarged liver. If deformities and kinking of the spine are severe, spinal cord

compression may occur with serious consequences that result in the lack of control of bladder and bowel.

Joint pains and developing arthritis are invariable, while hip dislocations may cause such severe joint

restriction that an affected person may be wheelchair bound.

Fortunately, Morquio disease is rare, various studies pointing to a birth prevalence ranging between one

in seventy-one thousand and one in three hundred thousand births.

While x-rays of the chest, spine, and long bones point to the likely diagnosis, additional tests of the urine

further help to nail down the specific diagnosis by measuring breakdown products of the

mucopolysaccharide. DNA diagnosis of the culprit gene (*GALNS*) clinches the diagnosis, confirms the

carrier status of both parents, enables the testing of the parents' siblings to determine their carrier status,

and provides future opportunity for precise prenatal diagnosis or preimplantation genetic diagnosis to

avoid a recurrence of this disorder.

Questions

- Given the known spine deformity that Kenneth had, why was a novice anesthesiologist allowed to perform the epidural anesthesia procedure?

Commentary

Most of us by far will encounter a surgeon in our lifetime. If you have already had a significant surgical

operation, did you happen to ask the surgeon if he had done your particular procedure before, and how

many times? Most people, in my experience, are hesitant to put the surgeon on the spot, recognizing that

their fate lies in his or her hands, and embarrassing him or her would not help. Notwithstanding this natural hesitancy, one would encourage discussion on this point in the office or other setting, not while lying on the operating table just prior to the initiation of anesthesia.

At some point, all surgeons will be performing a particular procedure for the first time. The answer we, as patients, would seek is an honest answer plus the admission that another more senior surgeon will be assisting the surgeon and providing any necessary guidance.

We would all wish that any physician performing any procedure on our bodies is competent and able to perform properly, having the necessary knowledge, skills, attitudes, and personal qualities. The more challenging or complicated a procedure is, the greater the training and duration expected. For epidural anesthesia, various studies have concluded that trainees should, on average, complete at least fifty obstetric epidurals to ensure that they are competent. Some programs do not allow novice trainee anesthetists to work alone until they have completed ten or more epidurals.

All that sounds reassuring, but how is competence determined? Once upon a time, there was the apprenticeship, now replaced by oversight, required number of procedures, cognitive assessments, and, more recently, simulation-based assessments. Both the Accreditation Council of Graduate Medical Education and the Royal College of Physicians of Canada are fully engaged in all aspects of professional competency including assessment.

The specialty of anesthesiology has seen major improvements in patient safety over many decades. Complications do however continue to occur (as in all specialties), despite practice guidelines developed by the American Society of Anesthesiologists. A closed claims analysis of cases between 2007 and 2012 examined complications of anesthesia in 607 cases. The authors reported that the most frequent injuries (other than damaged teeth) were death (18.3 percent), nerve damage (13.5 percent), organ damage (12.7 percent), pain (10.9 percent), and cardiac arrest (10.7 percent).

The performance of a lumbar puncture, for either diagnostic purposes (to sample the cerebrospinal fluid) or using the same technique to administer an epidural anesthetic, is a common and largely straightforward procedure. With careful attention to aseptic technique to avoid infection and with proper training, there should rarely be any complicating issue. However, when there is malalignment of the vertebrae of the spine, very careful preparation would be called for. Precise identification of the vertebral landmarks and the precise place to be plumbed requires preparation, planning, and experience. The lack of the latter should absolutely prohibit a novice performing an epidural without oversight for the first time on a malaligned, deformed spine. Such was the unfortunate experience to which Kenneth was subjected.

Neither the family nor the anesthesiologist didn't know, they didn't know.

LOOKING AND SEEING

Mark was three years of age, and his parents were very much aware that he was very loose jointed and had flat feet and knock-knees. In addition, his parents had noticed multiple tiny lumps on his tongue and lip. Their primary-care doctor was unimpressed and said that as long as they were not bothering him, nothing more should be done. By ten years of age, he had been seen many times by the family doctor for repeated problems with allergies but also for problems with his feet, arches, and knock-knees. At ten, he required surgery on his right hip, following a fall off his bicycle. The surgery was not successful and led eventually to a discrepancy in the length of his legs.

At twelve years of age, after bitterly complaining about back pain, a diagnosis of scoliosis was made. Once again, nodules on his tongue and mucous membranes of his mouth were noted, and this time biopsies were performed. At fourteen, the pathology report indicated that the tongue lesions were tiny neurofibromas. Notwithstanding the fact that he had no other diagnostic features of neurofibromatosis, the conclusion was made that this was the diagnosis. At that time, gene analysis was not available. He also had no family history of neurofibromatosis. He was noted to be strikingly tall at fourteen years of age (six feet) but weighed only 125 pounds. He had difficulty gaining weight, was depressed, and complained about back pain, abdominal pain, and distention.

At fifteen, still complaining about hip pain, he was referred to a geneticist because the family doctor thought that he might have Marfan syndrome (see chapter 9). The geneticist concluded that, although he had the general body-build seen in Marfan syndrome, the diagnosis was probably neurofibromatosis (given the tongue and mucous-membrane biopsy report) and that Mark's depression related to difficulties with his body image or that he had an adjustment disorder. He recommended no further follow-up but urged a greater calorie intake to increase his weight and physical training. He also recommended that Mark have a mental-health evaluation.

Mark was then referred to a neurologist who had a special interest in neurofibromatosis. He simply "confirmed the diagnosis clinically" and did no other tests.

Subsequently, his care was transferred to an internist in his health plan when he was almost sixteen years of age. He only saw Mark about one and a half years later. He never reviewed his patient's chart and was unaware of Mark's history of tongue, mouth, and lip lesions.

Over a year later, a medical resident training with this internist discovered a lump in Mark's thyroid gland. A thyroid scan revealed a cold (inactive) nodule in the left lobe of the thyroid gland. Because a cold nodule in the thyroid may be cancerous, the recommendation was made for the removal of his thyroid gland. The pathology report that followed revealed that Mark had a medullary thyroid cancer. Only then did that doctor, to whom Mark had been referred, recognize that Mark's body habitus resembled Marfan syndrome (a Marfanoid body habitus), with lax ligaments and other connective-tissue signs that pointed directly to a disorder called multiple endocrine neoplasia IIB (MEN IIB). A specific biochemical test for serum calcitonin was done, and an exceptionally high level was determined, consistent with that diagnosis.

Mark had his cancer surgery at Sloan Kettering Memorial Hospital, at which time multiple positive cancerous lymph nodes were found in his neck. The surgeons did a block dissection on the left side of his neck in an attempt to remove all the affected lymph nodes. The Sloan Kettering Memorial Hospital staff obtained the previous pathology slides from his tongue biopsy and recognized that the actual diagnosis was a mucosal neuroma, not a neurofibroma.

When Mark's mother asked after the thyroid cancer was diagnosed whether there was any connection between the cancer and the tongue nodules, Mark's internist responded, "What tongue nodules?" Apparently, having not read the patient's chart, he presumed that the diagnosis was neurofibromatosis.

Mark's distraught parents were informed about his very grim prognosis.

Mark received thyroid hormone replacement but steadily deteriorated from the metastatic thyroid cancer. He died at twenty-one years of age.

His parents sued the health-maintenance organization and the physicians who had so poorly taken care of Mark.

Pertinent Medical Facts

Multiple endocrine neoplasia is a disorder in which tumors, both benign and malignant, may occur in any of the endocrine (hormone-producing) glands (such as the thyroid, pituitary, pancreas, and adrenal glands). There are various subtypes of this remarkable disorder, Mark being affected by a type abbreviated MEN IIB. Children born with this subtype are usually identified in infancy or early childhood because of the presence of lumps on the tongue, palate, throat, or lips. These nodules may also line the eyelids, making them appear thicker or even everted. While the child grows, the lips tend to become more prominent.

Remarkably, type MEN IIB only accounts for about 5 percent of cases of MEN II. Unfortunately, risk of an aggressive medullary thyroid cancer approximates 100 percent; hence the exhortation to make a very early diagnosis even before the age of one year and to remove the thyroid gland as early as that. Without surgical intervention, the average age of death of those affected is twenty years. This was the age Mark died.

Almost 40 percent of those with MEN IIB have those nodules also growing along the gastrointestinal tract. As a consequence, symptoms experienced include abdominal pain, bloating, indigestion, or diarrhea. Mark, in fact, experienced abdominal pain, a complaint that was ignored. At least 84 percent of those affected have these gastrointestinal symptoms that begin in infancy or early childhood.

Mark's body-build that resembled Marfan syndrome is typical in some 75 percent of affected individuals. Additionally, clinical findings include spinal curvature (scoliosis), lax joints, and being extremely thin without any obvious fat. All of these features were obvious in Mark for many years. Moreover, he frequently fell off his bicycle or simply fell down, reflecting muscle wasting and weakness, also typical in this disorder.

A remarkable 50 percent of patients with MEN IIB may develop another tumor in the adrenal glands (called pheochromocytoma). These tumors occur in about 50 percent of those affected and cause a sudden, even fatal, rise in blood pressure.

When Mark was being studied, DNA analysis for the culprit gene (*RET*) was not available. Today, routine sequencing of the *RET* gene enables a diagnosis from a single teaspoon of blood from which DNA is extracted. We now know about 50 percent of those with MEN IIB inherited the disorder from an affected parent. Neither of Mark's parents was affected. Those who have not inherited the disorder are unfortunately born with a brand-new mutation in the *RET* gene. Curiously, the vast majority of brand-new mutations in the *RET* gene that cause MEN IIB are of paternal origin. In other words, the mutation occurred in a gene on a chromosome that derived from the father.

Once a mutation has been discovered, if a parent is affected, future prenatal diagnosis or preimplantation diagnosis is available. If a parent is known to have been affected, then mutation analysis should also be performed on that parent's siblings and, where appropriate, their children. While Mark was deprived of his life, those who have been diagnosed and treated early grow up and have the opportunity of having children. They will need to realize that there is a 50 percent risk of transmitting the *RET* gene and its mutation to each of their future offspring. Once again, the disorder can be avoided or prevented by prenatal diagnosis or preimplantation genetic diagnosis.

Medullary thyroid cancer may be suspected when the level of the hormone called calcitonin is markedly elevated. This hormone is produced by the thyroid gland and is normally involved in controlling the level of blood calcium.

Questions

- How was it possible for an overt genetic disorder, already evident by three years of age, to have been missed by so many doctors for seventeen years?

- With Mark in his teens, how was it possible for a geneticist to miss the diagnosis of a disorder, the fatal outcome of which could have been averted?

Commentary

Mark was seen by more than a dozen physicians over his truncated life. Involvement of multiple organ systems was reflected by a wide range of symptoms and signs. These included loose joints that generated aches and pains, knock-knees, flat feet, and weak muscles that led to repeated falls and bone injuries. Nodules on his tongue, mucous membranes, and lips were evident from the age of three. Current and intermittent eye infections were problematic while he was also noted to have excess tissue (called papillary hypertrophy) under his eyelids. His body-build resembled the lankiness features of Marfan syndrome (chapter 9), described as Marfanoid. He was markedly thin, had difficulty gaining weight, complained of abdominal pain, and was severely depressed.

His care involved the following physicians: primary-care doctor, internist, orthopedic surgeon, ophthalmologist, dermatologist, geneticist, psychiatrist, dental surgeon, neurologist, and eventually an endocrinologist.

It is both startling and worrisome that none of his providers, until the very end, saw the whole picture. A critical pitfall in the practice of medicine is the very nature of rushed appointments, which invites close attention to the symptom or sign of the day. Efforts to remedy the presenting concern have the unwanted consequence of not considering the entire patient. The limited time spent compounds the problem.

There are over seven thousand rare genetic disorders, a large number having multisystem involvement. Physicians are certainly not omniscient, and as patients, we constantly hope that our caregiver is aware of our clinical history, present complaints, and any possible overarching diagnosis. We all have the expectation that we will be referred to a relevant expert when our own doctor recognizes his or her limitations. This sadly was not what happened in the care of Mark when he first presented at the age of three and frequently thereafter.

Already obvious at that age were his connective-tissue disorder and nodules on his tongue. That was the first time he should have been referred for other opinions. Multiple other opportunities arose over time for various physicians to have also seen the whole patient and referred Mark for more expert opinions.

Anxious and concerned by Mark's obvious medical problems and worried about the nodules on Mark's tongue, his mother went outside the health-maintenance organization to seek the care of a dental surgeon. Remarkably, this resulted in the first biopsy of his tongue, which concluded with the false diagnosis of "neurofibroma." The dental surgeon was not the appropriate person to either question or understand that the pathology report was incorrect and that, in particular, neurofibromatosis does not present with lumps on the tongue, a connective-tissue disorder, or the other features already mentioned. Unfortunately, that incorrect diagnosis led to a referral to a neurologist who "specialized" in neurofibromatosis. Needless to say, with blinders, he too failed to see the whole patient and even failed to recognize the lack of the fundamental criteria required to make a formal diagnosis of neurofibromatosis.

The National Institutes of Health criteria for the clinical diagnosis of neurofibromatosis type I (a disorder of the nervous system with skin and bone abnormalities) require the presence of two of the following:

- Six or more café au lait spots (brown skin "stains")

- Freckles in the armpits and groins

- Two or more lumps (neurofibromas) in the skin (from benign growths along peripheral nerves)

- Two or more tiny nodules along the edge of the iris (in the eye)

- A benign tumor of the nerves (optic) to the eyes

- Bone abnormalities (such as scoliosis, knee or skull defects)

- One first-degree affected relative (a parent or sibling)

A suspected diagnosis can be clinched by analysis of the *neurofibromatosis type I* gene (*NF-1*). About 50 percent of those affected are due to new mutations (de novo) but will then have a 50 percent risk of transmitting the disorder to each of their children. About one in three thousand has this disorder (also see chapter 27).

The failure to make a diagnosis was compounded by the geneticist, who was also misled by the biopsy report that stated "neurofibroma" and "plexiform neuroma." He too had the responsibility of evaluating Mark's history and physical features in their entirety and especially recognizing that Mark's signs did not meet the criteria necessary for the diagnosis of neurofibromatosis.

All of the physicians who saw Mark for seventeen years of his life fell below the expected standard of care. The tragedy is that early diagnosis would have enabled a thyroidectomy, even when he was three years of age, and would have saved his life. The surgical removal of the thyroid gland in the face of the diagnosis of MEN IIB may be done before one year of age. While today the *RET* gene is known, together with the 100 percent risk of developing medullary thyroid cancer, that DNA test was not available at that time. However, the sensitive analysis of plasma calcitonin was available but was neither considered nor done, until it was too late.

Further compounding the miserable care meted out to Mark was the health-maintenance organization's failure that allowed physicians' reports and test results to be filed before being seen and initialed by the primary-care physician. The internist who undertook Mark's care when he was sixteen years of age was not aware of previous consult reports in his thick file, nor did he bother to look.

Mark's death was one of 250,000 who die as a consequence of medical negligence as "inpatients" and "outpatients." The Physicians Insurers Association of America established a registry of closed medical professional-liability claims. An analysis of the data collected between 1985 and 2008 was reported by the Department of Legal Medicine of the Armed Forces Institute of Pathology in Maryland. Among the 239,756 closed claims were 27,556 (11.5 percent) that involved primary-care physicians. Payments were made for 8,797 (31.9 percent) claims. The most common claim made against primary-care physicians was because of diagnostic error. Other studies have echoed this conclusion. Missed heart attacks and a failure to diagnose cancer were the most prevalent errors.

Despite being seen by so many primary-care physicians and specialists in a health-maintenance organization, no timely diagnosis was ever made. Mark died as a consequence of compounded errors, negligence, carelessness, and above all, ignorance. This did not have to happen. Yet another shame and disgrace!

The case was eventually settled.

THE HAT TRICK

Iris and Cam lived on a farm with a bucolic setting. Their lives, however, were not as peaceful and were about to undergo a severe change.

Cam had a dominantly inherited disorder called neurofibromatosis (see chapter 26), which had left him with dozens of tiny lumps all over his skin and face. In association with that disorder, he had experienced learning difficulties in school and opted to live and work on a farm, where he could use his skills unimpeded. Iris and Cam were aware that they had a 50 percent risk of transmitting the neurofibromatosis gene mutation to each of any children they might have. They did indeed already have one son, who inherited neurofibromatosis from Cam.

Iris was concerned about the 50 percent risk of having an affected child again and sought a consultation with her primary-care doctor. After considering various options, that discussion concluded with a plan to offer Cam a vasectomy. At home, Cam readily accepted the proposal to have a vasectomy. Accordingly, he made an appointment, underwent the procedure, and was relieved that a future recurrence of neurofibromatosis would be averted.

About nine months later, Iris found herself pregnant again despite Cam's vasectomy. She quickly made an appointment to see her primary-care doctor, who blithely told her that occasionally vasectomy fails. Nevertheless, he said, he would arrange a pregnancy termination forthwith by D and C (dilatation and curettage). Desperate to avoid any potential future recurrence of neurofibromatosis, she readily agreed and came in the next day for a D and C.

A few months later, she noticed a striking weight gain, and in particular, not only had her belly expanded, but also her menstrual periods had not returned since the abortion. She had been reassured in a phone call by her primary-care doctor that the failure of her menstrual periods to return after an abortion would occasionally happen. Obvious movements in her abdomen confirmed her suspicions that she was indeed pregnant and at that stage already at eighteen weeks. Despite the 50 percent risk of having another child with neurofibromatosis, they could not bring themselves to terminate the pregnancy at that stage.

In due course, Iris delivered their daughter, who was very premature, weighing just three pounds at birth. Those early weeks in the neonatal intensive-care unit were difficult and touch and go. Over eight weeks, their daughter slowly improved, gained weight, was weaned off oxygen, and could breathe room air.

By eighteen months of age, with delayed milestones, it had become clear that their daughter had cerebral palsy. Moreover, more than six café au lait spots (brown skin patches) had appeared on her limbs and trunk. Their daughter also had neurofibromatosis.

Cam and Iris had experienced a failed vasectomy and a failed abortion and had a second unplanned child with neurofibromatosis and cerebral palsy.

Iris and Cam sued her primary-care doctor and the pathologist.

Pertinent Medical Facts

Many men choose to have a vasectomy because it offers a permanent and safe method of contraception. Over 525,000 vasectomies are performed each year in the United States, with family doctors performing about 13 percent. Various methods and procedures are available, including a no-scalpel technique. In addition, the use of a jet injector to provide local anesthesia without the need for a needle appeals to many, since it may reduce pain. Bleeding and infection may occur, and occasionally a postvasectomy pain syndrome emerges. The overall failure rate appears to be less than 1 percent.

Prior to the procedure, careful counseling is usually provided, not only about the procedural risks but also about the requirements for subsequent semen analysis and of course the possibility of failure. The need for consent is obvious.

After vasectomy, there are strict guidelines that require analysis of semen to determine the presence especially of motile sperm. Guidelines indicate that one single semen analysis showing no sperm after an analysis be performed three months after the procedure *and* twenty ejaculations are considered sufficient to establish sterility. Furthermore, the guidelines require that the semen sample be obtained after a period of abstinence of at least two days. The sample should be transported while kept at body temperature and sent within sixty minutes of collection to be analyzed in a laboratory within four hours of ejaculation. Clearly, compliance with these guidelines is a challenge.

Vasectomy failure may occur if the two ends of the *vas* reconnect (recanalization), or in rare cases, there is a duplicate, unrecognized second *vas*, a collateral track. The likelihood of recanalization following vasectomy is small (0.4 percent) with pregnancy occurring in only about 0.07 percent.

Pregnancy termination in the first three months is common and can be accomplished by specific medications or surgical dilatation and curettage. Prior to any procedure, counseling outlining possible options and procedural risks is necessary. A vacuum aspiration is also a commonly performed procedure. Complications that occur after dilatation and curettage occur in about 0.5 percent of pregnancies undergoing this procedure and include failed abortion, incomplete abortion, bleeding, infection, and perforation of the uterus.

There are standard rules that require the submission of all tissues removed at surgery to be sent to the pathology laboratory. Visual examination of the tissue submitted should enable recognition of fetal structures. Microscopic examination that follows would further enable precise confirmation of embryonic/fetal-tissue origins.

Questions

- Why did the vasectomy fail?

- How did the dilatation and curettage fail to terminate the pregnancy?

- Why did the pathologist who received the uterine-tissue scrapings fail to recognize that the tissue was not fetal?

Commentary

Iris and Cam were extremely unlucky. The primary-care doctor failed to counsel Cam about the possibility of vasectomy failure. Moreover, he did not follow guidelines that required careful compliance with semen examination three months after the procedure and the twenty ejaculations necessary to establish sterility. The doctor also failed to fully explain the potential risks of dilation and curettage and especially the possibility of failure to achieve a successful pregnancy termination. Remarkably, the statistical likelihood that Iris and Cam would experience a failed vasectomy and a failed abortion procedure approximated one in twenty thousand!

Compounding their abysmal luck, the tissues thought to be fetal that were submitted to the pathologist were completely misdiagnosed and not recognized as not being embryonic or fetal in origin. Medical-negligence claims against pathologists approximate 8.3 percent and are almost always concerning tissues other than those submitted following pregnancy termination.

The primary-care doctor's failure to appropriately counsel prior to both the vasectomy and pregnancy termination and to document the discussion made for difficulties in defense. The fact that vasectomy may fail and that on occasion dilatation and curettage may also fail to achieve pregnancy termination makes careful counseling and documentation necessary. The primary-care doctor's failure compounded the incompetence of the pathologist, who had relied on the cytopathologist technician. Incompetence and bad luck make poor bedfellows.

The case was settled but only after five years of court arguments about the admissibility of a wrongful-birth claim.

FACTS, FAX, AND FAILURE

Doreen was extremely anxious when she arrived at her obstetrician's office, already at least eight weeks along in her first pregnancy. Her worry stemmed from her knowledge of her family history. Her sister had five living children, three boys and two girls. Two of the boys had died within weeks of birth. She also had three maternal uncles, all of whom had died within weeks of birth. While the cause of the uncles' death had not been absolutely established, new advances in genetic technology had enabled a precise diagnosis to be made in Doreen's sister's second boy. These advances in genetics led to the discovery of the specific gene with mutations that cause a fatal muscle disorder called myotubular myopathy. With this history in mind, her obstetrician immediately referred her to a clinical geneticist.

Doreen saw the clinical geneticist, who fully explained the X-linked pattern of inheritance for myotubular myopathy. She understood that her maternal grandmother must have been a carrier of the gene mutation, having had three affected sons, and that her mother had a 50 percent likelihood of being a carrier as well. Her mother must have also inherited the carrier status, given Doreen's sister had two affected boys. Therefore, Doreen realized that she herself had a 50 percent likelihood of also being a carrier. Therefore, if she was a carrier, she had a 50 percent risk of having an affected boy and a 50 percent likelihood of having a girl who would be a carrier but unaffected.

Since having experienced her sister's grief, Doreen was determined to not have a child with myotubular myopathy.

The clinical geneticist discussed the new advances in DNA analysis that enabled a precise prenatal diagnosis of myotubular myopathy by analyzing the culprit gene (*MTM1*). She emphasized that the only laboratory providing that analysis at that time was at the University of Chicago. Hence, when Doreen had the amniocentesis for the prenatal genetic diagnosis, the geneticist advised that the sample should be sent to the University of Chicago.

Doreen then sought out a maternal-fetal-medicine specialist to perform an amniocentesis with the specific aim of determining whether she was carrying an affected male. Her own obstetrician did not do that procedure. At about sixteen weeks of pregnancy, the amniocentesis was duly performed, and the amniotic fluid sample containing the fetal cells was dispatched to one of the country's largest commercial testing laboratories. The requisition form that accompanied the sample to the laboratory clearly stated as an indication for study "a history of myotubular myopathy" albeit spelled incorrectly. The space on the laboratory form for the specific indication of the test remained blank. A chromosome analysis was ordered on the requisition form.

Unfortunately, the clinical geneticist failed to ensure that the vital instruction to send the sample to the University of Chicago was conveyed to the maternal-fetal-medicine specialist who was to perform the amniocentesis. There was no indication in her formal genetic-counseling letter that a copy was being sent to the specialist, nor was there any record of a phone call about this vital information. She had apparently depended on her secretary to ensure that her note would also be sent to the specialist. The secretary maintained that she faxed a copy of the letter to the specialist, but there was no supporting paperwork in the medical record and none in Doreen's records at the specialist's office.

The maternal-fetal-medicine specialist gave no specific instruction to the laboratory to send the amniocentesis sample to the University of Chicago. In turn, the laboratory simply ignored the information on the requisition form that indicated a family history of myotubular myopathy. In due course, the laboratory analysis revealed a male fetus with a normal chromosome complement. There was no mention of myotubular myopathy in the report. Her regular obstetrician (who did receive the geneticist's letter about the University of Chicago) made the remarkable assumption, upon receiving the report, that a normal chromosome report excluded myotubular myopathy. He promptly conveyed the "happy information" that the genetic studies were normal! He was oblivious to the mode of inheritance of the X-linked form of myotubular myopathy and completely failed to note the instruction that the sample had been required to be sent to the University of Chicago. Moreover, neither of his two partners, who also saw Doreen, recognized the fatal error.

Doreen duly delivered her son, who immediately manifested extreme weakness, floppiness, and respiratory difficulty requiring assistance, reminiscent of the signs originally seen in her two deceased nephews. Analysis of the *MTM1* gene soon followed to confirm the diagnosis. Her son lingered on for some months before dying.

She sued the maternal-fetal-medicine specialist, the clinical geneticist, her own obstetrician, and the commercial laboratory for their negligence in not securing the correct sought-after prenatal diagnosis test that led to the suffering and death of her son.

Pertinent Medical Facts

X-linked myotubular myopathy (otherwise called centronuclear myopathy) may be severe, moderate, or mild in its manifestations. Doreen's son (and deceased relatives) had the severe form, which invariably leads to death in infancy. These boys are often dependent on a ventilator, and they have grossly delayed milestones. They never walk. Frequently they succumb to lung infection.

Today, known carriers, like Doreen, have the option of preimplantation genetic diagnosis, thereby avoiding the conception of an affected son, or of course, prenatal genetic diagnosis.

Questions

- How was it possible for a prenatal diagnosis of a known disorder with a known gene mutation to be missed, even though an invasive test had been done for that very purpose?

- Why was Doreen informed that prenatal studies were normal?

Commentary

Doreen had taken the correct steps and seen a clinical geneticist, received appropriate genetic counseling, was aware of her risks, and was knowledgeable about the test that was required. She was confident that the tragedies her sister had experienced would be averted, given the appropriate test. She was not aware, however, of the careless and thoughtless attitudes of the clinical geneticist, maternal-fetal-medicine specialist, obstetrician, and laboratory, whose failure led to Doreen having a child with a fatal genetic disorder. Compounding their carelessness was a demonstrable lack of knowledge by the obstetrician who did not recognize that a chromosome study had nothing to do with a gene analysis and that the test performed did not exclude, or even test for, myotubular myopathy.

The commercial laboratory, dealing simply in case volume, paid no attention to the information provided about myotubular myopathy. The lack of oversight in that laboratory meant that no question would be asked about the given family history of myotubular myopathy. Despite a precisely known disorder and the gene mutation, typical and multiple human factors yet again led to simple errors with grave consequences.

A similar discussion, with a slightly different causal path to negligence, can be found in chapter 46.

Every one of us will, at some point in our lifetime, have a blood sample drawn or a tissue sample sent for laboratory studies. We mostly give little thought to whether or not the results are actually accurate. The fact is that the myriad number of tests and analyses that are done are remarkably accurate. In addition to my clinical duties, I have also been the director of genetics laboratories for many decades and know firsthand about the potential for error. The vast majority of laboratory mistakes are usually due to human factor–related errors that include mix-ups of various types. These include wrong files being matched with different samples, numbering errors, labeling errors, tubes being placed in the wrong position on a testing rack, analytic errors, and a range of communication errors. One particular experience remains in the forefront of my mind.

We received two samples of blood from a clinic for cystic-fibrosis gene-mutation-carrier tests. Each tube had different names and birth dates. We duly performed the ordered tests and were startled to discover the same, very rare, cystic-fibrosis gene mutation in both samples. We of course first considered that our own technical staff could have used the same DNA twice from the same tube of one of the patients. We went back to the original tubes, repeated the assays, and used DNA markers to demonstrate that both of the original samples we analyzed came from different individuals.

Given the extraordinary unlikely coincidence of two unrelated patients harboring the same gene mutation, we requested that samples be drawn again from both patients. We were staggered to find that analysis of the second samples showed no mutation in either. Since it was certain that someone had this mutation, we insisted that the clinic determine which patients were present in the blood-drawing area at the time these samples were originally obtained. The clinic reported, on that very day in the clinic, there were three women present at roughly the same time having blood samples drawn. We insisted that all three women be called back to have blood samples drawn again. Needless to say, the third patient, whose blood was placed in the labeled tubes of the first two women, had the rare mutation. The other two did not. The error in this case was made by the phlebotomist, who labeled the tubes to be filled with blood *prior to* the samples being collected. She then absentmindedly picked up the wrong tubes without checking names and dates of birth. It is indeed a basic rule to label a tube with the patient's name and date of birth only *after* filling it with the blood sample.

The College of American Pathology accredits diagnostic laboratories and performs unannounced inspections. These valuable and rigorous steps, together with extensively provided guidelines for laboratories, serve to ensure the highest-possible performance standards. In addition, the College of American Pathology also provides a proficiency-testing system in which samples with known gene mutations or chromosome abnormalities are sent blind to laboratories for analysis. Laboratories are held to a high-performance standard, or they stand to lose their accreditation, and therefore their ability to exist, since insurance payments will only be made to accredited laboratories. Laboratories are licensed through the Clinical Laboratory Insurance Act, which operates in tandem with each state's Department of Health, which also performs unannounced inspections. It is therefore comforting to know that very high standards are expected and demanded.

There have been other claims of negligence where physicians, unaware of the technical challenges of chromosome analysis, for example, fail to alert genetics laboratories about a patient's previous subtle results that could otherwise be missed without prior warning. An example includes chromosomal translocations, in which two chromosomes break and the two pieces simply exchange places and reattach (a balanced translocation) mostly without eventuality (there is, in fact, about a 30 percent likelihood that breaks interrupt the integrity of a gene, with at least 6 percent of such cases resulting in either birth defects or intellectual disability). When one of the chromosome pieces is tiny and doesn't reattach and is lost (an unbalanced translocation), major birth defects and intellectual disability will be a likely consequence.

Brock and Rhea Wuth knew they had a 50 percent risk of having a child with a chromosomal translocation. Brock had discovered he was a carrier of a translocation following testing after he learnt about the cause of his severely disabled cousin. As reported by the *Seattle Times*, Rhea had prenatal genetic studies and received the report that fetal chromosomes were normal. At birth, it was immediately obvious that their son, Oliver, had abnormalities. Contrary to the prenatal report, Oliver was born with an unbalanced chromosomal translocation.

Court papers in this wrongful-birth case indicated that Valley Medical Center in Renton failed to provide Laboratory Corporation of America precise information about Brock's translocation. That laboratory also failed to make the diagnosis.

At five and a half years of age, Oliver had an IQ between fifty and seventy, a few dozen words, and was unable to walk upstairs or run. He would need care for the rest of his life.

The jury awarded Brock and Rhea $50 million because of the negligence of both the medical center and the laboratory, holding each equally responsible. Both defendants appealed, but the verdict was upheld.

Balanced translocations occur in about one in five hundred and unbalanced translocations in about one in sixteen hundred people.

Sample mix-ups in high-volume commercial laboratories have resulted, for example, in a failure to detect cystic-fibrosis gene-mutation carriers. In one negligence claim, the woman was a known cystic-fibrosis gene-mutation carrier. The carrier-test report for the husband indicated that he was not a carrier of a cystic-fibrosis gene mutation. In the subsequent lawsuit, laboratory records reflected a sample mix-up. The couple had gone ahead with a pregnancy only to give birth to an affected child. Many millions of dollars were paid for the lifetime care of that child.

In a university laboratory some years ago, amniotic fluid samples from three different pregnancies were submitted for the testing of the same biochemical genetic disorder, all at different times. They were all incorrectly diagnosed as being normal. Appropriate normal controls had not been used for the biochemical assays. In all of those pregnancies, the fetus was indeed abnormal. These pregnancies went to term, and the children were born seriously affected. That laboratory was closed down.

To avoid the ever-present risk of errors, constant attention to detail is necessary from each of us receiving medical care. We need to be involved in the details and make no assumptions that simple things will be done competently and efficiently. If a physician takes umbrage while you pursue the details, seek another doctor!

In Doreen's case, the letter from the clinical geneticist was crucial, and she should have called the maternal-fetal-medicine specialist herself given the high risk to ensure that he understood the unusual, but vital, information that the amniotic-fluid sample had to be sent to the University of Chicago. Her fateful reliance on a secretary to convey such vital information was the first error. Use of a fax message for such an important communication represented the second serious error. Faxed messages are notoriously unreliable. Inadvertently, wrong numbers can be used, messages may not be transmitted, they may not be received by the addressee, or they may be filed in the wrong record. Documentation of phone, fax, and written communications are absolutely necessary when important clinical communication is being transmitted. Where life-threatening information is to be communicated, direct phone contact with the caregiver (not a secretary) is required. Failure to notify vital clinical information has been associated with an increased risk of negligence litigation.

It was late on a Friday afternoon at yet another university clinic that a genetic counselor received a biochemical laboratory-test result. This communication concerned a sick inpatient—an infant, who was being treated for an infection. The report confirmed a suspicion that the child had a biochemical genetic disorder called galactosemia. These infants are especially vulnerable to infection by *E. coli* bacteria, for which treatment was not being provided.

The genetic counselor had made prior arrangements to have a weekend at a friend's place on the beach. She decided to call the result on Monday morning when she returned.

She duly made the call on Monday morning to hear that the child died the night before from *E. coli* sepsis, for which there was ready treatment!

The Joint Commission on Accreditation of Healthcare Organizations created a set of guiding principles for communicating abnormal test results. They recommended, inter alia, that there be polices that outlined responsibility, fail-safe communications of abnormal results, definition of critical tests, and timelines between the availability of test results and patient notification.

Once again, and discussed elsewhere in this book, is the risk of being cared for by three or more physicians during a pregnancy. Since no doctor can be on duty endlessly through a year, it is necessary for other physicians in practice to share the care of the pregnant patient. However, the natural tendency for each physician to rely on the other who saw the patient previously is an open invitation for trouble.

For patient safety, I believe that one physician in a group should be responsible for total oversight of a patient's care, regardless of how many times another physician in the group has seen that patient.

Doreen's lawsuit was eventually settled against all physicians for their carelessness, thoughtlessness, and lack of knowledge, as well as the laboratory for their negligent oversight. The settlement did nothing to ease the pain of burying her son.

HYPOXIC ENIGMA

It had been a distressing two years. Deena had lost both of her parents in an accident and subsequently had two pregnancy miscarriages. Her genital herpesvirus infection had flared, and, despite her generally happy disposition, she was having trouble shaking off her depression. Fortunately, she was buoyed by her two bright and lovely young daughters. She then discovered her unplanned pregnancy and, smack into her first three months, experienced a significant vaginal bleed. Her physician advised rest and absolutely no coitus. The bleed ceased, and all was well until the third trimester, when she again had a heavy vaginal bleed. At term, she went into labor, at which time she had a sudden and large vaginal bleed that continued through seven hours of labor. Her blood pressure dropped, and she became progressively anemic. There were discussions about a blood transfusion, but none was given.

At the end of seven hours of labor, the electronic fetal monitor began to indicate decelerations in the fetal heart rate down to 50–60 beats per minute (instead of 120–140 beats per minute). These very brief decelerations were followed by a recovery of the fetal heart rate to 120–140. Nevertheless, because they continued intermittently, the decision was made to perform a Cesarean section. Remarkably, this was performed under epidural rather than general anesthesia.

At delivery, Daniel was found to have his umbilical-cord wound three times around his neck. At birth, Daniel was not breathing, had no heart rate, and was floppy and blue, with no reflexes. To all intents and purposes, he was born dead. Immediate resuscitation progressively restored his vital functions and was assisted by placing him on a ventilator. He had begun breathing spontaneously at six minutes after birth. Blood tests at that time revealed that he too was severely anemic with many nucleated red blood cells in his circulation. This was due to his bone marrow working overtime to push out and supply the blood cells almost before they were ready to circulate. Moreover, because of the lack of oxygen, considerable acid had accumulated in his bloodstream (metabolic acidosis). To make matters even worse, the level of his blood platelets, so important for preventing bleeding (see chapter 2), dropped to a dangerous level. He required a platelet transfusion to avoid a catastrophic hemorrhage.

His blood pressure dropped precipitously, which led to intravenous treatment to remedy that dangerous complication. He was given the intravenous drug dopamine, which quickly raised his blood pressure and, in subsequent days, contributed to transient heart failure. Fortunately, he weighed seven pounds eight ounces and was twenty-one inches in length. Head circumference was normal, and he began to improve rapidly. Microscopic examination of the placenta revealed that certain cells (macrophages) contained meconium (usually the first stool). The placenta also tested negative for viral infection. However, within twenty-four hours it was clear that he was making hardly any urine. Blood tests that measured kidney function were found to be strikingly elevated, pointing to serious kidney failure. An ultrasound of his kidneys revealed echo-dense images, typical for cell death (acute tubular necrosis of the kidney).

Daniel received intravenous fluids, and his lungs rapidly became turgid with fluid (pulmonary edema), and he began to manifest respiratory failure again.

On day eight of life, he was placed on peritoneal dialysis because his kidneys had totally shut down. Ultrasound studies of his brain were performed repeatedly and were reported as normal. However, at about three weeks of age, an MRI of his brain raised the question of whether there was a little blood between his white and gray matter.

Notwithstanding this whole series of complications, Daniel slowly recovered, except for his kidney function. Both kidneys remained nonfunctional. The decision was then made to continue on peritoneal dialysis for as long as possible and then to seek kidney transplantation.

At four weeks of age, he was transferred to a teaching hospital and continued on peritoneal dialysis. During his stay at the tertiary-care hospital, he had an episode of hypertension, as well as infection due to his peritoneal catheter that drained the fluid from his abdomen. The kidney-ultrasound study at six weeks of life was reported with echogenic images consistent with injury due to a lack of oxygen (hypoxia). Daniel was eventually discharged home to continue his peritoneal dialysis, which went on for the first nine months of his life.

Inexplicably, his anemia returned despite no blood loss. Deena had also noticed that his belly seemed rather protuberant. This observation led to an MRI of his abdomen. To everyone's amazement, the MRI revealed a large tumor that seemed to originate from his left adrenal gland, also encompassing the kidney on that side. He was quickly prepared for surgery, at which a large tumor (a neuroblastoma) was found originating in the adrenal gland and enveloping the left kidney. The adrenal gland, the kidney, and the tumor were removed. His bone marrow was checked to be sure that there was no cancer, and a bone scan of his skeleton was performed for the same reason. He also had a total body MRI, which also proved normal. The cancer had not spread. Microscopic examination of the tumor revealed that it was a malignant neuroblastoma originating in the adrenal gland. The kidney, however, showed a well-known pathology called diffuse mesangial sclerosis, with about 95 percent of the functional kidney being destroyed.

By the time he was fifteen months of age, his father had been shown to be a match for a kidney transplant. This was duly done, but not without complications that included serious bleeding. In the year following his kidney transplant, Daniel improved dramatically. By the following year, he was running around, happy and with no intellectual disability. He was neurologically completely intact!

Deena and her husband sued her obstetrician for his delay in delivering Daniel that they claimed resulted in severe hypoxia that damaged and destroyed his kidneys.

Pertinent Medical Facts

A lack of oxygen to the child during labor and delivery, depending upon its severity, has the potential for damaging not only the brain but also the heart, bone marrow, liver, and kidneys, to mention the most important organs. The longer the hypoxia lasts, the greater the damage and the severity. Severe hypoxia has the effect of excess acid pouring into the circulation, causing metabolic acidosis, which in turn has the potential for causing more brain damage. Hypoxic exposure will typically lead to transient damage to the tubules of the kidney and mostly not the filters (glomeruli) leading to a drastic diminution of urine production.

The discovery of a malignant neuroblastoma tumor at nine months of age gave us so-called experts reason to rethink what happened to Daniel.

Neuroblastoma represents the most common solid tumor outside of the brain in childhood. Over seven hundred cases are diagnosed each year in the United States. Neuroblastoma is an embryonic tumor, which must have been slowly growing when Daniel was still a fetus. In fact, malignant neuroblastoma is known to have metastasized (spread) in the fetus even as early as seventeen-weeks gestation. This tumor finds its origin in the cells of the sympathetic nervous system, which includes certain cells in the adrenal glands. These special cells produce adrenaline-like substances called catecholamines, which have the effect of raising the blood pressure. The hypoxia also stimulated the kidney to produce a hormone called erythropoietin, which in turn stimulated the bone marrow to rapidly produce the prematurely delivered red blood cells, still with nuclei because of their early delivery into circulation. That explained the very high-nucleated red blood cell count Daniel had.

Further complicating the situation was the observation that the kidney's architecture was seriously disfigured with fibrous-like tissue, a condition called diffuse mesangial sclerosis. This disorder is considered an autosomal recessive condition, stemming from a gene mutation originating from each parent.

There was no family history of neuroblastoma in Deena's or her husband's families. This does, however, occur "out of the blue," and an affected person subsequently may have a 50 percent risk of transmitting this disorder to each of his or her children.

Questions

- Did Deena's doctor breach the expected standard of care required for the management of Deena's labor and delivery?

- Because of his management of her labor and delivery, did Daniel suffer a hypoxic injury that shut down and destroyed his kidneys?

Commentary

The American College of Obstetrics and Gynecology has clear guidelines that proscribe the use of epidural anesthesia in the face of significant maternal bleeds and abnormalities on the electronic fetal monitor. Deena's doctor, despite his experience, clearly departed from the expected standard of care in the management of her labor and delivery. Subsequent microscopic examination of Daniel's placenta revealed cells (macrophages) that contained traces of meconium. Since it takes at least twelve hours or more for cells to gobble up bits of meconium, the conclusion reached is that hypoxia was of a duration exceeding twelve hours. Meconium is a nonspecific indicator of fetal stress but may also occur normally, but not then found, within macrophages.

The enigma that confronted experts on behalf of Daniel and Deena was the total destruction of his kidneys while his brain remained intact. This was a remarkable discrepancy where the opposite virtually always rules. The plaintiff experts, including yours truly, had no useful information and concluded that Daniel experienced significant and prolonged hypoxia during labor and delivery, worsened by the umbilical cord around his neck. He was then effectively born dead, with no heart rate, no respiration, severely anemic (further diminishing his oxygen supply), and with low blood pressure. His hypotension was remedied by the use of the intravenous dopamine, which, like adrenaline, would raise the blood pressure by constricting vessels, which, in turn, would diminish the blood flow to the failing kidneys. Moreover, the growing tumor was almost certainly producing catecholamines, which, like dopamine, served to further constrict the blood vessels serving his kidneys and further diminish the oxygen supply to already-abnormal kidneys. All of these compounding factors ultimately explain why Daniel was fortunate enough to emerge intellectually intact despite a horrendous newborn period and an infancy that was almost devastated by a malignant tumor and complicated by kidney failure.

The case was settled.

We so-called experts didn't know, we didn't know.

YELLOWER

Lena and Christos met at a Hellenic festival. They had just graduated from college and found that they shared an in-depth appreciation of art. They became inseparable for the next two years as they both pursued a master's degree in history and art. Both of their parents had immigrated to the United States from Greece when they were infants. They married shortly after graduation, and an unplanned pregnancy soon followed.

Pregnancy was uneventful, until the last few weeks before Lena delivered. She developed a urinary-tract infection, for which she received a sulfa-containing medication. She was still on the medication at the time their son, Alexis, was born prematurely. He was born at thirty-six weeks gestation and weighed only four pounds fifteen ounces. Notwithstanding his weight, he was active and alert. On his second day of life, doctors in the nursery commented on his yellow color, explaining that this jaundice was almost certainly physiological due to the fact that his liver was still maturing. The color, they explained, was due to a substance called bilirubin, which produced this yellow pigmentation. They reassured Lena and Christos that as the liver matured, the color would disappear and that the level of indirect (unprocessed) bilirubin (which was then 8.9 mg/dL) would quickly return to a normal level (1.0 mg/dL).

Alexis was taking his feeds well, and the doctors decided to discharge him from the nursery thirty-three hours after delivery.

It took less than twenty-four hours for both grandmothers to begin hovering over their first grandchild. One of them used to be a nurse in her youth but had not lost the observational and caring skills most nurses retain. From the moment she saw Alexis, she had begun to express concern about his yellow color. When she returned to their tiny apartment at the end of Alexis's third day of life, she was insistent that he was "yellower and yellower." Not being of a reticent disposition, she loudly and forcefully insisted that they take Alexis directly back to the hospital. Yielding to her mother-in-law, Lena bundled Alexis up and took him to the hospital.

The emergency-room physician immediately became concerned about Alexis's marked yellow jaundice, took a blood sample, and admitted him to the nursery. There they gave him intravenous fluids and placed him under ultraviolet lights, which normally help decrease the bilirubin level. However, soon after admission to the neonatal intensive-care unit, Alexis was noted to be drowsy and that he had begun having brief episodes of not breathing (apnea). His doctors quickly realized the gravity of the situation and the serious implications of the high level of indirect bilirubin in his bloodstream, which had reached 30 mg/dL (equal to about thirty times the normal level). Moreover, Alexis began arching his back and stiffening up as though he was having a seizure.

Arrangements were quickly made to set up an exchange transfusion to rid his circulation of the excess bilirubin. In this community hospital, however, it took another twenty-one hours from the time of admission to begin the exchange transfusion. Only at that juncture did the doctors order a test for a genetic disorder called G6PD deficiency (glucose-6-phosphate dehydrogenase deficiency). They also began to worry that there was a risk that Alexis could sustain brain damage, especially when, on his sixth day of life, they heard his high-pitched cry. They then ordered an MRI of his brain on day seven of life. The imaging report showed a normal brain.

The exchange transfusion had to be repeated because his bilirubin level had not dropped sufficiently. The second exchange transfusion made a huge difference by dramatically decreasing his bilirubin level and also remedied the anemia he had developed.

Alexis was discharged at fifteen days of life, gaining weight and feeding well. He no longer had any stiffening of his limbs or arching of his back. There was a small concern about his hearing, leading to a recommendation that he return in a few weeks to have another hearing test. The second test revealed that he had significant hearing impairment.

By three months of age, it was clear that Alexis was not only hearing impaired, but also his development was lagging. Repeated neurological assessment through his first year of life concluded that he had the clinical signs similar to cerebral palsy, caused by the high levels of bilirubin that damaged a specific part of his brain (basal ganglia), a disorder called kernicterus.

Lena and Christos did their very best to help remedy Alexis's obvious disability (he could not even stand unsupported at two years of age). It was then that they decided to sue not only the physician who initially discharged him prematurely and the hospital for the delay in having the exchange transfusion available and set up for immediate use but also the nurse in charge who made no objection to Alexis's premature discharge in the face of significant jaundice.

<u>Pertinent Medical Facts</u>

It may be hard to believe, but G6PD deficiency affects more than four hundred million people worldwide! The majority of those affected live in malaria-infested areas of the world, including Africa, southern Europe, the Mediterranean, the Middle East, India, and China. This is an X-linked disorder, primarily affecting males, the known culprit gene, and its mutation being located on the X chromosome. Females are carriers with 50 percent of their sons at risk of being affected. *G6P*D is an enzyme that serves to protect the integrity of red blood cells.

Red blood cells have a life-span of about 120 days. They then break up, releasing heme, the iron-containing portion of the oxygen carrying protein hemoglobin. The liver processes the released heme into molecules called bilirubin and biliverdin, which in turn are discharged through the bile into the intestine. The yellow color derives from the bilirubin. When the red blood cells break up prematurely en masse, the immature liver of a premature infant is quickly overwhelmed, and bilirubin levels rise in the bloodstream. The process of red blood cells breaking up is termed "hemolysis." Given the breakup of the red blood cell, a hemolytic anemia follows. Hemolysis can be caused by a number of genetic and acquired factors. In the presence of G6PD deficiency, hemolysis is triggered by certain drugs, including sulfa-containing medications and antimalarials. In premature infants, the resulting hemolytic anemia with steeply rising bilirubin levels may have to be remedied by exchange blood transfusion.

Women who are carriers of a mutation in this gene may sometimes manifest signs of this disorder when exposed to these triggers.

The premature infant with G6PD deficiency is at special risk for developing brain damage because of the deposition of bilirubin in the basal ganglia of the brain. The only known remedy is timely exchange transfusion. When performed as soon as it is clear that the bilirubin level is rising continuously and quickly, exchange transfusion will prevent brain damage. Once normal levels of bilirubin have been achieved, no future brain damage will occur. The timing, therefore, is critical.

Questions

- Why did the physician discharge Alexis, who was jaundiced and premature, thirty-three hours after he was born?

- Why did it take so long to begin the exchange transfusion?

- Was the senior nurse responsible for not objecting to Alexis's discharge at thirty-three hours of age?

Commentary

There was an abysmal failure by the doctor to recognize the danger that premature infants have due to an elevated bilirubin level. Every newborn nursery has graphic nomograms that enable the level of bilirubin to be plotted over hours and days and that reflect not only the concentration of bilirubin but also the very important velocity of a rising level. Available graphic representation and algorithms with detailed published guidelines from the American Academy of Pediatrics in 2004 and 2009 serve as critical intervention thresholds. Simply plotting Alexis's level and recognizing his vulnerability as a premature infant should have halted any thought of discharge.

The actual level of Alexis's bilirubin at the time of his discharge was not the single factor that caused his kernicterus. Rather, as should have been anticipated, it was the velocity of the rise of his bilirubin level and the high level that it reached that caused his irreversible brain damage. Moreover, the physician also failed to recognize the Greek/Mediterranean ancestry of Alexis's parents (see chapter 20), a history that should have added further to anticipatory caution.

Lack of ready equipment in the neonatal intensive-care unit for exchange transfusion to be performed at very short notice reflected the hospital system's poor organization or an unwillingness to spend sufficient funds. This failure to have critical equipment and supplies in an intensive-care unit harkens back to the same problem discussed in chapters 2 and 17.

Difficult as it might seem, nurses have the responsibility and the knowledge to call out physicians if they witness medical negligence. The senior nurse who participated in the discharge of Alexis was well aware of the facts enunciated here. She failed to either observe or report any deviation from the expected standard of care. She should also have been fully aware of the implications and danger of a high and rapidly rising bilirubin level.

The very angry mother and mother-in-law, both of hot, fiery, Mediterranean disposition, brought to mind the awful and violent responses to perceived medical negligence reported in other cultures and countries. Global attention has been brought to the plight of physicians in China, Taiwan, and India. The problem in India is startling.

In 2017 in Mumbai, India's largest city, more than two thousand medical residents staged a strike for four days to protest violence against doctors. They were seeking better government security and protection. A 2015 survey by the Indian Medical Association determined that three out of four physicians have faced some form of violence at work due primarily to patient dissatisfaction.

In one remarkable incident in Kolkata, a private hospital was vandalized by an irate mob following the death of a patient allegedly due to medical negligence. One further remarkable consequence was the introduction of a new law with severe penalties that included criminal prosecution for medical negligence!

Thankfully, we do not have to bear this type of extreme response.

This case was eventually settled. Once again, we have a physician who didn't know, he didn't know; a nurse who did not act; and a hospital that did not care.

NURSES

Oona and Raj had spent their early years in the very attractive city of Delhi (when there was much less smog) in India. They were first cousins. They both attended different colleges in the United States, Oona becoming an engineer and Raj a computer programmer. In true Indian tradition, both of their parents decided that they were good for each other and, indeed, meant for each other. The parents then went about ensuring that relationship, which resulted in a fabulous Indian wedding back in Delhi.

Three years later, living in New York State, they decided to start a family. Other than having many family members on both sides with diabetes, there were no additional concerns or recognized risks. It didn't take long for Oona to become pregnant. The nine months passed without any problems.

During an extremely heavy snowstorm, Oona went into labor precisely at nine months of pregnancy. Oona was five feet tall and had a slight build. The baby, however, turned out to have a rather large head, just like Raj. Labor was prolonged and difficult and eventually assisted by vacuum extraction. They named their son Zoran after a deceased family member. At birth, Zoran was not breathing, was blue and floppy, but did have a heart rate of one hundred beats per minute. Vigorous resuscitation was necessary, and, together with oxygen given by bag and mask, Zoran slowly recovered.

Just over forty-eight hours later, the nurses caring for Zoran told the pediatric resident that they thought that Zoran's legs were not moving normally. The resident took a brief look, noted that Zoran's legs did move, and did nothing more. Some hours later, the nurses reported to the resident that they did not think that Zoran could move his legs at all. The resident, who was busy, said he would take a look later. By the time he did examine Zoran, it was clear that his legs appeared paralyzed. It took another couple of hours for imaging of Zoran's spine to be done, at which time he was found to have had a hemorrhage into his spinal canal. Concurrently, they found that the level of his blood platelets had dropped to an extremely dangerous level. The platelets have a key role in preventing bleeding (see discussion in chapter 2).

I saw Oona and Raj a couple of years later when they were planning to have another pregnancy. The reason for the consultation was their concern for having a child with a genetic disorder or congenital malformation. They were anxious because of the realization of their consanguineous relationship and the potential risk it posed for bearing a child with a birth defect, genetic disorder, or intellectual disability. It turned out that during the awful weeks immediately following Zoran's birth, he was noted to have dextrocardia. Fortunately, while his heart was on the right side of his chest, it was functionally normal and specifically without any structural abnormality. Nevertheless, they were especially anxious given that relatively rare occurrence.

They brought Zoran with them, and I vividly recall tearing up as I watched Zoran, paralyzed and incontinent, pull himself around the carpeted floor, bright, smiling, and paraplegic.

Subsequently I heard that Oona and Raj had filed a medical-negligence lawsuit against the obstetrician who delivered Zoran, the hospital, and the resident. Their claim against the obstetrician was for his negligence in managing her labor and not doing a timely Cesarean section and against the hospital and resident for failure to make a timely diagnosis that could have prevented the destruction of his spinal cord.

Pertinent Medical Facts

On average, all couples have a 3–4 percent risk of bearing a child with intellectual disability, a major birth defect, or a genetic disorder. First cousins have about double that risk, especially due to autosomal recessive disorders, characterized by each parent carrying a mutation in the same gene and the child receiving a double *dose*. Since we all carry two hundred to three hundred gene mutations, a couple with many of their genes being derived from a common ancestor will both have an increased risk for receiving and transmitting the same harmful mutation. In the Middle East especially, and also in India and Asia, the rates of consanguinity range between 50–70 percent of marriages!

Oona and Raj had been informed about Zoran's heart being on the right side of his chest while he was still in the nursery. At that time, the cardiologist was not certain that another structural defect was present. Subsequently, further studies, including an echocardiogram, revealed no additional abnormalities. However, it became clear that not only was his heart on the right side of his chest but also that his liver was on the left side and his spleen on the right (a condition called situs inversus totalis). It was not surprising when they learned that this was a recognized disorder of development due to a gene mutation they both shared. Namely, this was an autosomal recessive disorder, and they would have a 25 percent risk of having another child with the same multiorgan asymmetry.

The frequency of this disorder approximates one in ten thousand births. There is a 5–10 percent incidence of actual heart defects (congenital heart disease) in patients with this total inversion. The population frequency of congenital heart defects approximates 0.8 percent of all births. These cardiac defects include a range of structural abnormalities, including open communications between the atria or the ventricles or much more complex defects.

Elegant scientific studies have revealed the remarkable mechanism by which the heart and the organs may end up on opposite sides to their usual location. The basic mechanism has to do with tiny hairlike protrusions found on the surface of cells that line parts of many organs. These hairlike structures are called cilia. Seen by electron microscopy, there appear to be about two hundred cilia per cell. Each of the cilia is composed of about 250 proteins organized like escalators within the cell. Thus far, at least twenty-nine different genes have been recognized that contribute to the structure and function of cilia. The cilia, when motile, wave back and forth like a wheat field swaying in the wind, influencing the direction of developing cells in an embryo to move one way or another. A mutation in a key gene may cause ciliary dysfunction, resulting in the heart, liver, and spleen ending up in completely different positions than one would ordinarily find.

Not unexpectedly, the motile cilia are also found lining the entire respiratory tract, the lining of the ventricles within the brain, and the tubes (fallopian) that carry eggs down to the uterus. In addition, the tail (flagellum) that propels sperm has a similar structure to organ cilia. From this, you could guess that genes with mutations that disrupt ciliary movement will invariably cause serious problems. In the respiratory tract, for example, ciliary failure would lead to the inability to expel mucus, which then remains in place, becomes infected, and causes very serious lung disease (bronchiectasis). The same problem exists in the sinuses, where infection settles permanently. When the ciliary propeller is a problem for the sperm, infertility is the result. In fact, when the lungs, sinuses, and sperm are all affected by an autosomal recessive gene mutation, a well-known syndrome (Kartagener) emerges, which has been known for over one hundred years. When cilia do not function in the lining of the brain, the cerebrospinal fluid may not circulate and expansion of the ventricles may occur, causing brain damage due to a condition called hydrocephalus.

Questions

- Why did Zoran have a hemorrhage into his spinal canal?

- Why was there no timely diagnosis and action to manage the disastrous complication?

- Why were the observations by the nurses effectively ignored?

Commentary

Hemorrhage into the spinal canal has the potential for devastating consequences by damaging the spinal cord. Realization that a bleed has occurred should automatically be managed with urgent surgical decompression of the spinal canal. Absent that intervention, there will almost invariably be permanent damage to the spinal cord, resulting in paraplegia often with lack of control of the bladder and, not infrequently, the bowel. Failure of the resident to pay attention to the opinion of the nurses regarding Zoran's diminished and eventually absent movement of his legs was a fundamental error. For an alert resident, aware of the long and difficult labor preceding the birth, Zoran's perilous entry into the world should have alerted him to the possibility that oxygen lack could have been at the root of possible complications. More specifically, a lack of oxygen during a long labor, or the final stage of labor, may be followed within forty-eight hours by a precipitous drop in the level of platelets in Zoran's circulation. The lower the platelet count, the more likely serious hemorrhage could eventuate (see chapter 2). Immediate attention to the nurse's report should have directly prompted imaging of Zoran's spine. This would have enabled early diagnosis of the hemorrhage and provided the opportunity to avert the subsequent catastrophe by timely surgical intervention.

Who knows whether inexperience, arrogance, hubris, ignorance, fatigue, or a mixture of these factors had a role in the faulty decision making by the resident. An unanswered question is why the nurses did not simply seek out the attending physician, especially if they felt confident in their observations. Nurses are the ones who care and stay with the patients, not the physicians. I have always looked to the nursing staff when I needed to know how the patient was doing. In relative time spent, the nurses are constants, while the residents are transients with reference to patient care. Ultimately, the hospital must educate and make it clear to the nursing staff that they too have responsibilities to break rank and reach more senior personnel. The primary fault was of course that of the resident physician and not the nurses. There are state-defined standards of supervision for physicians supervising nonphysician care providers. First, however, where was the attending pediatrician whose duty was to oversee the resident? Direct liability accrues to that doctor, just as vicarious liability attaches to oversight of nonphysician clinicians. A clear escalation of vicarious liability has occurred with physicians being held responsible for the errors of nurse practitioners, nurses, and genetic counselors.

The obvious difficulty small-statured Oona had in labor was pushing Zoran, with his big head, through her small pelvis. Large head size (macrocephaly) is not uncommon and is very often a dominantly inherited characteristic, transmitted usually from one parent. Familial isolated macrocephaly is not a birth defect and is not associated with any neurological consequences. There are, as an aside, multiple genetic syndromes in which macrocephaly may be a factor. Mothers with diabetes may deliver large babies who also may have macrocephaly, but then they often weigh nine or ten pounds at birth. When I saw Zoran, he had already had one episode of pneumonia but had otherwise been generally well except for his paraplegia. He required catheterization of his bladder multiple times per day when an indwelling catheter in his bladder was not in use.

Zoran, who has a permanent colostomy bag, will inevitably experience repeated urinary-tract infections from the lifelong need for catheterization. This will lead to chronic kidney infection and eventually failure and his death. He is unlikely to be considered for renal transplantation because of the bladder paralysis. Various pharmacological treatments will be tried and possibly surgical urinary diversion. Whichever management effort is tried, Zoran faces a lifetime of fecal and urinary incontinence—a sentence compounded by dual medical negligence.

The case was eventually settled.

TOO EARLY, TOO LATE

Irene was twenty years of age when, at full term, she delivered Julia without any problem. She had a previous pregnancy that ended with a miscarriage. Tests performed upon admission when she was in labor showed that she was not infected with the common β-streptococcal bacteria, but that she did have an elevated white-blood-cell count, with at least a proportion of cells that typically point to bacterial infection. Julia weighed almost six pounds at birth and was alert and vigorous. Four hours after birth, Julia was noted to be breathing rapidly (eighty-two/minute), her nostrils were flaring, and she was grunting with her increased respiratory rate. This was all resolved within two hours. The attending physician decided that Julia had "transient tachypnea (fast breathing) of the newborn" and that it would resolve spontaneously. Some feeding difficulty was noted, and her mother expressed concern that Julia seemed unable to properly latch on to her breast. Notwithstanding Irene's concern, Julia was discharged by the attending physician some thirty-four to thirty-five hours after birth. Instructions were provided to Irene to call if there was any concern and to return for a checkup when Julia was four days of age.

The very next day, Irene called the hospital to report that she felt that Irene had a fever. The advice she got was to remove the blankets and allow Julia to cool down. Her temperature did indeed recede. However, about thirty-two hours after her early discharge, Irene and her husband brought Julia back to the emergency department, concerned about her fever. They also noted, as did the emergency-department physician, that Julia's eyeballs were wobbling back and forth (nystagmus). Multiple residents, nurses, and attending physicians noted the nystagmus.

Because of a cough, an increased heart rate, and an increased respiratory rate, urine and blood samples were collected to detect any infection, and a chest x-ray was ordered. All test results were normal or negative, except the white-blood-cell count that was strikingly low at 1.9 (normal values 4.9–21.0). The low white-blood-cell count (which normally signals infection when it is elevated) was noted by three residents and reported to the attending physician. Her interpretation was that the low white-blood-cell count was probably a laboratory error. A repeat blood count was ordered, which yielded an even lower white-blood-cell count (1.0). However, the medical record also indicated that the residents who ordered the second blood count did not request that the test be expedited.

At this point, a temperature of 102.6°F was noted, and the decision was made to perform a lumbar puncture. Incredibly, there were three unsuccessful attempts to perform the lumbar puncture aimed at examining the cerebrospinal fluid for the presence of infection. The decision was then made simply to administer antibiotics. Even after the decision was made to administer antibiotics, it took an hour and a half for Julia to receive her first dose. The antibiotics were administered almost seven hours after Julia was admitted with the main concern of fever. Arrangements were then made to transfer Julia to a teaching hospital. Before transfer, a nursing note recorded that Julia was listless, pale, whimpering, and that she had a bulging fontanel (soft spot). At the tertiary-care hospital, the lumbar puncture was performed, and a diagnosis was positively made of meningitis. The blood culture obtained at the birth hospital yielded a positive result with bacteria found in the bloodstream.

At two weeks of life, brain imaging by both CT scans and MRI revealed enormous destruction of brain tissue from the meningitis. Julia's parents were advised of the grim long-term prognosis and the possibility that Julia would not survive.

Due to the remarkable care provided at the tertiary-care hospital, Julia did survive. However, the devastation to her brain resulted in profound global developmental delay, expanding ventricles (hydrocephalus) that required a permanent shunt to relieve the pressure on the brain, epilepsy, spastic quadriplegic cerebral palsy, and a breathing tube through her windpipe (because she needed a tracheostomy). She remained on a ventilator. In addition, feeding was done through a tube into her abdomen (G-tube). She was nonverbal, had hearing loss, and could not see. She eventually required a wheelchair.

Irene and her husband sued all of the physicians and the birth hospital for their failure to make a timely diagnosis and initiate appropriate treatment, which left Julia completely and totally disabled.

Pertinent Medical Facts

In chapter 16, I discussed the crucial importance of recognizing signs in the newborn that could herald infection. The reader is referred to the section under pertinent medical facts, wherein the critical need to administer antibiotics to the newborn is discussed, under the assumption, without proof, that an infection is ongoing until proved otherwise. Deviations from the expected standard of care in this case are different to those discussed in chapter 16.

Doctors caring for newborns are well schooled about the nonspecific signs of cryptic infection and are usually aware of the need to treat until there is proof that infection is not present. Infection in the newborn is a leading cause of death worldwide in children under five years of age. Even with proven infection and on treatment, death rates in Western countries can be as high as 30 percent.

Questions

- Why was Julia discharged early from hospital after birth?
- How was the diagnosis of meningitis missed?
- Why was treatment not initiated immediately upon admission, even without a definitive diagnosis of infection?

Commentary

Clearly defined policies at the birth hospital were available. Established procedures govern the early discharge of a newborn. To begin with, there is a requirement for there to be a request from the parent for early discharge. Not only was there no such documentation, but Julia's parents also clearly stated that

they did not request an early discharge, given that Julia was not feeding well. Failure to recognize the

importance of Irene's reporting that Julia seemed to have a fever was the next error. It was incumbent

upon the physician taking Irene's call to recommend she immediately return to the hospital with Julia.

The next grave error was perpetrated by the attending physician, who decided that the very low white-

blood-cell count was a laboratory error. As discussed elsewhere (see chapter 20), errors at the lab bench,

especially of such simple tests as a white-blood-cell count, are highly unlikely. Moreover, recognition of a

low white-blood-cell count in a newborn provides an important, albeit nonspecific, signal for the presence

of infection.

Again, in this sad case, the opportunity was lost to administer critical and effective treatment. The awful

realization is that some seven hours passed from the time Julia was admitted into the emergency

department to the time that she received antibiotics. The fact that three efforts failed to perform a lumbar

puncture for cerebral spinal fluid to obtain the diagnosis of meningitis again speaks to the incompetence

of the medical team. The failure to initiate timely therapy was compounded by the realization that Julia

had abnormal eye movements, cough, poor feeding, and a history of fever.

Evidence-based medical literature and guidelines from the American Academy for Pediatrics are

unequivocal about the standards of expected care in the face of suspicion of infection in a baby less than

twenty-eight days of age. The requirement is to immediately obtain the necessary blood and urine tests,

perform a lumbar puncture, obtain a chest x-ray, and immediately begin empirical treatment with

antibiotics. Presence or absence of fever is irrelevant in this age group.

Pediatricians are sued much less often than many other specialties. Malpractice claims against physicians

covered by a nationwide liability insurer between 1991 and 2005 included 40,916 doctors. Among them

were 1,630 pediatricians. The annual percentage of pediatricians facing negligence claims was reported to

be 3.1 percent compared to the 7.4 percent for other physicians.

***

In England, in a case that is unfortunately not a rare exception, a pediatrician was found guilty of manslaughter following a boy's death from septic shock. This youngster had Down syndrome and was given appropriate diagnostic tests that revealed serious bacterial infection, for which he was placed on antibiotic treatment. The physician, however, failed to notice the test results that pointed to kidney failure. Hours after the administration of antibiotics had started, the patient had a cardiac arrest. While efforts were being made to resuscitate him, the doctor in question instructed that resuscitation be stopped immediately, after mistaking this patient for another who had a "Do Not Resuscitate" notice in his record!

***

The residents in training were subject to simply awful guidance by a hopelessly inadequate attending pediatrician. Ignorance and incompetence in the care of a seriously ill patient is a recipe for disability and death. This pediatrician, who would receive no sanction, will not have to care for the profoundly disabled Julia.

This case was settled.

PLOTTING

Jose was the third child of his parents, Ilena and Jorge, who respectively worked as a pharmacist and as an engineer. Pregnancy had been uneventful, until the second trimester when a routine maternal-serum screen for chromosomal abnormalities revealed that Ilena had one in two hundred odds for having a child with Down syndrome. She was offered an amniocentesis for prenatal chromosome studies but declined because of the risk (less than 0.5 percent) of a procedure-related miscarriage. Detailed ultrasound analysis at fifteen weeks showed that fetal measurements, including his heart, head circumference, and abdominal circumference, were all normal. In particular, the ultrasound report indicated that the brain, cerebral ventricles, their internal vascular lining (choroid plexus), the posterior part of the brain, the midline, and the cerebellum, as well as all other features, were perfectly normal.

Pregnancy continued uneventfully, and a final ultrasound at just over thirty-seven weeks of gestation was again reported as normal, in particular with a head circumference in the twenty-fifth percentile for gestational age. Almost exactly on her expected delivery date at forty weeks, Jose's mother went into labor and was admitted to hospital. Labor was augmented with a uterine stimulus (Pitocin). During labor, she developed a fever, and Jose's heart rate sped up to two hundred beats per minute. Given a lack of progress, the decision was made to perform a Cesarean section. Jose weighed eight pounds four ounces at birth and needed a little mask and bag resuscitation but was quickly active, with a normal heart and respiratory rate. At birth, his head circumference was in the sixty-sixth percentile. Jose did well after birth but did have slight jaundice, treated with ultraviolet light. He was discharged from hospital on the fourth day of life.

At his first-month checkup, he was seen by a nurse practitioner and his doctor. His head circumference was measured by his doctor and found to be 41.9 cm (ninety-seventh percentile). The doctor's note indicated that Jose's parents expressed concern that he didn't seem to cry but did make sounds. Ilena was also concerned, because she thought Jose did not see her at a distance. Examination by the doctor revealed no abnormalities and certainly none about Jose's eyesight. The doctor's notes stated that Jose was a well baby with a head circumference greater than ninety-fifth percentile. At two months he exceeded the one-hundredth percentile, and over the next five months, Jose's head circumference skyrocketed to reach a level equivalent to 11.48 standard deviations above the mean (right off the chart), as shown in Figure 1. During that period, Jose was seen by four different board-certified physicians, including a pediatrician, ophthalmologist, and a neurologist. The primary-care doctor stated that he had benign familial macrocephaly (big head).

Despite Jose's mother's concern about the size of his head and his vision, she was reassured without any brain ultrasounds or MRIs being ordered. She was asked to return in two months with Jose.

Two months later, she switched her care of Jose to a board-certified pediatrician, to whom she again expressed the same concerns she had about his vision and his failure to roll over as expected for his age. At that visit, the pediatrician's staff documented that Jose's head circumference had reached the one-hundredth percentile, his height at the one-hundredth percentile, and his weight at the ninety-fifth percentile. Examination by that pediatrician concluded, in his notes, that Jose's vision and neuromuscular system were entirely normal. He did not document that Jose had macrocephaly. That pediatrician concluded that Jose was simply a large child in weight, length, and head size. He did not, however, look back to determine Jose's head circumference at birth, graph the head measurement, or note the trajectory of his head growth. At that point, Jose's head circumference was far above the one-hundredth percentile. His parents were asked to bring him back for his fourth-month checkup. No brain imaging by ultrasound or MRI was done.

At his fourth-month checkup, Jose's head circumference far exceeded the one-hundredth percentile, as did his weight, while his height was in the ninety-second percentile. Jose's parents again expressed their concern about his lagging development and his inability to track or fix with his eyes, as well as make eye contact. In particular, he seemed to have trouble holding his head steady or raising his body with his hands while prone. Nor was he rolling from his stomach to his back or following objects with his eyes. He was not smiling, cooing, laughing, or squealing.

The board-certified pediatrician wrote in his notes that Jose had limited tracking ability with his eyes, did respond to light, and had a large head. He made no note of Jose's large anterior fontanel (soft spot). Because of Jose's delayed milestones, he planned to refer him to a neurologist. Jose's parents had great difficulty obtaining an appointment and received little assistance from the pediatrician. Eventually, from the doctor who worked in the same clinic as she did, they obtained a referral to an ophthalmologist, who eventually saw Jose. He was then five months of age. The ophthalmologist reported that he had a vision problem and searching nystagmus (eyes moving back and forth constantly). Examination of the back of his eyes showed that his optic nerves were pale but normally developed. His large head was noted.

Jose's mother then called the pediatrician yet again to ask if he could order an MRI meanwhile while waiting for an appointment for a neurologist. He declined, stating that insurance would be unlikely to pay for an MRI before Jose was seen by a neurologist!

At five and a half months of age, Jose was found to have a developmental level equal to an infant of one to two months of age. At almost six months of age, he was eventually seen at a teaching hospital when his head circumference was 54.5 cm, 9.29 standard deviations above the mean. This teaching-hospital neurologist concluded, after a totally incompetent examination, that Jose, at five months, had macrocephaly, hypotonia (lack of tone), and developmental delay. Incredibly, he went on to state that Jose's head circumference was parallel to the growth curve (which he obviously never looked at or constructed) and that his neurological examination was normal! He did recommend that a brain MRI be done "in the next few months." Even though a routine MRI could only be arranged for six weeks later, this doctor failed to even order a brain ultrasound, which could have revealed the diagnosis. In fact, an urgently ordered MRI was possible immediately. Even when Jose's mother called to express her concern that his soft spot was bulging, she was unable to achieve an appointment for an urgent MRI. She was continuously shunted between the various physicians and the teaching hospital.

Eventually at seven months of age, an MRI was done. Imaging revealed severe enlargement of the ventricles (hydrocephalus) and thinning of the compressed cortex of the brain due to a blockage or narrowing in the canal connecting his lateral (frontal) ventricles (spaces) to his third ventricle (called aqueductal stenosis). In addition, the optic nerves were thin and displaced and the hydrocephalus so massive that there was very little white matter left in the cerebral cortex. Two days later, with his head circumference at 58.5 cm, equivalent to 11.48 standard deviations above the mean, Jose, with his very large ventricles and a remaining thin rim of cortex, had neurosurgery to place a ventriculo-peritoneal shunt to decompress the intracranial pressure.

The neurosurgeon insisted that a resident perform the surgery with him in attendance. Jose's parents were informed that this was a teaching hospital and that they had no choice. Their fears were realized the next day when it was determined that the shunt catheter placed by the resident had been malpositioned. This required Jose to undergo a second neurosurgical operation, at which time a new catheter was repositioned.

Extensive genetic testing, including a microarray to determine any microdeletion or microduplication in his genome (see chapter 38), as well as a thorough gene analysis called whole exome sequencing to seek out a gene with a mutation that could possibly explain the hydrocephalus, failed to identify a genetic cause. The putative cause was thought to possibly be a small hemorrhage or defect that obstructed the aqueduct. However, the possibility of X-linked aqueductal stenosis due to an undetected gene mutation could not be excluded. Jose has been left with profound neurodevelopmental defects and is legally blind.

Jose's parents sued all the physicians and hospital for not recognizing his hydrocephalus, not performing the urgently required brain imaging, and not providing timely brain-saving ventriculo-peritoneal shunting, which left him with profound disability and blindness.

Pertinent Medical Facts

Hydrocephalus is a disorder that results from progressive accumulation of excess cerebrospinal fluid within the ventricles of the brain, resulting in increased intracranial pressure on brain tissue, which can damage the brain and lead to coma and death if untreated. This is not a rare condition, occurring in approximately one in one thousand births. Any obstruction that interferes with the natural flow of cerebrospinal fluid through the ventricles of the brain and into the spinal canal has the potential to cause hydrocephalus. Hemorrhage into the ventricles (as commonly seen in premature infants) is one not-uncommon cause. In a recent study of 137 patients with hydrocephalus, the causes were hemorrhage into the ventricles (31.4 percent), spina bifida (25.5 percent), infection (11.7 percent), congenital (present at birth) (10.2 percent), a cyst in the posterior part of the brain (8.8 percent), narrowing in the canal between the lateral ventricles and the third ventricle (called aqueductal stenosis) (8.0 percent), and other miscellaneous causes such as a tumor (4.4 percent).

Undiagnosed hydrocephalus in the first few months of life conveys a high risk of developmental delay, resulting in lifelong intellectual disability, which can be severe, and possible blindness.

In another recent study of 236 children with hydrocephalus, 59 (25.0 percent) had aqueductal stenosis. Often, however, hydrocephalus may occur without any evident extrinsic cause. Aqueductal obstruction, leading to hydrocephalus of early onset, is known to be associated with the most severe developmental problems.

By far the most common cause of aqueductal stenosis is due to a mutation in a gene (*L1CAM*) located on one X chromosome. This gene is known to have a key role in influencing brain-cell migration during development. Transmission of this gene and its mutation is via X-linked inheritance. This means that a female (who is not affected) who has two X chromosomes and is a carrier will transmit one of her X chromosomes with this culprit gene to 50 percent of her boys (who will be affected) and 50 percent of her girls (who will be carriers but not affected). A family history of affected males on the mother's side provides an immediate clue to the cause of hydrocephalus. Absent any history, a brand-new mutation may have to be invoked, unless the mother harbors this mutation in some of her eggs (called germline mosaicism).

The treatment of hydrocephalus is surgical and is often very urgent with rising intracranial pressure. A tube is placed into the largest ventricles and threaded down into the abdomen so the cerebrospinal fluid can drain into the abdominal cavity (called a ventriculo-peritoneal shunt). This is a lifesaving and maintaining treatment, which unfortunately is not free of trouble. Shunt infection is not uncommon and may lead to meningitis and, even with treatment, may be fatal. Acute shunt dysfunction may occur from leaking or blockage of the tube or some other indiscernible problem, leading to a cessation of cerebrospinal-fluid flow. Such an event is an emergency and, if not promptly relieved, may cause death.

Questions

- How was it possible for multiple physicians, who all recognized his large head size, to fail to order brain imaging and make a diagnosis?

- What system of care and what kind of physicians allowed extremely worried parents to be ignored and messed around for seven months while their child's brain was destroyed?

- What was the relevance of Ilena's routine screen during her pregnancy that reported her odds of one in two hundred for having a child with Down syndrome.

Commentary

This case represents an abysmal breach of the standard of expected care. The physicians, including a board-certified pediatrician, a neurologist, and an ophthalmologist, all failed miserably, demonstrating a profound lack of knowledge and a carelessness that, in a better system, should have resulted in the loss of their medical licenses. The management provided for this family can only be regarded as a disgrace! This view extends to the care and management at the teaching hospital. Here was a child with an eminently treatable disorder, the timely treatment of which would have enabled normal intellectual development, rather than an outcome characterized by severe neurological damage and blindness.

The awful truth reflected by the careless, thoughtless, and callous treatment of this family was that all could have been avoided by simply plotting the head circumference systematically on a head- circumference graph clearly showing the rapid and dramatic escalation in the growth of Jose's head (see Figure 1). The simple failure to graph measurements of the head contributed to the root cause of the grievous harm visited on this innocent patient and family. A simple order for a brain ultrasound (an inexpensive, noninvasive test) would have immediately revealed the hydrocephalus. The fact that this case was settled for millions of dollars in mediation, without a trial, speaks volumes about the recognized incompetence of all of Jose's doctors. What a dreadful shame!

These physicians have apparently been reported to the state Board of Registration in Medicine. Don't expect any punitive action!

Today in all pregnancies, a routine blood test is offered to all mothers around eleven weeks of pregnancy as a noninvasive screen for at least three chromosomal abnormalities (Down syndrome, trisomy 18, and trisomy 13). While Down syndrome is well known, trisomies 13 and 18 are characterized by severe malformations and very unlikely survival through pregnancy or the first year of life. The use of the screening test is to determine pregnancies at risk if the fetus has these chromosomal abnormalities. Note that the test *does not detect about 50 percent of all chromosome abnormalities*. A positive result is followed by a *diagnostic* amniocentesis. A different screening test that Ilena had employs hormonal and protein biomarkers that can be offered in the first or second trimester of pregnancy with lower detection rates.

For that test, which Ilena had, results are expressed as likely odds for that pregnancy having an affected fetus. Laboratories have different cut-off action lines, some reporting that the results are abnormal if the odds are 1 in 270 or worse. Others may use 1 in 250 or 1 in 200 as odds that lead to a recommendation for precise prenatal diagnosis studies by chorionic villus sampling (in the first trimester) or amniocentesis (in the second trimester). This screening test is mostly not used now if insurance coverage is available for the noninvasive test.

Ilena, in this pregnancy under discussion, advised of the odds of Down syndrome, declined to have an amniocentesis.

Both we and others have published studies that showed when screening revealed increased odds for Down syndrome, and a subsequent amniocentesis result as actually normal, a significant risk of complications existed for that pregnancy. These risks included other fetal defects, premature delivery, fetal death, stillbirth, emergency Cesarean section, and newborn death. Increased odds, therefore, may simply flag a pregnancy that has increased risk and provides an early warning that requires attention in the care of the patient for the ensuing months of that pregnancy. This, of course, was ignored by those who undertook the care of the newly born Jose. They not only failed to look at the screening result but also had no idea of its implications.

A failure to graph serial measurements is not unique. In a different lawsuit in which I was involved, three physicians in a group practice all saw a child during his first four years of life. Measurements of his growth were systematically made at his "well child" visits, but his height was never graphed. Finally, the parents, and then one of those three physicians, noticed what appeared to be a buckling of his lower limbs. They suspected a diagnosis of rickets, which they then confirmed on an x-ray. Rickets is among the most frequent childhood diseases in third-world countries, where the usual cause is vitamin D deficiency or lack of adequate calcium in the diet. The disorder results in poor mineralization or calcification of a child's bones, resulting in fractures and deformity. However, this little boy lived in a prosperous state in the United States, and his rickets was not due to vitamin D deficiency.

An urgent series of tests initiated by a specialist revealed that this little boy had severe chronic kidney disease. His bone disease was the result of kidney failure, due to the condition called renal osteodystrophy. The failure to graph his failing growth, which for two years had fallen below the third percentile, resulted in then-untreatable kidney failure, which eventually ended with kidney transplantation.

In yet another case, repeated routine ultrasound studies in what was thought to be a normal pregnancy documented precise measurements of the fetal head circumference and the abdominal circumference. Progressively through the pregnancy, the abdominal circumference exceeded the head circumference, which is normally quite the opposite. The serial measurements were not plotted on the same graph. The progressive discrepancy was not recognized. Consequently, the child was born with microcephaly (a small head) and intellectual disability.

All measurements made in pregnancy and in children in particular should be graphed systematically. Failure to keep a graph of growth parameters up front in the medical chart invites serious, if not catastrophic, consequences.

Inexperienced physicians and those who do not care may fail to listen and pay attention to mothers who have had previous children. When these mothers, as in the case of Ilena, report observations they have made about their baby or child, close attention and sometimes immediate action by the physician are required. Ilena's very early complaints about Jose's vision and subsequent psychomotor delays were systematically ignored, even by a board-certified pediatrician. The doctors who failed Jose and his parents will not have to live through the pain and suffering this family must entail. It is bad enough they didn't know, they didn't know. What is so awful is that they didn't care either!

Birth to 36 months: Boys
Head circumference-for-age and
Weight-for-length percentiles

NAME ___

RECORD # _____

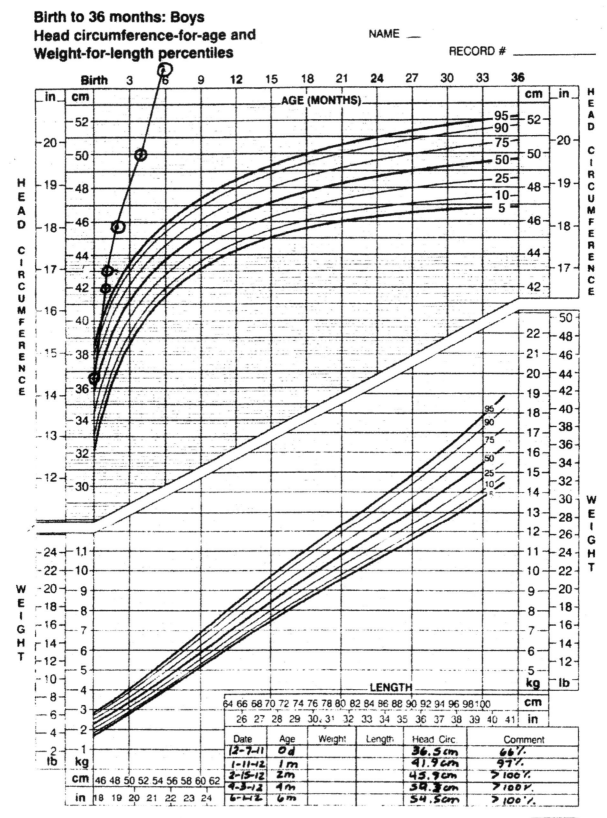

Date	Age	Weight	Length	Head Circ.	Comment
12-7-11	0 d			36.5 cm	66%
1-11-12	1 m			41.9 cm	97%
2-15-12	2 m			45.9 cm	>100%
4-3-12	4 m			59.3 cm	>100%
6-1-12	6 m			54.5 cm	>100%

http: www.cdc gov growthcharts

CDC

SAFER · HEALTHIER · PEOPLE

ARRESTED

Angela was born after an uneventful pregnancy when her mother was twenty-one years of age. Angela was alert and vigorous; weighed six pounds ten ounces; was nineteen inches in length; and had a normal head circumference. Hospital discharge was arranged some forty-eight hours after birth, with Angela feeding well and all usual routine screening tests yielding normal results. A required checkup two weeks later showed that she had gained weight and was doing well. The next few months were characterized by frequent colds and some wheezing. Developmental milestones were normal. She had continued to gain weight but had recurrent ear infections. At thirteen months, she had a five-day period of vomiting three times a day, being extremely fussy, and not sleeping. She continued to cry throughout the night and for almost twenty-four hours, after which twitching of her left leg and arm was noted. This observation led to her emergency-room visit, where she was found to be lethargic and floppy. Because of neurological signs and a likely seizure, a CT scan was ordered. The images obtained revealed low-density areas in the frontal portion of the brain, suggesting possible injury due to a lack of oxygen.

Angela was admitted to the hospital, at which time she had a fixed, glassy gaze; was making no sounds; was making no purposeful movements; and was unable to grasp any object in her left hand. A small 1 cm scar on her forehead was noted with some discoloration, raising the question of possible head trauma. This observation was coupled with the CT scan, which had shown possible brain injury due to a lack of oxygen.

As part of the routine evaluation, blood and urine samples were obtained and studied for a range of biochemical tests. The laboratory reported an elevated white-blood-cell count and a twice-repeated elevated level of ammonia in her bloodstream. The interpretation by the attending physicians was that these elevated levels of ammonia were due to hypoxic (lack of oxygen) injury also damaging the liver (the site for ammonia production). Review of the CT scan of her brain the following morning showed

swelling of her brain (cerebral edema), once again, "suspicious for non-accidental head trauma."

Another CT scan the next day showed diffuse brain damage and swelling, concluding that the findings

provided evidence of "significant destruction consistent with hypoxia." At that point, and under duress,

the father confessed to having placed a pillow over Angela's head to stop her ceaseless crying!

Angela's father was promptly arrested.

During the next four days in hospital, Angela began to do very much better than her CT scans would have

predicted. She was awake, responsive, and able to eat and swallow. However, she had no purposeful

movements, was not vocalizing, and did not fix on an object and follow with her eyes.

During that admission, Angela had another period in which she was agitated, crying inconsolably, became

lethargic and less responsive, and was unable to sit or feed. A feeding tube was placed to avoid her

aspirating fluid and food into her lungs. She remained in hospital for about a month, after which she was

discharged with the diagnosis of asphyxia secondary to suffocation.

At nineteen months of age, she was rushed to the hospital because of bleeding gums and drowsiness.

Biochemical tests suggested possible liver failure. Once again, she recovered, following specific

treatment with fresh-frozen plasma to control her unexplained bleeding. The consulting physicians

ordered urine samples for testing her amino acids because they had previously noted elevated levels of

ammonia in her blood. Specifically, they asked for analysis of orotic acid that had to be sent to a distant

laboratory. The urine sample obtained was considered inadequate for the required tests, and a new sample

was requested but never obtained.

A month later, she was readmitted to hospital, again with continued bleeding gums. Once again, fresh-

frozen plasma was administered, and the bleeding was controlled. This time, they noted that her ammonia levels were again increased, and samples were sent to a distant laboratory. The results of the analyses showed that Angela had a rare biochemical disorder called ornithine transcarbamylase (OTC) deficiency.

Angela's father was released by the police, and he and his wife sued Angela's physicians for failing to make a diagnosis of a disorder that was initially treatable and which left Angela with irreversible brain damage.

Pertinent Medical Facts

Ornithine transcarbamylase (OTC) deficiency is an X-linked disorder that manifests within two to three days after birth, usually with catastrophic consequences. I discussed the X-linked mode of inheritance elsewhere (chapters 7 and 13) and how females who are carriers of a gene mutation may also be variably symptomatic, presenting later in infancy, childhood, adolescence, or adulthood. In fact, some males, who, like females, may be partially deficient, may also present later in childhood or even in adulthood (see below). In the male presenting within a few days of birth, rapidly rising levels of ammonia are followed by drowsiness, then coma, and then often death if not diagnosed immediately. If the male survives, brain damage may have occurred, depending on how long the ammonia level was elevated. He may also have seizures. Very rapid diagnosis enables rescue, but by six months of age, liver transplantation is required.

Females who are effectively partially deficient frequently display symptoms when switched from breast milk to formula or whole milk. Quickly, episodes of vomiting, lethargy, irritability, and delay in attaining milestones are invariably seen. The incessant crying by Angela was eventually understood once the diagnosis was established. All of the symptoms are due to elevated levels of blood ammonia.

The amount of the *OTC* enzyme activity in the liver dictates the severity of symptoms in an affected female. The actual level of enzyme activity in liver cells depends in turn upon which of the two X chromosomes in a female is active. Located on the long arm of one of every female's X chromosome is a functional gene that inactivates (puts to sleep) gene functions on that chromosome. That inactivation is random and would therefore not be predictable, for example, for the function of the *OTC* enzyme in the liver. Angela's symptoms and signs were typical for an affected female carrier. These included the bleeding episodes, which resulted from diminished production of clotting factors manufactured by the liver and diminished during episodes of high ammonia levels. Angela's recurrent infections served as a stressor on liver functions, precipitating symptoms due to increasing levels of ammonia.

OTC deficiency is estimated to occur in about one in fourteen thousand live births in the United States. In other countries, estimates range from one in sixty-two thousand to one in seventy-seven thousand live births. Not unexpectedly, failure to include or ignore carrier females will obviously affect the estimates, let alone diagnostic accuracy.

Ammonia is toxic to the brain. The longer it is elevated, the worse the brain damage. The fastest method to decrease the ammonia level is dialysis. In addition, there is also a very specific intravenous infusion that requires management by a biochemical geneticist. In addition, protein intake is drastically cut, and calories are provided from sugar and fat. Protein restriction for life is necessary, but so is the use of an essential amino-acid mixture to ensure growth and development. Lifetime care with a biochemical geneticist and a nutritionist is vitally important. Unfortunately, at any age, high levels of ammonia may be precipitated by liver stressors, such as infections. Various drugs are also proscribed and include Valproate (which should not be used for seizure control) or steroids. Fasting and physical stress may precipitate a steep and sudden rise in ammonia levels, sparking a hyperammonemic crisis.

The diagnosis for Angela was made by the finding of the typical increased level of orotic acid. However, a precise diagnosis of *OTC* enzyme deficiency can be made by analysis of the specific gene (*OTC*). Just as for other X-linked disorders, family history of deaths among male newborns on the mother's side or females with symptoms as described above may be an important clue. Once diagnosis by molecular testing is made, future preimplantation genetic diagnosis or prenatal diagnosis becomes available for any subsequent pregnancy.

Questions

- How did the physicians caring for Angela miss the diagnosis of a biochemical disorder that was treatable?

- Why did Angela not manifest signs of this disorder before fourteen months of age?

Commentary

The common pathway to medical error and missed diagnosis was faithfully traveled once again. Ignoring the history, disregarding and misinterpreting the laboratory results, and drawing a conclusion to fit a preconceived diagnosis once again set the stage for error. One month prior to their rush to the emergency department, Angela's mother switched from breast milk to whole-milk bottle feeds. This switch prompted five days of vomiting at least three times per day. From that time, she continued to exhibit irritability, poor appetite, and respiratory infection. This was followed in the hours prior to coming to the emergency department by Angela sleeping all day. It was the twitching of her left eye and arm that precipitated the rush to the emergency department. There, they noted that she had been sleeping excessively for two days prior to admission and, upon examination, was drowsy and floppy. She responded only to painful stimuli.

Upon transfer to a tertiary-care hospital, she was noted to be irritable, to have an intermittent fixed glassy gaze, was not vocalizing, had no purposeful movements, and was unable to grasp objects in her left hand. One physician noted a 1 cm scar on her forehead with a fading bruise, and a CT scan showed changes that were consistent with injury due to a lack of oxygen. At the same time, blood samples had shown elevated levels of ammonia. They also ascribed her increased liver-enzyme levels and her elevated ammonia levels to the effects of hypoxia, despite a history of illness for four weeks prior to the emergency-department visit.

Their error was to ignore the chronic history, the accumulating acidity in her blood, the elevated ammonia levels (which they never sought to repeat again), and their failure to consider other explanations for the CT-scan findings.

The physicians' thought processes sought to couple the CT-scan findings suggesting a lack of oxygen to the brain with the small scar on Angela's forehead. Since she had an otherwise normally developing year, they concluded that child abuse was a possibility. Confronting the father and him confessing that he had used a pillow to quiet her crying, they concluded that this was a straightforward situation of abuse, and the father was arrested.

These physicians systematically ignored an initial blood sample at the community hospital that showed that her level of carbon dioxide was 16 (normal 22–35 mmol/L), long after any putative suffocation. They ignored her recent history of five days of vomiting and, of course, the two elevated levels of ammonia. Finally, they did not consider that the findings of the CT scan of her brain could be mimicked by a number of different biochemical genetic disorders.

It took twenty months and another hospital admission for a clinical geneticist to make the diagnosis of OTC. By then, Angela was permanently brain damaged due to a disorder that, if treated promptly, could have spared her from intellectual disability and becoming profoundly disabled. The CT scan of her brain at twenty months showed severe atrophy of her brain.

***

Women who are *OTC* gene carriers almost always develop an aversion for meat and often proteins. I recall the report of one patient who was taken to a steakhouse for her birthday. Against her better instincts, she had a steak for dinner and, upon emerging from the restaurant, became completely psychotic with increasingly bizarre behavior. Immediate admission to hospital led to quick recognition of her elevated ammonia levels. Once appropriate treatment was ongoing, a diagnosis of OTC was made within forty-eight hours. Her ammonia level returned to normal as did her behavior and mental state.

A rare clinical presentation was the basis of yet another lawsuit in which I was involved. Sam, then fifty years of age, developed a severe cough on top of his asthma and was diagnosed in the emergency department as having pneumonia. He was treated with antibiotics as well as cortisone for his associated asthma. He was seen the following day by his primary-care doctor who, after checking him thoroughly, had him continue his medication. That treatment continued for seven days, and Sam, the director of operations in a major retail chain, complained of being excessively tired. His wife noted that he became lethargic and seemed confused. When he began asking where his shoes were (which were on his feet), his wife promptly took him to the emergency department because of his disorientation and confusion.

Of interest in his past history was the curious diagnosis of attention deficit disorder, made at the age of forty-four! Many years before, the mild yellow appearance of his eyes (jaundice) led to the assumed diagnosis of Gilbert's syndrome (a benign disorder of the liver that interferes with the processing of pigments released following the breakup of red blood cells).

Upon entry to the emergency department, he was examined by a nurse practitioner, who reported his findings to the primary-care doctor by telephone. Given his confusional state, an MRI of his brain and a CT scan of his head were ordered immediately. By morning, and with a normal brain-imaging report, Sam had begun to have seizures. Attention turned to other possible causes of his mental confusion and seizures.

Laboratory results revealed a markedly elevated level of ammonia, implying severe decompensation of liver function. While the reason for his hyperammonemia was unclear, treatment was promptly initiated with the aim of reducing his ammonia level. During his stay in the community hospital, Sam was seen and examined by a nurse practitioner, his primary-care doctor, a neurologist, and a gastroenterologist. None came up with a diagnosis, and in the face of seizures not responding to treatment and a rapidly deteriorating level of consciousness, Sam was transferred to a major Boston teaching hospital. Despite additional treatment to lower his ammonia level, which was by then astronomically elevated, Sam continued to deteriorate, lapsed into coma, and was determined to be brain-dead. He had developed severe brain swelling (cerebral edema) due to the hyperammonemia, which proved only slowly responsive to treatment. His family requested withdrawal of further treatment.

Subsequent postmortem DNA studies established the diagnosis of OTC, which had been present since birth and, incredibly, never diagnosed.

Sam's wife sued the doctors in the emergency department and the community hospital for failing to make a diagnosis and institute lifesaving treatment.

Sam's presentation at fifty years of age with OTC was extremely rare. One important clinical clue was his jaundice. That, however, was explained away by the assumed diagnosis made years before of his benign Gilbert's syndrome. His doctors, including the neurologist, quickly focused on the potential cause of his mental confusion by imaging his brain. Only after no pathology was found did they turn attention to metabolic or biochemical reasons for his mental state. Sam's sad case illustrated once again the danger of preconceived diagnostic thinking without covering a wider field of disorders that may interfere with brain function. However, late-onset OTC is well known to have a very high mortality rate despite appropriate treatment.

Faulty reasoning in Angela's profoundly sad case was the root cause of the subsequent tragedy. The common precursors of clinical error that include inattention, distraction, preoccupation, memory lapse, fatigue, and stress were not operative factors. Rather, the physicians concluded that the symptoms and signs were consistent with their preconceived diagnosis (confirmation bias), especially because they had suffocation in mind (availability bias). Moreover, by ignoring the acidosis in the community hospital (occurring so long *after* the *suffocation*), they failed to adjust their initial putative diagnosis (anchoring bias).

These various biases, so well known in cognitive psychology, together with failure to synthesize the clinical data and consider a differential diagnosis, proved disastrous for Angela. Psychologists point to the need for physicians to be aware of their thinking process and of these biases (situational awareness) to avoid flaws in their diagnostic reasoning.

Published studies showed that cognitive errors are due to failures to synthesize information (50 percent), to verify data (33 percent), or to accurately collect data (14 percent). A lack of knowledge accounted for only 3 percent. Swiss authors have emphasized that errors in how doctors think (or don't) are involved in 75 percent of cases.

Professor James Reason of Manchester University in England, and an authority on the psychology of human error, pointed out that accidents in hazardous technologies were due to human error in over 90 percent of cases. Over two decades ago, he too stressed that accidents (errors) were the product of multiple factors: "personal, task related, situational and organizational."

Understanding the pathogenesis of errors provides vital opportunities to anticipate, avoid, and prevent mistakes. Sadly, the chances were lost for both Angela and Sam.

Sam's case was settled. While Angela's case also reached settlement, her father and mother were left to cope with their daughter's irreversible, irremediable brain damage and his painful memory of being in prison.

PICKLED

Ellen and Bill were the first college graduates in each of their families. They were both Native Americans and met one summer working on an Indian reservation. They had much in common and soon married, with Ellen giving birth to her first child at the age of twenty-one. Except for a minor vaginal bleed around eight weeks, pregnancy progressed normally until around thirty weeks, when she suddenly experienced the contractions of early labor. An immediate admission to hospital and application of a fetal electronic monitor showed a nonreassuring fetal-heart tracing plus an increased heart rate. An ultrasound showed that the placenta was small (less than tenth percentile). The decision was quickly made for an emergency Cesarean section.

Their son, Marty, born prematurely, weighed only 860 grams (1.89 lbs) and had a normal length and head circumference for gestational age. He was surprisingly vigorous despite his size. He soon, however, developed respiratory distress, was resuscitated, and was connected to a ventilator. Later he had episodes of a dramatically slowing heart rate. Over the ensuing few weeks, Marty developed the expected jaundice so frequently seen in premature infants (see chapter 30). Other than receiving ultraviolet-light exposure, no further treatment for his jaundice was required. However, because a heart murmur had been detected, an echocardiogram was done, which showed a few tiny holes between the left and right ventricles of his heart (ventricular septal defect), each measuring only 1 mm–2 mm in size. The neonatologist felt that these lesions would close spontaneously. There was some concern about his low blood pressure, but this was not unexpected in a tiny, premature infant. This was readily managed.

At birth, Marty was noted to have unusual-looking genitals, which included the exit from his penis to be located way down the underside of the shaft (called hypospadias), close to his scrotum, which had a bifid appearance. His testes were still located in his groins and had not yet migrated into his scrotum. Given his limited oral intake, he had been continued on intravenous fluids. Because of his low blood pressure and anemia, secondary to his prematurity and repeated blood sampling, he also received a transfusion of packed red blood cells. Typical of severe prematurity, he also had brief periods of not breathing (apnea of prematurity). His penis was small. Hormonal and genetic studies during that admission revealed no abnormality. Given his limited oral intake, he had been continued on intravenous fluids. The chromosomal microarray that was done revealed that Marty, like all of us, had twenty-three matching pairs of chromosomes, one contributed from each parent. There were no tiny bits missing or duplicated (microdeletions or microduplications) (see chapter 38). The report did show that there were chromosome pairs with identical blocks of genes even though they were derived from each parent (technically called runs of homozygosity).

At five weeks of age, Marty had continued to receive intravenous fluids. The neonatologist noted that his electrolyte values showed an unexpectedly low potassium and chloride level. He therefore ordered a change in the formulation of Marty's intravenous fluids, requesting that the intravenous bags be made up precisely with specified amounts of sodium chloride, potassium chloride, and calcium gluconate.

Within twenty-four hours of receiving the new intravenous fluid formula, compounded by the hospital pharmacy, Marty began to have severe respiratory problems. At almost six weeks of age, his caregivers noted that not only was he having difficulty breathing but also that his anterior and posterior fontanels (soft spots) had begun to bulge, signaling massive brain swelling. They quickly discovered that the blood levels of his various electrolytes had skyrocketed, with his sodium level at an astronomical 204 mmol/L (normal range 139–146 mmol/L) and a chloride level of 155 (normal 98–107 mmol/L). It didn't take long to discover that the intravenous fluids that had been prepared by the pharmacy were improperly formulated, resulting in the extreme levels of sodium and chloride (salt) that was inadvertently administered to Marty intravenously.

Previous to this dreadful incident, Marty had been gaining weight, breathing room air, and was stable. After this incident, he relapsed to require intubation and conventional ventilation. Soon thereafter, he began twitching and having seizures. A brain-ultrasound examination revealed no hemorrhage or stroke.

Marty quickly deteriorated, lapsed into coma, and his family gathered for Last Rights. These were administered, and the parents requested cessation of further care. Marty was allowed to die peacefully. The autopsy showed the tiny holes between the ventricles of his heart and one found between his atria, all being insignificant. Examination of his brain revealed extensive swelling. His brain had effectively been pickled.

The parents sued the medical center and the associated health-care system for their negligence, which resulted in the death of their son.

Pertinent Medical Facts

Markedly premature infants face an uphill struggle. Marty was not only seriously premature but also small for his gestational age, suggesting intrauterine growth restriction. Even today, a significant proportion die in the first three months of life, while close to 50 percent are left with widely varying degrees of disability, including intellectual disability, epilepsy, vision problems, and stunted growth—all of these despite often remarkable and outstanding neonatal care.

Intravenous administration of a high sodium and chloride mixture is highly likely to be fatal. Despite urgent efforts to ameliorate the salt load, the overwhelming brain swelling indicated that the die was cast.

The genital abnormalities that Marty had were of unclear origin. Given that hormone and genetic studies were unrevealing, a final diagnosis was not made. However, the runs of homozygosity noted on the chromosomal microarray results raised the possibility that Marty inherited a single mutated gene in one of the paired blocks of genes contributed by each parent and transmitted to him as an autosomal recessive disorder. This remains speculative. His parents may well have been unwittingly related. However, his minor genital anomalies had nothing to do with his iatrogenic death.

The congenital cardiac abnormalities noted were tiny and not uncommon in extremely premature infants. These lesions would almost certainly have closed spontaneously and did not contribute to Marty's death.

The American Association of Hospital Pharmacists has published extensive guidelines on intravenous infusions, which you will see in chapter 41.

Question

- What protocol was in place in the pharmacy to ensure that the order for precise compounding of a solution for infusion was correctly prepared and with appropriate oversight?

Commentary

The pharmacy personnel who compounded the infusion that had been required to elevate Marty's low levels of potassium and chloride used a concentration of sodium chloride over twenty times the required level. The pharmacy admitted that its employees fell below the applicable standard of expected care in compounding, preparing, and dispensing the ordered infusion, and further, that the infusion administered to Marty was the cause of his death.

Experts testified that Marty would have been expected to be discharged from the hospital within three weeks of his last treatment. They opined that he would have had an otherwise normal life expectancy, since he did not have life-threatening or life-shortening disorders. Moreover, autopsy revealed no brain abnormality and therefore no evidence that he would have had neurodevelopmental delay.

Incidents of damage or injury caused by medical care are termed "iatrogenic events." Newborns, especially those born prematurely, are especially vulnerable given the complex care necessary. Infections due to indwelling intravenous catheters, tenfold drug-dosing errors, and intravenous fluid dose and rate errors and unplanned disconnection (extubation) from a ventilator occupy the top of the list of iatrogenic events.

The family distress, the future suffering of the patient, the inevitable financial burden, and the medicolegal consequences are self-evident. The pity is that the vast majority of these errors are preventable by systematic, disciplined care by both physicians and nurses, proper training, and required incident reporting.

Failure of oversight of the pharmacy technician compounding the intravenous solution represents the sad and tragic error that caused Marty's death.

The case was settled.

NOT SWEET

Shakela had reached the bottom of her personal pit. She was depressed and homeless, and her husband was in jail. She suffered from asthma, hypertension, and weighed 286 pounds. The last straw was when she discovered her unplanned pregnancy and that she was carrying twins, having already had five pregnancies and four births. Because of multiple previous Cesarean sections, this latest pregnancy was also scheduled for a surgical delivery at thirty-eight weeks. The day before surgery, her blood sugar (glucose) was noted to be elevated, consistent with the fact that she had developed gestational diabetes.

Both babies were vigorous at birth; Baby A delivered first with a weight of five pounds ten ounces, and Baby B, named Ashton, weighed five pounds eleven ounces. Both had normal measurements for their lengths and head circumferences. They were first fed about three and a half hours after birth, and the records indicated that their next feed was seven and a half hours later. Initial blood-glucose levels from both were within the normal range but were not tested again for the next twenty hours. It was then that Ashton was noted to have become hypothermic and "was twitching." A blood-glucose-level test strip was used and revealed a startlingly low concentration, subsequently confirmed by a blood sample, from which a result was provided with an incredulous zero glucose concentration!

The physician was notified, and he gave a telephone order for additional formula after each breast feed and to check the blood glucose before each of the next three feeds. About thirty minutes later, a glucose level was 19 mmol/L and three hours later was the same. Only at that point, the doctor ordered intravenous sugar water (at a concentration of dextrose 5 percent), which took more than another ninety minutes to begin.

Meanwhile, Ashton's heart rate had reached 180 beats per minute, and she began having jerky movements of her head, leg, and toes. Once again, the nurses reported a second episode of seizure-like activity, and fifteen minutes later her blood-sugar level was 19 mmol/L. This time, the doctor ordered an immediate direct intravenous administration of 10 percent dextrose water (equal to one teaspoon). Then, with a blood-sugar level of only 23 mmol/L did the doctor order a continuous intravenous infusion of 10 percent dextrose water. Ten minutes later, a change to dextrose 12.5 percent followed, as well as the administration of the hormone glucagon in a desperate effort to raise her blood-glucose concentration. Ashton's blood sugar rose very slowly to thirty-five, while she still had additional episodes of seizures. An hour later, the doctor ordered that Ashton be transferred to the university hospital. At the time Ashton was transferred, her blood-glucose level had reached fifty.

On admission to the university hospital, imaging by MRI showed changes that were similar to brain injuries seen following severe hypoglycemia. A subsequent MRI of her brain revealed diffuse brain injury with loss of brain substance mimicking the findings usually seen following asphyxia.

During the next four days in the university hospital, Ashton underwent extensive genetic and metabolic tests, all of which yielded normal results. Her hypoglycemia completely resolved and was no longer a problem.

At three years of age, Ashton was microcephalic with a head circumference in the second percentile. She could not walk, had no speech, was visually impaired, and continued to have seizures. An MRI at that time revealed layers of dead brain cells (laminar necrosis), brain atrophy, and scarring of her posterior brain (occipital lobes) as well as layers of her cortex, all typical findings seen as a consequence of severe hypoglycemia.

Ashton's mother sued the physician and the birth hospital for their negligence and failure to properly treat Ashton, resulting in permanent and irreversible brain damage.

Pertinent Medical Facts

The brain depends upon an adequate supply of glucose, which provides more than 90 percent of the energy used by brain cells. A blood-glucose level of less than forty-five defines "hypoglycemia." Severe hypoglycemia occurs with levels of blood glucose less than or equal to fifteen. There is, however, no universal exact level to which severity can be pinned. A range of factors has a potential impact on the consequences of low blood-glucose levels. These factors include individual susceptibility, the cause(s) of the hypoglycemia, the gestational weight and age of the baby, duration and severity of the hypoglycemia, presence of other issues (such as a lack of oxygen), the time the initial feed was provided, and the type of feed and volume given. It is clear, however, and universally accepted that prolonged and severe hypoglycemia, rather than transient hypoglycemia, can have serious to devastating consequences to the baby's brain.

Every doctor caring for tiny babies is aware of the often-nonspecific signs that suggest the possibility of hypoglycemia. These include poor feeding, a drop in body temperature, jitteriness, irritability, drowsiness, floppiness, respiratory problems, and seizures.

As every diabetic knows, insulin drives down the level of blood glucose. In the newly born, a mother with diabetes or gestational diabetes with associated elevated levels of blood glucose will stimulate the baby's pancreas to produce a significant and unnecessary amount of insulin that can dramatically lower the blood-glucose level, causing potentially disastrous effects. This continuing secretion of insulin may last for days on end; hence, the importance of anticipation and the recognized urgency to diagnose and treat hypoglycemia immediately upon diagnosis. Babies who have not gained sufficient weight during pregnancy (called intrauterine growth restriction) may already have an inadequate store of glucose and be even more susceptible to secreted insulin. Rarely there is a diagnosis of the disorder called congenital hyperinsulinism, which is an autosomal recessive disorder, in which both parents carry a mutation in a gene they share.

Imaging of a baby's brain by six weeks of age following serious hypoglycemia will usually reveal a pattern of brain damage appreciably different, but equally devastating, to the effect of oxygen lack (hypoxia). Neurodevelopmental defects are well-known consequences of significant hypoglycemia in premature and newly born infants. In time, cognitive problems and even seizures are likely and even include the clinical appearance of cerebral palsy.

Questions

- Why did this hospital appoint a physician to care for premature infants who lacked the basic necessary knowledge of how to treat newborns with hypoglycemia?

- Why did the nurses not break ranks and report this overt malpractice to the head of nursing on duty?

Commentary

The care provided for Ashton by her doctor was simply dreadful. Given that Ashton's mother was a gestational diabetic, he was on notice but clearly oblivious to the real possibility of hypoglycemia in Ashton. Even though Ashton was asymptomatic initially, anticipatory caution should have led to checking her blood glucose after feeding. The real catastrophe, however, was even after a zero level of glucose was determined, the physician prescribed feeding and checking blood glucose after three feeds. This, however, was a medical emergency, not recognized by this doctor. The absolute requirement was to immediately and directly administer intravenous dextrose. This was an emergency equal to asphyxia! Notwithstanding this crisis, at least one and a half hours more elapsed before intravenous dextrose was administered. Incredibly, only 5 percent dextrose water was used rather than the required 10 percent or 12.5 percent for that infusion. To all intents and purposes, this effectively meant that Ashton was suffering the equivalent of asphyxiation, during which her brain was being destroyed. It took even more time and the appearance of more seizures for this physician to order direct intravenous administration of 10 percent dextrose solution.

The series of failures in the diagnosis and treatment of Ashton were profoundly distressing. Failure to recognize that Shakela's gestational diabetes represented a risk of hypoglycemia for her newborn was the first departure from the expected standard of care. Not testing Ashton's blood-sugar level after her second feed was next. Then at about thirty-one hours of life, discovery of a zero blood-sugar level should have led to a direct intravenous push of at least 10 percent dextrose and initiation of continuous intravenous 10 percent or 12.5 percent dextrose infusion. Use of a 5 percent dextrose infusion was totally inadequate.

The American Academy of Pediatrics (AAP) and the Pediatric Endocrine Society (PES) have similar but not identical guidelines for the diagnosis and treatment of hypoglycemia. The differences are not unlike splitting hairs. The AAP guidelines require blood glucose to be maintained at forty for the first four to twenty-four hours. The PES recommends a level of at least fifty for the first forty-eight hours of life. Regardless, Ashton's levels were desperately far from what was required, resulting in lifelong profound handicap, and for a mother whose misfortune saw no end.

A further disturbing aspect was the failure of nurses to recognize a clinical emergency and to call the head of nursing for immediate intervention. Medical residents, trainees, or nurses are guided by principles of ethics and professionalism, captured at least for doctors in the Physician Charter on Medical Professionalism. Three of the fundamental principles focus on the primacy of patients' welfare, their autonomy, and social justice. As pointedly emphasized by a Mayo Clinic report, nurses may fear retaliation, verbal abuse, threats, confrontation, pressure from supervisors, and of being ostracized or simply lack confidence.

All institutions should endeavor to develop and maintain a culture conducive to speaking up and moreover to provide instruction about how to fulfill this important duty, so desperately absent in the sadness described in chapter 17.

The case was settled without a trial, leaving this homeless mother with an even deeper personal pit.

CAUSE AND CONSEQUENCE

Arthur was the second child of Victoria, a university professor. At thirty-nine years of age, she had one previous child, born prematurely, and except for attention deficit hyperactivity disorder (ADHD), was apparently doing well. Arthur, however, was extremely premature, having been born at about twenty-six weeks of pregnancy, weighing less than two pounds at birth. When Victoria suddenly developed uterine contractions and rushed to the emergency department in a nearby hospital, her contractions decreased in their intensity and frequency, and she was allowed to go home. No medication was provided to stop the contractions. Within twelve hours, she was back in the hospital, where, yet again, no effort was made to still the contractions. The electronic fetal monitor showed a fetal-heart tracing that was unremarkable initially but within hours recorded a marked decrease in the heart rate with prolonged periods of heart-rate decelerations, dropping from 130 beats per minute into the 60s. Earlier in the pregnancy, Victoria had reported some vaginal bleeding.

Arthur was delivered vaginally without difficulty but quickly developed respiratory distress, not unexpected for such a tiny baby. He was placed on a ventilator, on which he remained for some three months, during which time he had multiple episodes when his heart slowed dramatically and he appeared blue. An effort was made to discontinue the ventilator, but it became clear immediately that even after three months, he could not maintain a normal respiratory rate, and he was placed back on the ventilator in the pediatric intensive-care unit, connected via his required tracheostomy.

During this period, a host of complications typical for such tiny infants occurred in waves. First, because of concerns for his future cognitive status, an ultrasound of his brain was done that revealed a small hemorrhage within his ventricles. This was followed by a fearsome, bloody diarrhea (called necrotizing enterocolitis). Shortly after, an ophthalmologist diagnosed that he had the severe retinopathy of prematurity (a vascular abnormality at the back of the eyes eventually remedied by laser therapy). His neurological status raised concern because of his tendency to arch his body. By eight months of age, his bones were thin and poorly mineralized, their low density and strength leading to a rib fracture. Meanwhile, the cardiologist had reported a marked narrowing of his pulmonary artery where it exits the heart (pulmonic stenosis). The neonatologist recorded some unusual facial features that included wide-set eyes, low-set ears, a broad nasal bridge, down-slanting palpebral fissures, and a small head.

At four months of age, he still had pulmonary stenosis, and brain imaging raised the question of possible damage to his basal ganglia. The long period on the ventilator caused severe lung damage (bronchopulmonary dysplasia) and was associated with growth failure, compounded by an episode of pneumonia. Because he had been unable to feed, his calories were provided by a tube from his nose into his stomach initially but then replaced by a tube directly into his stomach through his abdomen (G-tube).

At about one year of age, Arthur was noted to have low levels of immunoglobulins, indicating that his immune system was not functioning well. He was treated with intravenous immunoglobulins. Developmental delay was already obvious, some four months after coming off the ventilator. For the next few years, he had difficulty chewing, was mostly nonverbal, and remained tiny with a low weight and small head circumference. He walked eventually at four years of age.

Notwithstanding the rough start to his life, he did make some progress despite additional challenges. He required eye surgery for cross-eyes (strabismus) and a bilateral groin-hernia repair. He also needed medication for an underacting thyroid (hypothyroidism) and spectacles for marked astigmatism. He continued to receive monthly intravenous immunoglobulins, which appeared to stave off infections. Unexpectedly, he manifested unexplained precocious puberty. Developmental delay resulted in the need for special-education classes when he was ten years of age.

At the age of ten, Arthur was noted to have white lesions on his scrotum and the following year had puffy skin to his scrotum that leaked lymphatic fluid. His physicians concluded that he had been born with abnormally developed lymphatic ducts that drained his groin and genitals. In addition to his short stature, he had hunched shoulders (kyphosis) and marked incurving of his lower back (lumbar lordosis).

Remarkably, when Arthur was seventeen years of age, Victoria sued the obstetrician who delivered Arthur and the neonatologists who cared for him in the early months of his life, for not preventing his early delivery, not recognizing fetal distress, and failing to prevent hypoxia (oxygen lack) during the critical early months of his life that resulted in brain damage.

Pertinent Medical Facts

Birth at twenty-six weeks is fraught with life-threatening complications and a mortality rate of 30–50 percent. The long list of potentially lifelong complications commonly includes intellectual disability, seizures, blindness, deafness, speech and language delays, stunted growth, cataracts, susceptibility to infections, severe jaundice, bone fractures, and on and on. The risk of cerebral palsy increases the more premature the baby. That risk approximates 1 percent at thirty-four weeks of gestational age at birth to 20 percent at or earlier than twenty-six weeks.

The use of medications such as Terbutaline to stop premature contractions is usually advised. Precisely why it was not used in this pregnancy remains uncertain. Care in the neonatal intensive-care unit and the subsequent pediatric intensive-care unit did not appear to fall below the standard of expected care. The perilous state Arthur was in, not unexpectedly, was punctuated by episodes of diminished oxygen saturation (due to apneic episodes when he would stop breathing) and a slow heart rate. Arthur's survival was a compliment to the neonatal staff.

Because of Arthur's dysmorphic facial features, a chromosome study was ordered that yielded a normal result. His doctor also considered whether he had a particular syndrome in which there was a tiny deletion in chromosome 22. This test also proved negative.

Questions

- Did the care rendered by Arthur's obstetrician and neonatologists meet the expected standard of care?

- Did any lack of care lead to Arthur's subsequent delayed development and other permanent deficits?

Commentary

Arthur came into the world as an extremely premature infant, weighing only 850 grams (1 pound 14 ounces) and facing daunting morbidity and mortality rates. While the prematurity rate approximates 9.5 percent (2014 data), the likelihood of death at this weight and gestational age ranges between 30 and 50 percent. As noted above, Arthur suffered many of the well-known complications of severe prematurity. The claim that he suffered a lack of oxygen causing brain damage was supported by the fact that he had a small intraventricular hemorrhage in the brain and that a CT scan subsequently showed an area deep in his brain (basal ganglia) that raised the question of hypoxia-induced brain damage.

Developmental delay and intellectual disability are common sequelae of severe prematurity, but then again, hypoxia could produce a similar outcome.

Expert obstetricians on both sides of this case argued strenuously about the electronic fetal monitor tracings and their potential significance with reference to fetal distress. There was also argument about the use of Terbutaline aimed at stopping Victoria's preterm labor. The American College of Obstetricians and Gynecologists discourages the use of Terbutaline specifically for the prevention of preterm labor. Some obstetricians will use the Tocolytic (anticontraction medication) for a period of up to forty-eight hours to prevent preterm labor. Significant maternal side effects include a drop in blood pressure, fast heart rate, anxiety, tremors, headaches, fluid in the lungs (pulmonary edema), and even death. The Food and Drug Administration required that a boxed warning be placed on the drug's label because of these side effects. The fetus, subject to the maternal Terbutaline, may develop a fast heart rate and may have very low blood-sugar levels at birth.

Because Arthur was born with a few unusual facial features, I was asked to review the case, obviously to determine if there was a genetic basis that could explain Arthur's problems.

Arthur was clearly dysmorphic. In particular, he had wide-spaced eyes, low-set ears, a broad nasal bridge, and down-slanting palpebral fissures. Subsequently, it became clear that he had a heart defect (pulmonary valve stenosis as well as narrowing of some of the branches of the pulmonary arteries). It also soon became evident that he had very short stature, developmental delay, and in particular, expressive and receptive language deficiency. He was also noted to develop cross-eyes (strabismus). Around eleven years of age, the medical records reflected the observation that he had tiny, white lesions on his scrotum. At fourteen years of age, his scrotum was apparently swollen and leaking lymphatic fluid, with the physicians concluding that he had a congenital abnormality of his lymphatic ducts in his groin and genitals.

This entire clinical presentation immediately brought to mind (with the wisdom of hindsight) that a likely diagnosis was Noonan syndrome. Literally all of the features just mentioned above are seen in this condition that occurs in about one in one thousand to one in twenty-five hundred people. Somewhere between 30 and 75 percent of cases arise from transmission from one affected parent. The rest are brand-new (de novo) mutations that occur in one of at least eleven different genes that cause this autosomal dominant disorder. This means that an affected individual has a 50 percent risk of transmitting this disorder to each of his or her offspring. There are a number of other features of this condition, but suffice it to say that over time it was clinically obvious that Arthur had Noonan syndrome.

I requested that a blood sample be obtained for analysis of the eleven Noonan syndrome genes at our nonprofit Center for Human Genetics in Cambridge, Massachusetts. We duly performed the sequencing of these genes and found that indeed Arthur has a mutation in the *PTPN11* gene, which occurs in about 50 percent of those with Noonan syndrome.

As is so often the case, multiple factors required consideration in determining whether any culpability existed in the management of Arthur's birth and neonatal care. Extreme prematurity has a high rate of disability (in survivors!), and mild hemorrhage in the brain is extremely common in the severely premature infant, even in the absence of any known hypoxia.

This case highlights the surprisingly common compounding of causal factors. These included obstetrical-management issues, use of Terbutaline, prematurity, neonatal-care problems, and a definitive genetic disorder. Fetuses with genetic disorders have a greater frequency of being born prematurely and even at normal gestational age may be more susceptible to the stresses of labor and delivery. Routine consideration should always be given to the possibility of a genetic basis for an unexpected adverse outcome to pregnancy. Plaintiff attorneys, in particular, should pause and consider genetic causation, even when they think they have a straightforward case of negligence that led to hypoxic brain damage. I have heard them echo, "I didn't know, I didn't know."

DELETED

Tanya was born amid a huge crisis. Pregnancy was near term and her mother, who had sought prenatal care late in pregnancy, had developed preeclamptic toxemia with hypertension and had suddenly become extremely ill and anemic and had begun bleeding through her bowel as well as vomiting blood. Liver enzymes had begun to leak out of her liver cells, and her kidneys began to fail. Her lungs became congested from accumulated fluid, and there was a distinct possibility that she would die before delivering Tanya. An urgent Cesarean section at thirty-five weeks of pregnancy concluded with the birth of Tanya and her twin. Other than prematurity, her nonidentical twin did well.

Tanya, however, was noted to have an umbilical cord with two instead of three blood vessels. She weighed twenty-three hundred grams (in the fiftieth percentile for gestational age) and was otherwise vigorous, not requiring resuscitation. However, alerted by the findings in the umbilical cord, a search for any birth defect was initiated. A diagnosis of a congenital heart defect was suspected and soon confirmed in the neonatal intensive-care unit, to which she was admitted. She was found to have a complete atrioventricular defect (a complete communication between both ventricles and both atria) at the *center* of the heart, as well as abnormalities of her aorta, which had a severe constriction (called coarctation). At surgery, the constriction was cut out, and the two ends of the aorta were rejoined (called end-to-end anastomosis). Limited heart repair was also accomplished. A perilous four weeks ensued, during which she slowly recovered and was discharged with continuing treatment.

Unfortunately, within a few days, she was back in hospital, having breathing difficulty, vomiting, and still being fed by a nasogastric tube. She was again discharged a few days later but was back again to replace her nasogastric tube as well as to determine why she was still having respiratory distress and a rapid heart rate. Diagnosis of a viral infection was made, and home care continued. Some three weeks later, at the age of two months, she had marked reflux and constant gagging. At two and a half months, she was again seen in the emergency room at the teaching hospital, for vomiting, choking, gagging, and with a low-grade fever. The emergency-medicine physician decided that she had a viral infection, given that her twin was also coughing and vomiting, and sent her home without a specific medication. Four hours later, Tanya's mother called the emergency 911 number because she was clearly not doing well and had become pale, and her lips appeared blue. While she was on the phone, Tanya ceased breathing. Her mother began CPR and continued until the emergency crew arrived to take over. However, back at the teaching-hospital emergency department, although they had reestablished her heart function, imaging of her brain as well as the electrical recording (electroencephalogram) indicated brain death from lack of oxygen. Autopsy confirmed the viral-infection diagnosis and the severe brain damage from lack of oxygen.

In an effort to find the cause of Tanya's heart defects, a chromosomal microarray was done to determine if Tanya had any structural abnormalities in her chromosomes. The results showed she had a tiny sliver sliced out of the long arm of chromosome 10 (called a microdeletion) that involved the absence of ten different genes, which included one that related to cardiac structure. It was also clear that Tanya, in addition to her heart abnormalities, would also have had serious intellectual disability should she have survived.

Tanya's mother sued the hospital and the emergency medicine doctor because of the alleged failure to admit Tanya to hospital in time to save her life.

The lawsuit was not successful.

The history of Amelia's case represents a second illustrative example. Amelia was the first child of her parents, who were second cousins. Her mother, who was obese, developed gestational diabetes. About seven weeks prior to delivery, she had experienced a vaginal bleed, which, upon ultrasound study, revealed that the placenta literally covered the exit to the uterus (called placenta previa).

When she returned in labor at forty weeks, the placenta had moved away from the uterine exit due to the expanding muscular wall of the uterus. Notwithstanding the access to the vaginal canal, the cervix did not dilate adequately, and progress was arrested. A Cesarean section at forty weeks resulted in Amelia's birth, at which time she was vigorous and, as expected, a large baby weighing eight and a half pounds with a large head circumference. Her newborn period was uneventful.

It soon became clear, however, that Amelia was not rolling over from back to stomach or the reverse. At six months of age, she could not even sit supported. No specific diagnosis was made at that time, and Amelia's mother began to suspect that she must have sustained brain damage because of some delay in performing the necessary Cesarean section. At ten months of age, in addition to Amelia's obvious muscle weakness, Amelia's mother noticed a tendency to shake and jerk. The doctor observed that these jerks (myoclonic seizures) seemed to occur every thirty seconds and in clusters. Amelia did not babble and also tended to drool. She was floppy and had difficulty controlling her large head. An MRI of her brain revealed some mild changes in one or two areas but no diffuse or generalized abnormality. No definite cause was offered to explain the findings seen on imaging.

Given the serious developmental delay, the myoclonic epilepsy, and the MRI observations, Amelia's mother brought a lawsuit against the obstetrician for failure to perform a timely Cesarean section, which she claimed would have avoided the brain damage Amelia sustained.

Further investigation using a chromosomal microarray revealed that Amelia had a microdeletion on the long arm of chromosome 14, but not in all cells. This implied that this microdeletion had occurred sometime after she had been conceived and that she was a mosaic for this microdeletion. In other words, only some of her cells had this deletion, while others did not. Clearly, there were a sufficient number of cells with a microdeletion in her brain to cause irreversible abnormality, along with the fact that her head and brain were of a large size. Not unexpectedly, neither of her parents had this deletion, consistent with the fact she was a mosaic. Moreover, the original microarray revealed large blocks of genes clearly shared by her parents (called long runs of homozygosity) involving about three hundred genes they had in common. It was likely that a harmful recessive gene mutation shared or contributed by both parents caused the neurological disorder. A study from the Middle East of 227 individuals from a highly consanguineous population revealed runs of homozygosity in 32 (14 percent), containing disease-causing genes and their mutations.

The lawsuit failed, due primarily to the discovery of the de novo microdeletion, albeit in the mosaic form.

Pertinent Medical Facts

Each of us has a number of glitches in our genomes. Needless to say, above and beyond the two hundred to three hundred variants (mutations) we have in our genome, there are many tiny deletions and duplications, each with one or many genes involved. These glitches, which are usually inherited from one parent, may be inconsequential as long as the parent of origin is in fact healthy. Worse still, a microdeletion may wipe out an entire gene, a portion of a gene, and not infrequently, simultaneously delete a large number of contiguous genes. Curiously, there are also syndromes due to duplications of a set of genes at the same location that create different consequences, compared with the same genes when deleted.

Chromosomal microdeletions and microduplications are described as copy number variants (CNVs). A gain or loss of a stretch of DNA made up of our building blocks (nucleotides) is described as a CNV, of which there are thousands. The size of the deletions and duplications is important. The larger the CNV, the more likely a serious clinical disorder will emerge. While many CNVs throughout the genome are recognized, there are now over twenty that keep on recurring, resulting in recognizable syndromes (a collection of characteristic symptoms and signs). These disorders result in a wide range of symptoms and signs and are especially characterized by intellectual disability, autism, epilepsy, heart defects, hydrocephalus, microcephaly, abnormal facial appearance (dysmorphism), speech defects, and on and on. It seems that there are specific hot spots for deletions and duplications to occur and recur. In very extensive studies on intellectual disability, about 14 percent of cases have been reported to have a microdeletion/duplication syndrome.

While we all have CNVs in our genomes, both in autism and schizophrenia, repeated studies show an increased number of microdeletions/microduplications. The same applies to those with epilepsy.

CNVs may occur spontaneously or be inherited from one parent. When inherited, it is highly likely that the transmitting parent has a similar, but not necessarily identical, clinical finding. Discovery of a brand- new (de novo) CNV is more likely than an inherited CNV to result in a serious or severe disorder. Testing for CNVs is done by a microarray analysis, which has largely replaced routine chromosome analysis for the investigation of intellectual disability, birth defects, or autism. In a study of 21,698 patients with these three categories of disorders, the diagnostic yield reported was 15–20 percent compared to the approximate 3 percent detection of cause using routine chromosome analysis.

The realization that microdeletions and microduplications are not rare, and may contribute to otherwise-inexplicable symptoms and signs, not infrequently bedevils legal claims of medical malpractice.

Questions

- Was it possible to have diagnosed Tanya's congenital heart defect and the microdeletion she had prenatally?

- Could Amelia's myoclonic epilepsy disorder have been detected prenatally, given that only some of her cells had a chromosome 14 microdeletion?

- Were Amelia's developmental delay and epilepsy due to hypoxia caused by a failure to perform a Cesarean section in time?

- Did Amelia's mother's gestational diabetes cause or contribute to her developmental problems and her epilepsy?

Commentary

Tanya's mother went for prenatal care late in pregnancy. If she had been more caring and attended earlier, an ultrasound examination would have revealed the serious heart defect between sixteen and eighteen weeks. Moreover, an immediate amniocentesis study, indicated because of the cardiac abnormality, would have led to a microarray test that would have revealed the microdeletion that Tanya had. The only options that she had at that point were (1) to continue pregnancy with knowledge that serious intellectual disability and possible death would occur, (2) to request pregnancy reduction of the affected twin, and (3) to terminate the pregnancy.

Selective pregnancy reduction in the case of twins with one having a known abnormality is a well-established procedure. Mostly an amniocentesis needle is used to inject potassium chloride into the fetal heart of the affected twin causing death. Possible complications include loss of the pregnancy (including the healthy twin), premature labor, premature delivery, infection, a serious clotting disorder in the mother, and psychological problems. Even combined, all of these risks are low. In pregnancies with nonidentical twins, the risks of total loss approximate 8 percent in some reports. Success is highly unlikely if the twins are identical and in the same amniotic sac.

In Amelia's case, a microarray test would have diagnosed the microdeletion, even in the mosaic form, as early as eleven weeks of pregnancy. There was, however, no specific indication to do a prenatal genetic test. Previously, amniocentesis was recommended for all women at thirty-five or more years of age. Today, *all* women should be routinely offered an amniocentesis at fifteen to sixteen weeks of pregnancy. A test that *biopsies* the placenta at eleven weeks (called chorion villus sampling or CVS) has a slightly higher risk of procedure-related loss and should be reserved for those with significant risks of a fetal genetic disorder.

The risk of pregnancy loss from amniocentesis ranges from 0.1 to 0.2 percent in experienced hands, while the loss rate for CVS is less than 0.5 percent. Many women are choosing the noninvasive prenatal blood-screening test available from at least ten weeks of pregnancy and aimed especially at detecting Down syndrome and two other even more serious chromosome abnormalities (trisomies 18 and 13). Some also choose detection of sex-chromosome abnormalities. *Few realize, and even fewer are told, that this screening test will miss about half of all chromosome abnormalities.* There is also a low false positive rate and an unknown false negative rate (thus far). Hence, the need for all women to consider prenatal diagnosis via amniocentesis or CVS was indicated.

Amelia's parents' consanguinity (second cousins) may well have resulted in transmission of a mutated recessive gene that caused her neurodevelopmental delay and epilepsy. Further studies to examine all her coding genes (by a test called whole exome sequencing) were not done. Her mosaicism for the microdeletion in the long arm of chromosome 14 likely occurred when she was still an embryo and did not originate from either parent. This microdeletion quite separately from any recessive gene could also have caused her disabilities.

Her mother's gestational diabetes almost certainly resulted in her increased birth weight. Fortunately, the known association of pre-pregnancy obesity with cerebral palsy as well as birth defects (such as spina bifida, congenital heart defects) did not apply to Amelia.

It is much more likely than not that the microdeletions of both Tanya and Amelia were the root cause of their respective disabilities. Their lawyers would have saved their money and not caused physicians' grief if they would simply have first sought a genetics consultation. They didn't know then, but now they do!

EXPOSURE

Jillian was a quality control laboratory technician who worked at a company that manufactured a chemical powder used to coat shelves. Some four months after beginning her new job, Jillian unexpectedly became pregnant. Given the short time she had been employed, she decided to wait out the first three months before informing the human resources department. She informed her immediate supervisors and was suddenly required to wear a dust mask and special gloves when working with the powder. She was also restricted from certain areas of the plant. In addition, she was not allowed to spray samples or even handle the powder. Unfortunately, wearing the mask made her nauseous and light- headed. After repeated complaints, she was placed on disability for the rest of her pregnancy and through the six weeks postpartum.

When she was at work, she and others had experienced headaches, congestion, nosebleeds, hoarseness, and throat and eye irritation as well as skin sensitivity. Chemicals in the manufactured powder were known to cause respiratory symptoms, skin irritation, and eye inflammation. Prolonged inhalation of the dusk powder was thought to be harmful with a potential risk of causing fibrosis of the lung. Jillian did have a pulmonary test, the results of which were perfectly normal. The printed written materials made no reference to pregnancy in humans. Studies apparently did show, for some of the chemicals, that overexposure could affect testicular function adversely. At least two of the chemicals were regarded by the state of California as having the potential to cause both cancer and birth defects. Chemicals used in the manufacturing process included epichlorohydrin and epoxy resin, titanium dioxide, tin oxide, and the mineral mica.

Ryan was born at almost thirty-eight weeks of pregnancy by Cesarean section, because Jillian had had a previous son by surgical delivery. Surgery had been uneventful, except that Jillian had noted that, in comparison to her first son, Ryan seemed to move very little. He weighed eight pounds six ounces and had a normal head circumference. Immediately noted was the larger right compared to left leg, with the right having a large, purple birthmark. In addition, his right ear was flat and pointed. He and his mother left hospital on day three of life, both doing well. However, by day five, he had not yet had a bowel movement and was fussy. A suppository temporarily solved the problem, which recurred immediately, requiring continuous use of laxatives.

Over the ensuing months, it became clear that Ryan was hypotonic and had delayed milestones. He also seemed to have difficulty moving his jaw and swallowing. He had impaired speech and visual-perception problems and was highly sensitive to sound.

Imaging of his brain by MRI showed a few areas that were not fully myelinated but without any specific diagnosis. Jillian noticed that he seemed largely oblivious to pain and actually stated, "We have to teach him what pain is."

Ryan did slowly progress, learned to walk and talk, but remained with some difficulties in swallowing and diminished sensitivity to pain. No definitive diagnosis was actually made.

Jillian and her husband sued the paint-and-powder plant at which she worked for their failure to protect her and her developing fetus from the developmental issues he subsequently manifested.

Pertinent Medical Facts

I was sent this case for review with the express purpose of trying to determine whether Jillian's exposure to toxic chemicals caused Ryan's problems. No specific diagnosis had yet been made by his caregivers. I was immediately struck by clinical observations that had been made since he was born. Immediately at birth, Ryan was noticed to have his right leg larger than his left. Almost immediately, severe constipation emerged and became a continuing problem. He was also noted to have low tone (hypotonia). He also had some swallowing difficulty, and as the months progressed, he clearly manifested developmental delay. His mother also made the remarkable statement that "we have to teach him what pain is."

The series of clinical observations just mentioned made for a diagnosis of congenital insensitivity to pain or hereditary sensory and autonomic neuropathy. This is a mostly autosomal recessive disorder due to a gene mutation that originated from both parents equally.

This is an extremely rare genetic disorder with at least half of cases occurring in the offspring of consanguineous couples. Jillian denied that there was any possibility that she and her husband were related. They each did have Irish ancestors.

In some cases, there is a lack of sweating and quite often, because of the lack of pain perception, injuries to various body parts. While Ryan's manifestations were relatively modest thus far, time will tell once he has all his teeth, whether he will bite part of his tongue off, bite his lip, or bite or mutilate his fingers!

The MRI imaging of his brain showed some areas with a lack of myelination, which is consistent with this disorder. At the time this case occurred, we did not yet know the two culprit genes that were subsequently discovered. Today it is possible to achieve a precise diagnosis and provide carrier tests with future prenatal diagnosis or preimplantation genetic diagnosis in mind.

Questions

- Why was the diagnosis of congenital insensitivity to pain not made?

Commentary

Clearly, the toxic chemicals that Jillian was exposed to had nothing to do with the autosomal recessive genetic disorder that Ryan inherited. Once the diagnosis was made, Jillian and her husband were advised of the 25 percent risk of recurrence in a subsequent pregnancy. In addition, of course, the options of prenatal diagnosis and preimplantation genetic diagnosis would have been explained.

There was no expectation that physicians in primary-care practice would be faulted for not making a diagnosis of such an extremely rare condition. The hope is that when faced with unusual signs and symptoms in children and in adults, referral for a consultation with a clinical geneticist is recommended. Proof that an environmental toxin or a specific medication is the cause of intellectual disability or a birth defect is extremely difficult and not often taken up by plaintiff attorneys.

Despite there being no connection between the toxic exposure and Ryan's disorder, because of a lack of safety measures at the powder plant, a small settlement was made in this case.

BIG AND BLAME

It was a fresh, beautiful spring day when I was called to consult on a patient in one of the residential wards of a very large children's hospital, Queen Mary's Carshalton in Sutton, Surrey, in the south of London. Upon entry to the old-styled English hospital ward, one could see all thirty beds, since there were no individual patient rooms. The child I was to see was located in the far right-hand corner of the ward. I vividly recall strolling down the center of the ward and halfway down seeing a child jumping up and down on her bed as if it was a trampoline. Her nurse was having trouble controlling her. When I reached the patient for whom the consult was requested, I remember blinking and wondering if my mind was playing tricks on me. I could have sworn that the child I saw halfway down the ward looked exactly the same as the patient I came to see.

To cut a long story short, that was precisely the case. Both had large heads (macrocephaly) and flushed cheeks, were about twice the height for their age, and had intellectual disability.

The condition that I had recognized had been described the year before and was called cerebral gigantism, subsequently named Sotos syndrome after the descriptor.

Many years later while working at Boston University School of Medicine, I was called to another state to perform an independent medical examination (IME) on an eight-year-old girl whose parents had sued their daughter's pediatrician and the small community hospital. Her mother who brought her in for the IME was none too pleased and projected a defensive, surly attitude.

Wanda had been delivered by repeat Cesarean section and was reasonably vigorous at birth. However, very soon after, she began displaying poor tone and poor color and clearly had respiratory difficulties. After applying positive-pressure ventilation with 100 percent oxygen, a blood sample showed that Wanda had become acidotic (an increasing acid concentration in her blood) indicating a drop in oxygen saturation. Arrangements were made to transfer Wanda to a larger hospital, but that request was not made for an urgent, immediate transfer.

The transfer was affected some seven hours after Wanda was born. The transfer team was concerned about her respiratory problem, so they intubated her and connected her to a ventilator.

Wanda remained in hospital for some forty-six days, during which time the physicians noted that she had a long, narrow face; excess skin in the nape of her neck; underdeveloped nails; and a heart murmur that turned out to be a patent ductus arteriosus (the fetal blood vessel that transmits blood from the aorta to the pulmonary artery and that normally closes at or soon after birth).

During that hospitalization, a series of chromosome and biochemical genetic tests were done, all of which yielded normal results. MRI imaging of her brain showed that the folds of her brain (gyri) were less prominent than usual and that the ventricles were more prominent. There was also some brain atrophy and slight changes in the basal ganglia and brain stem.

After a stormy start, Wanda recovered nicely, and by the time she was discharged, measurements of her head circumference, weight, and length all exceeded the ninety-fifth percentile! She remained, however, with low tone. At the age of six months, her head circumference was over the one-hundredth percentile and way off the head-circumference graph. At that time, she was noted to also have a rather prominent forehead, widely spaced eyes, a bell-shaped chest, low tone, and delayed milestones. Repeat imaging of her brain by MRI at fourteen months of age showed decreased volume of her white matter in her frontal lobes and some thinning of the corpus callosum (the bundle of nerve fibers that connect the two cerebral hemispheres). During her initial hospital stay, she had heart surgery, and the patent ductus had been tied off.

I got to see Wanda when she was eight years of age. She walked into the room with her mother, and yes, I blinked again. Although it was many years later, I had a distinct sense of déjà vu dating all the way back to the hospital ward in London. In the intervening decades, I had seen a number of children with Sotos syndrome. Her history and physical signs made it all but certain that she had Sotos syndrome. Notwithstanding my immediate impression, I took a thorough history and did a detailed examination, confirming that she was way ahead of her age-expected height and head circumference.

Wanda's mother told of her limited vocabulary and that she functioned at about a three-year level, with limited abilities both intellectually and motorically. She could not really run, because she would fall, and she had to hold on to stairs when climbing. Temper tantrums occurred at least once a day. Toilet training was still seriously problematic, despite her age.

At that point, Wanda's mother suddenly refused to answer any more questions, left the room with her daughter, and went "to confer with her lawyer." She returned ten minutes later and without apology allowed me to continue the IME.

My examination confirmed that her head circumference was greater than the one-hundredth percentile and that she was very tall for her age, but she wouldn't stand still for a measurement. Head and neck examination revealed some facial asymmetry, widely spaced eyes, strabismus (cross-eyes), a prominent jaw, some missing teeth, and some teeth with enamel defects. A bell-shaped chest with some mild curvature of her spine was evident. She had low tone and clearly had some balance issues.

At that point, I asked if it would be possible to get a blood sample for further genetic studies. Wanda's mother asked me if I did not agree that she had cerebral palsy due to a lack of oxygen following the failure of her doctors to care for her in the hospital where she was born. When I responded that I thought that Wanda had Sotos syndrome, explaining the signs of that disorder, Wanda's mother became furious and charged out of the room again. She returned fifteen minutes later fuming but provided permission to obtain a blood sample for a chromosomal microarray and gene sequencing if necessary.

Later in the laboratories at our nonprofit Center for Human Genetics, we determined that the culprit gene (*NSD1*) was completely deleted from the genome, clinching the absolute diagnosis of Sotos syndrome.

Pertinent Medical Facts

Wanda had the classical features of Sotos syndrome that included a broad and prominent forehead, down-slanting eyes, flushed cheeks, a long and narrow face with a prominent chin, intellectual disability, overgrowth in height and head circumference, behavioral problems, a heart defect, lax joints, scoliosis, and typical findings on the brain imaging noted above.

About 95 percent of children born with this disorder have either a gene deletion or a mutation in the *NSD1* gene that is de novo (brand new and not inherited). About 5 percent of children inherit the mutated gene from one parent who invariably has some of the intellectual, behavioral, and physical signs of Sotos syndrome. The estimated frequency of this disorder is one in fourteen thousand live births.

Questions

- Why did it take seven hours to recognize that Wanda needed ventilator assistance because of her respiratory difficulties?

- Did the delay in transferring her to the tertiary-care hospital result in oxygen lack that damaged her brain?

- How much of her intellectual disability was due to Sotos syndrome?

Commentary

Wanda had the classical signs of Sotos syndrome. Her initial vigorous state at birth, subsequent blood tests, and brain imaging provided no basis to ascribe hypoxia as a cause of her intellectual disability. And, of course, none of her physical features or ailments could be ascribed to hypoxia either. Because of this genetic disorder, she will require care for the rest of her life.

Growth acceleration in Sotos syndrome makes a five-year-old look as tall as a ten-year-old. The reason for this growth velocity, which only continues into the early teens, is not known. However, it occurred to me when faced with the two affected children in London that this growth acceleration might well have begun in the developing fetus. In searching for some indicator of early and rapid growth, I thought about our fingerprints. I knew by fourteen weeks of pregnancy that the tiny ridges and whorls that constitute our fingerprints are already clearly established. Since there is a significant genetic element to the development of our fingerprints, I wondered whether counting the ridges of the prints on our fingers could possibly reflect advanced growth of the fetus so early in pregnancy.

There was one problem, however. I knew essentially nothing about counting the ridges of fingerprints or what was normal. Being young and naïve, I simply picked up the telephone and called Sir Lionel Penrose. Professor Penrose was a world-famous psychiatrist, geneticist, scientist, and mathematician and head of the famous Galton Genetics Laboratory in London. Among his amazing attributes, he was also an authority on dermatoglyphics, the science of fingerprinting.

I almost fell off my chair when he personally answered the phone. I quickly recounted my story while he listened intently to the then-inexperienced pediatrician. He instructed me on the method to obtain the fingerprints of the two children and to bring them to him. I followed his instructions and took the prints to Professor Penrose, who did the ridge counts. I was fascinated to learn that the normal range of ridge counts had been established and that the number of ridge counts for both children clearly exceeded two standard deviations above the mean. This finding was consistent with already-evident growth acceleration in the early-developing fetus. I thanked Professor Penrose then and in the publication in 1969 of my paper in *Pediatrics* that followed.

Genetic disorders are common and not infrequently occur in the same child subject to problems encountered during labor and delivery or in the newly born. Considerable time, effort, and expertise are often expended in teasing apart the relative contributions of acquired and genetic problems. Clinically Wanda displayed none of the multiple systemic signs seen in newborns suffering from oxygen deprivation. Fortunately, she had been delivered by repeat Cesarean section, so her macrocephaly couldn't be held accountable for being stuck in the birth canal and subject to hypoxia. We do know that a large head in the fetus is more likely to lead to operative delivery than one less than the ninety-fifth

percentile. At no time after Wanda's birth was she without oxygen supplementation. Her initial

respiratory difficulties after birth were not unusual for Sotos syndrome, which ultimately was the cause of

her intellectual disability and dysmorphic features.

Delay in transferring Wanda to the larger hospital lit the fire of litigation and reflected poor judgment, but

not negligence. Wanda had not been deprived of oxygen during those seven hours, and brain imaging

showed no evidence of damage due to hypoxia. Nevertheless, some minor settlement was reached in this

case because of the delay in transfer.

BRAIN FOG

Marian was twenty years of age and excited about her first pregnancy. She had been an insulin-dependent diabetic since childhood but, with good care, had her diabetes under excellent control. Pregnancy had been uneventful, except near term she had a slight vaginal bacterial infection (β streptococcus). This was quickly treated with penicillin. At thirty-eight weeks gestation, because of the diabetes, she was admitted for elective induction of labor. Contractions began and progressed normally.

She had been cared for throughout her pregnancy by a certified midwife, which had been her preference. The midwife and a registered nurse assistant tended to her during her labor, ministering to her needs. They had applied the electronic fetal monitor, which initially yielded a completely normal tracing, which was reassuring. After about five hours of labor and good progress, augmentation with intravenous Pitocin to stimulate the uterine contractions was initiated.

While sitting up in preparation for the placement of an epidural anesthesia, the midwife noted that the fetal heart rate dropped momentarily into the 80s from the previous normal rate of 120 beats per minute. Two more marked decelerations occurred, and the intravenous Pitocin was turned off, and oxygen was administered to Marian. At that point, the midwife ordered additional standard intravenous fluid solution. Repetitive variable decelerations continued, and the obstetrician was promptly informed. He immediately ordered the preparation for an immediate Cesarean section. An attempt was also made to push the fetal head inward in an attempt to relieve any possible hidden umbilical cord compression.

The Cesarean section was performed expeditiously. Jim and Marian's baby, whom they named Jenna, was delivered within twenty-five minutes of the decision having been made. Unfortunately, the electronic fetal monitor reflected serious fetal distress for a period of close to twenty minutes, prior to the incision.

Jenna was born requiring immediate resuscitation with a heart rate down to 70 bpm but not breathing, blue, and floppy. Shortly thereafter, the anesthesiology staff noted that Marian had received an infusion of normal saline with Pitocin instead of the simple lactated ringer solution the midwife had ordered. A serious excess of Pitocin had inadvertently been given intravenously. The nurse had turned on the infusion from the wrong fluid bag that contained Pitocin.

That bag was completely drained out.

Jenna required intubation and connection to a ventilator. After ten minutes, her heart rate had risen to 170 bpm, and she had pinked up. She took her first breath at eight minutes after birth, and it took up to twenty-four minutes to establish regular breathing. Jenna remained completely flaccid and for a good while did not move her arms or legs. Meanwhile, the pediatric team learned that the blood drawn from the umbilical cord at birth showed that Jenna had become seriously acidotic, implying severe oxygen lack prior to delivery. Jenna recovered within thirty minutes, self-correcting the acidosis. Later that first day of life, she had a seizure. She was also started on intravenous 10 percent dextrose infusion. Given her respiratory difficulties, a chest x-ray was obtained, which also revealed an incidental hemivertebra in her lower spine. The pediatricians also thought that she had atypical facial features and ordered chromosome studies as well as biochemical genetic testing. All results were normal.

By five months of age, it had become abundantly clear that Jenna was seriously delayed in her milestones.

Imaging of her brain by MRI revealed diffuse abnormalities consistent with severe hypoxia with specific damage to the basal ganglia. Over the ensuing months, Jenna became increasingly spastic and was diagnosed as having cerebral palsy. She also began having severe gastroesophageal reflux that required surgery. At one year of age, a repeat imaging of her brain showed cortical atrophy due to the oxygen lack. It became clear that Jenna would require care for the rest of her life and would not be able to fend for herself.

Jim and Marian sued the hospital facility and the midwife for the failure in the management of Marian's pregnancy that resulted in Jenna's irreversible brain damage that would never allow her to care for herself.

Pertinent Medical Facts

Medication errors are among the most common causes of morbidity and mortality in hospital patients. The Institute of Medicine estimated that medical errors cause 1 in 131 outpatient deaths and 1 in 854 inpatient deaths. There is little doubt that these estimates are on the seriously low side. In some studies, the range of chemotherapy errors ranged from 7 to 18.8 percent of clinic visits. Remarkably, administration errors occurred in 56 percent and ordering errors in 36 percent. The problems involving administration of all forms of medication go well beyond the use and misuse of Pitocin.

The American Society of Hospital Pharmacists (ASHP) issued critically important guidelines concerning medication errors, especially from chemotherapy, in 2015. The nationally coordinating Council on Medication Error Reporting and Prevention stated that medication errors may be related to "professional practice, health-care products, procedures, and systems that include prescribing, order communication, product labeling, packaging, nomenclature, compounding, dispensing, distributing, administration, education, monitoring, and use." The ASHP, recognizing human fallibility and system failures, urged that their guidelines extend to patients so that they can participate in securing their own safety.

ASHP insisted that all personnel who prescribe, prepare, dispense, administer, and handle hazardous drugs or contaminated materials complete appropriate training and evaluation. Moreover, expected competencies should be reassessed annually or more frequently if required. The guidelines specify an exhaustive list of requirements for pharmacists to dispense chemotherapeutic agents. Since verbal orders for chemotherapeutic drugs are strictly disallowed, they have advocated computerized chemotherapy entry. This has been adopted increasingly by hospital pharmacists. While this system has clearly prevented prescribing errors, there is still a requirement for due diligence and independent checking. The

American Society of Clinical Oncologists has stressed the importance of standardized calculations and

has also produced guidelines for dosing chemotherapeutic agents in obese patients. All abbreviations for

drug names, scheduling information, and directions for administration should be prohibited.

There are also rules, regulations, and guidelines for the use of intravenous infusions for medications.

Intravenous therapy for hospitalized patients is often complicated, and errors may occur. Such errors have

included problems with the infusion rate, incorrect dosage, wrong patient, or wrong drugs. A Cleveland

clinic study of the use of a robotic device for compounding patient-specific chemotherapy doses was very

instructive. The robot was used to create 7,384 medication doses. Only 1.2 percent were found to be

outside the desired accuracy range and were manually modified by the pharmacy staff. Not unexpectedly, a

notable finding was that human error, such as the loading of an incorrect vial or bag into the machine, was

a problem!

Questions

- How was it possible for the assistant to use the wrong infusion bag that allowed an overdose of
  Pitocin?

- What was the effect of the Pitocin overdose?

- How did a hospital physician training program allow Betsy Lehman to receive a massive
  overdose of chemotherapeutic drugs that killed her?

- How could a simple preparation of heparin through an intravenous line result in a one thousand
  times overdose?

Commentary

The invaluable care midwives provide has not come without inevitable litigation after the occurrence of

adverse events. One report on 162 closed claims involving midwives provided an analysis by members of

the Professional Liability Section of the American College of Nurse-Midwives Division of Standards and

Practice.

Fetal death, stillbirth, and newborn death or injury ranked highest in their evaluation. Negligent management of pregnancy, labor, and delivery was next and included maternal injury. Failure to make a timely diagnosis that the baby could not traverse the birth canal (called shoulder dystocia) due to size, position, or pelvic anatomy, resulting in injury or death, fulfilled a third category. Even failure to anticipate or provide genetic information or testing was noted.

Accurate documentation, timely consultation, practiced simulation, referral, and informed consent, all emerged as key strategies to avoid litigation.

The simple, but catastrophic, error that ruined Jenna and her family's lives was sadly not unique. Unfortunately, many cases of medication errors have been reported. I will briefly describe four illustrative cases.

The Betsy Lehman Tragedy

Betsy Lehman was an award-winning health columnist at the *Boston Globe*. At thirty-nine years of age and a mother of two children, seven and three years of age, she was diagnosed with advanced breast cancer. Given her training, she carefully researched her treatment options and chose the use of certain standard drugs but with an experimental protocol. This plan was offered by the Dana Farber Cancer Institute affiliated to the Harvard Medical School. The medication involved high-dose chemotherapy preceded by removal of her own blood cells for storage and, after chemotherapy, infusing them back into her circulation. The purpose was to have the treatment with the cell-destroying chemotherapy, by harvesting the stem cells from her own blood, which would then be used to repopulate her blood and bone marrow and also reconstitute her immune system. That was her plan. That was her hope.

The chemotherapy dose was to be calculated by the amount of her body-surface area. The dose she was to have received was 1,630 milligrams each day for four consecutive days. Instead, she received 6,520 milligrams/day for four days. It was four times the correct dose!

Betsy began vomiting and telling her caregivers that something was seriously wrong. Apparently, they failed to pay close attention, and she rapidly deteriorated and died.

Only much later, as part of a routine data check on the experimental drug protocol, it was realized she had been given a massive overdose.

The original prescription had been written by a research fellow in training (see chapter 19), who apparently misinterpreted the protocol. However, at least five other physicians and nurses countersigned the experimental drug order as reported by the *Boston Globe*. None of the pharmacists noticed the error either.

At autopsy, no visible signs of cancer were found!

At about the same time, another fifty-two-year-old patient was also given an overdose using the same experimental protocol. That woman suffered permanent and irreversible damage.

Time magazine characterized these awful events with a heading "The Cure That Killed the Patient." The Dana Farber Institute recognized their grievous errors and immediately apologized. Later, the Betsy Lehman Center for Patient Safety was founded.

All of this happened in 1994, and, as you would expect, all manner of systems changes and computer fixes were organized and set in place. We would have expected real change as a consequence of such steps. The discussion below may reorient your opinions.

The Quaid Twins

The actor Dennis Quaid and his wife, Kimberly, with the help of a surrogate, had biological twins in 2008. Thomas and Zoe went home from the hospital after three days and were doing well. Several days later, they both developed streptococcal infections, obviously picked up at the birth hospital. This potentially serious development led to immediate hospitalization at Cedars Sinai Medical Center, specifically for intravenous treatment with antibiotics.

During the night, nurses administered Heparin (a blood thinner) through the intravenous line for the routine purpose of avoiding clots, which would block the infusion of antibiotics. Unfortunately, the dose of heparin given, twice, was one thousand times the recommended dose. Remarkably, only Zoe showed any sign of bleeding, with blood oozing from the intravenous entry site, her heel, and from the umbilical cord stump. No one at Cedar Sinai Medical Center called the parents, who learned about this error the next day at 6:30 a.m.

Upon discovery of the error, a heparin antidote was administered. No further bleeding occurred.

Subsequently, state regulators discovered that the pharmacists who prepared the vials of heparin had made a mistake. Each vial contained a concentration of ten thousand units per milliliter instead of ten units per milliliter.

The twins spent eleven days in the intensive-care unit and recovered fully. At eight years of age, they were perfectly healthy. The parents subsequently founded the Quaid Foundation devoted to patient safety and combined with TMIT (Texas Medical Institute of Technology), a nonprofit medical-result foundation dedicated to saving lives. They also sued Baxter Healthcare Corporation, one of the manufacturers of heparin, claiming that the manufacturing and design of the product led to the error.

The case was dismissed.

Errors have also persisted in the use of intravenous medications controlled by smart pumps. A 2017 study focused on 478 patients who received 1,164 medications by intravenous infusions. A startling 60 percent had one or more errors associated with their administration. Errors included incorrect labeling and bypassing the smart pump.

Another distressing arena of medication errors is that occur during emergency resuscitation or emergencies generally. It is well known that due to the chaos of the resuscitation environment, errors occur in dosing, preparing, labeling, and administering the urgently needed drugs.

A British study concluded that 19.2 percent of morphine infusions prepared for newborns in the intensive-care unit were outside the required limit. These especially involved dilutions of small volumes in a syringe.

Many potential human and system vulnerabilities impact the possibilities of medication errors. Prominent among the human errors are inattention, fatigue, haste, poor communication, "brain fog," and "maths anxiety" (in calculating dosage). Many of us have transitory moments (some call them "senior moments") where, for example, one might enter a room and forget what you came to do or get. We also see more prominent "brain fog" in conditions such as the connective-tissue disorder, Ehlers-Danlos syndrome of the hypermobility type. Many people with very flexible joints are often unaware of this diagnosis, which I have also seen in nurses! System factors are well recognized, and multiple solutions have been recommended. Unfortunately, not all recommendations have been adopted. These steps to avoid medication errors include the use of bar codes, other codes, distinct packaging, larger print, the manufacture of ampules that look different for different medications, better drug labeling, and computerized provider-order entries. The latter has become critical because of the required complex dose calculations needed for chemotherapy. The tendency for dilution errors, especially when tiny volumes are involved, needs to be carefully avoided and repeatedly checked, preferably by a second trained individual.

Other system-based strategies include bar-code management, establishment of infusion pump policies, and a reduction of the nursing workload in intensive-care units.

Efforts to avoid medication errors have to be made on multiple fronts. Triaging by physicians, pharmacists, and nurses comes first, with additional instruction about the avoidance of errors and pitfalls. Second comes the system's changes discussed here. Third, every patient, if not too sick, needs to question what is being administered every time, and, fourth, every patient needs to bring to the hospital an advocate who could stay for as many hours as possible and act as another set of eyes watching and caring. Fifth, especially important is the need for senior constant oversight, both in the hospital pharmacy and at the bedside when particularly lethal medications are to be used. We will never know whether "brain fog," inattention, distraction, or something else made the nurse use the Pitocin-containing infusion bag instead of the lactated ringer's solution. The effect was to cause the uterine muscle to contract for a prolonged period, cutting off the blood supply and hence the oxygen to the child.

Having a research fellow not fully dedicated to patient care, and simply dabbling part-time in such a critical-care situation, represented a seriously flawed arrangement. Betsy Lehman fell victim to an ill-conceived system that allowed someone in training to end her life. Teaching hospitals, in their effort to train specialty fellows, frequently allow those pursuing research projects to spend a portion of their time seeing patients. I believe that a much better system is to allow fellows in training to pursue aspects of their training in uninterrupted blocks of time and not piecemeal. This would be especially important if the fellow's involvement had to do with critical patient-care responsibilities, such as chemotherapy-care administration, surgery, obstetrics, and so on.

The Quaid twins were incredibly fortunate to have not had a fatal hemorrhage. Others have not been as fortunate.

I have repeatedly emphasized in this book that good doctors also make mistakes. One noteworthy example involved failure to monitor the use of a powerful drug (methotrexate) that was being used by a patient who then sustained irreversible liver damage and died. The highly respected physician was Dr. Peter Wheeler, as reported in 2017 by the *Sunday Telegraph* in London. He was the former private physician to Diana, the Princess of Wales. He admitted to a "catalogue of serious failings" that led to the premature death of a leading city banker.

A fourth example involved a forty-five-year-old businessman who was seen for his annual physical examination. Among the routine laboratory tests that were ordered by his physician was the PSA (prostate-specific antigen) analysis to monitor for prostate cancer. His doctor had his secretary call for the result, as reported in *Medical Economics*. She was told his PSA value was 2.1, and the secretary duly wrote that into his file, and his doctor informed him of the normal result.

Two years later, again at his annual checkup, his PSA level was found to be very high. On questioning his doctor, she reviewed his file to discover that she had never received a printed report of the PSA test result. A request to the laboratory yielded a copy of the report that showed a PSA level of 21 (very high). Either the laboratory or the secretary omitted the decimal point! Once again, we see compounding errors.

He was referred to a urologist who biopsied his prostate gland. The pathology report revealed he had an adenocarcinoma. A bone scan showed that the cancer had spread. Nevertheless, he underwent a radical prostatectomy followed by radiation and hormone therapy. He was left impotent and incontinent!

The errors made in this case are desperately simple but are unfortunately not rare. No report should be filed without being initialed by the physician. A running log should be maintained to be sure that a report is actually received. As discussed in chapter 24, whoever has a life- or health-threatening report (e.g., a laboratory, pathologist, or radiologist) must make voice contact with a patient's care provider.

This businessman sued his physician. The case was settled before trial.

One final point. The Quaid twins almost certainly picked up their infection from their birth hospital. In 2017, a report in the *New England Journal of Medicine* noted that infection causing illness and death affected more than one and a half million Americans each year. The Centers for Disease Control and Prevention report that almost 650,000 patients acquire an infection while in hospital each year. About 75,000 of them die!

Stay out of hospital unless absolutely necessary!

SUCKED OUT

Millie and Joe met in high school. They never dated but had friends in common. Joe became a carpenter

and Millie a nurse. Years later, both still single, they met again at a July 4 celebration on the public

common at a fireworks show. They were both sports minded and began attending ball games together and

eventually married. They had one healthy son, and years later, when Millie was thirty-six years of age,

they had a second pregnancy.

The second pregnancy progressed well, except Millie, while having difficulty remembering, thought that

toward the end of the pregnancy, there was less movement compared to her first pregnancy years ago. At

sixteen weeks of pregnancy, she had an amniocentesis because of her increased risks for having a child

with a chromosomal abnormality (such as Down syndrome) in view of her age. The laboratory reported a

normal chromosomal complement and a normal alpha-fetoprotein level in the amniotic fluid. At that time,

a routine ultrasound study of the fetus showed no abnormalities, nor did another at twenty-four weeks of

pregnancy.

She delivered vaginally without incident. However, it was immediately obvious that their newborn son,

Joshua, was not moving one side of his body. He otherwise had normal facies and no structural

abnormalities of his limbs or trunk. An immediate cranial ultrasound revealed a startling observation.

Much of the one side of his brain was missing! A tiny sliver of brain was present anteriorly and

posteriorly on that side of the skull. An MRI of the brain soon confirmed these findings.

They sought out their obstetrician and confronted him with their belief that the amniocentesis he had

performed, apparently with some difficulty (he needled the amniotic sac twice after failing to aspirate

amniotic fluid the first time), must have pierced the skull and sucked out part of the fetal brain or caused

destruction in some way by entering it with the needle. Millie and Joe were certain that their obstetrician did something wrong with the procedure. Moreover, they had never liked his offhand manner and lack of sensitivity. His attitude to them in this confrontation was characterized by Joe as a "brush-off." After that consultation, they were angry, distressed, and eager to seek legal redress.

Millie and Joe sought out a well-known medical-malpractice lawyer and sued their doctor for having caused irreparable damage to their child's brain. I was asked to review this case with special reference to genetic studies performed on the amniotic fluid and cells.

Pertinent Medical Facts

At that time, amniocentesis even with ultrasound guidance was regarded as having a 0.5–1.0 percent risk of pregnancy loss as a consequence of the procedure. Nowadays, in good hands and with experience, that risk is 0.1–0.2 percent. I confirmed that the genetic chromosome studies had been correct and that the alpha-fetoprotein levels were perfectly normal and that in particular, there were no brain cells in the amniotic fluid that had been examined. I went on to point out that Joshua must have suffered a stroke in utero.

"Fetal stroke" is defined as occurring between fourteen weeks of pregnancy and the onset of labor that results in delivery. Stroke that occurs just before, during, or immediately after delivery is defined as "perinatal stroke." The rates of perinatal stroke are estimated to be at least one in thirty-five hundred live births. Indeed, stroke is more likely to occur in the perinatal period than any other time in childhood. It is the most common cause of hemiparetic (weakness in one side) cerebral palsy, which Joshua manifested. Fetal stroke may be caused by hemorrhage, a lack of blood flow (ischemia), thrombosis, or a combination of these factors. The incidence of ischemic stroke is relatively high in identical twins and less so for fraternal twins.

The causes or contributing factors to fetal stroke may be due to maternal conditions, pregnancy-related disorders, or actually fetal disorders. Among the maternal conditions, one can include severe uncontrolled diabetes, trauma, fever with infections, medications including anticonvulsants and anticoagulants, and immune thrombocytopenic purpura (low platelets). Preeclampsia is a recognized maternal risk factor that causes problems by reducing placental blood flow. This in turn results in fetal-brain underperfusion, leading to possible ischemic brain injury. Other maternal factors include a history of infertility, no previous pregnancy, prolonged rupture of membranes, and placental infection (chorioamnionitis). Use of cocaine during pregnancy is a potential risk factor, causing arterial stroke attributable to blood vessels constricting and going into spasm. Women who smoke also have an increased risk. Among the pregnancy-related disorders, brain hemorrhage might occur as a consequence of alloimmune thrombocytopenia (see chapter 2). Hemorrhage or thrombosis within a placenta appears to be important factors as does the complication of the placenta peeling off the wall of the uterus (placental abruption).

The opening in the septum between the right and the left atrium of the heart may allow the passage of clots from the placenta or the venous circulation and may lead to a clot shooting into the brain arteries, resulting in a stroke. I already mentioned twins, especially in a situation where one twin is stealing blood supply from the other (twin-twin transfusion syndrome). Rare genetic disorders may also be a contributing cause of fetal stroke. Certainly, viral infections (such as cytomegalovirus infection) are potentially important as are genetic disorders that predispose to clotting. An estimated 15 percent of infants with stroke have inherited clotting disorders.

Infants with perinatal stroke, if not detected soon after birth, usually show signs within the first forty-eight to seventy-two hours following birth. Seizures are by far the most common, but subtler signs may be noted and include periods of not breathing (apnea), lethargy, feeding difficulties, and breathing problems. Unfortunately, outcomes are invariably sad. They include hemiparetic cerebral palsy (unilateral), serious developmental delay, behavioral problems, vision abnormalities, and continuing epilepsy.

Questions

- Was the claim rational that the amniocentesis needle caused the destruction of most of one side of the fetal brain?

Commentary

Joshua as a fetus clearly had a major stroke involving his middle-cerebral artery that resulted in the destruction of much of one side of his brain. An amniocentesis needle that punctures a major artery (such as the middle-cerebral artery that supplies a large area of the brain) would inevitably result in a hemorrhage. Imaging of the brain after birth would reveal evidence of prior hemorrhage. Certainly, clotting in that artery would cut off the oxygen supply to the area of brain served and result in dead brain tissue being resorbed. (Note that after an early fetal death of a twin, no evidence of that twin's existence may be found at birth, the tissue having been absorbed.)

The fact that much of the brain was missing and so clearly seen immediately after birth indicated that the stroke must have occurred many weeks or months prior to delivery. The cause in this case was not established, which, even today, remains the case in close to 50 percent of fetal strokes. There is no good reason to believe that the amniocentesis needle had anything to do with Joshua's stroke. However, during legal discovery, the plaintiff attorney determined that the same doctor, in another case, had performed an amniocentesis, and the needle had pierced the fetal brain. In that case, the fetus died. Once this information became known, and with the realization that the information would be presented to the jury, the case was settled.

Information about previous lawsuits almost invariably comes to attention in the courtroom. Unfortunately in this case, there was no evidence that the doctor did anything wrong. Nevertheless, the insurance company carrying his liability coverage decided not to risk jury consideration.

CONGENITAL

Mica was born at thirty-seven weeks of gestation through a routine vaginal delivery without complications. She weighed six pounds eleven ounces and was vigorous but was noted to have low blood glucose. This hypoglycemia was ascribed to her prematurity and slowly resolved on treatment with intravenous dextrose. The neonatologist noted that she had rather high red blood cell counts (polycythemia) and a red birthmark on her forehead just above her nose. She went home after about ten days in hospital without further issues related to her blood glucose.

At seven and a half weeks, during a routine checkup with her pediatrician, he observed that her right leg was larger and longer than her left. This observation prompted a referral to an orthopedic surgeon. He in turn diagnosed hemihypertrophy of the right side, this time including the right arm. The x-rays he ordered confirmed the increased lengths of the right arm and leg. To his credit, he recalled an association between hemihypertrophy and kidney tumor (called Wilms tumor). The ultrasound he ordered was primarily focused on the kidney, but some (but not all) of the liver was seen in that imaging. The study revealed no abnormality.

At six months of age, during a routine visit, her mother complained that Mica's tongue was cracked and bleeding. Also, her tongue protruded out of her mouth all the time (review of Mica's photographs as a newborn revealed that even then her tongue protruded through her mouth). At eight months of age, she was obviously ill. She was pale, having diarrhea and vomiting, and "sleeping a lot." Notwithstanding these symptoms, no specific treatment was pursued. Scheduled visits to the orthopedic surgeon for a follow-up of her hemihypertrophy also resulted in no further tests. Less than two months later, Mica's mother returned to the pediatrician concerned about the bulging right side of her abdomen. She had pointed out Mica's prominent belly previously but had been effectively ignored.

Mica was immediately referred to a surgeon, who ordered a CT scan of Mica's belly. A huge tumor occupying 70 percent of the entire abdominal cavity was detected. A blood sample was obtained to measure a liver-produced protein, alpha-fetoprotein. Not unexpectedly, the level was extremely elevated.

Immediate surgery was recommended for Mica, then only forty-two weeks old. The surgeon attempted to resect the tumor, which she inadvertently ruptured, resulting in seeding the cancer cells throughout the abdominal cavity. She also perforated the colon (the cecum) in an attempt to remove the huge tumor.

Mica survived the surgery and the complicating peritonitis from the bowel perforation. The diagnosis was hepatoblastoma, a tumor that had had its origins prior to birth, a so-called embryonal tumor. A chemotherapy schedule was initiated some three weeks after and continued until she was nineteen months of age. At that point, because of a continuous cough, an x-ray revealed metastatic cancer in the left lobe of her lung. Further surgery was indicated, and about 8 percent of her right lung was resected with the tumor. A new schedule of chemotherapy began and continued for the following three months.

A consultation with a geneticist at the time the hepatoblastoma was detected concluded with the diagnosis of a rare congenital disorder called the Beckwith-Wiedemann syndrome. Mica had the diagnostic features of this rare but well-known disorder evident from birth.

Mica's parents sued all of the physicians who had seen and failed to diagnose and monitor Mica's disorder, which could have initiated timely and proper lifesaving surveillance and treatment.

Pertinent Medical Facts

The Beckwith-Wiedemann syndrome is a remarkable disorder that variably and unpredictably interferes with growth in the womb. At delivery, infants are often large for their gestational age. This congenital disorder is recognized by a characteristic combination of signs (a syndrome) that include newborn hypoglycemia; a large tongue that protrudes; an increased size and length of the body on one side (hemihypertrophy); not infrequently an opening in the abdominal wall, allowing some bowel to extrude through the gap around the belly button (called omphalocele); tumors of the liver, kidney, and adrenal glands among others that have embryonic origins; and increased size of organs within the abdominal cavity (kidney, adrenal, etc.). A curious unexplained finding is a linear crease in the lobes of the ears. This syndrome occurs in about one in ten thousand live births.

Mica manifested the combination of hypoglycemia, large tongue, and hemihypertrophy. In addition, there was also a typical red birthmark on the forehead just above the nose.

The clinical signs would alert the pediatrician to check for hypoglycemia and initiate a surveillance plan. The follow-up includes ultrasound scanning of the liver and kidney at the time of diagnosis and every three months until eight years of age. In addition, a blood sample should be examined for a liver protein, alpha-fetoprotein, every three months for the first four years of life, aiming to detect early development of a liver cancer (hepatoblastoma). An elevated or rising level of alpha-fetoprotein would spark an immediate and detailed search for the site within the liver of the developing cancer. Surgical intervention, with excision of the tumor and chemotherapy, could be lifesaving. Ultrasound of the kidney is recommended from the age of eight to midadolescence, with special reference to kidney stones.

This syndrome appears out of the blue in about 85 percent of cases. About 15 percent have a family history, with one parent possibly having been affected or a child having been conceived by assisted reproductive technology (ART). A 2017 Italian study of 379,872 live births concluded that the Beckwith-Wiedemann syndrome occurred about ten times more often in children born following ART compared with those conceived naturally. Earlier English studies suggested a five times increased risk. The frequency in the Italian study was 1 in 1,126 live births and 1 in 3,724 in the English study. Another disorder with intellectual disability and other neurological signs (Angelman syndrome) is also thought to occur with increased frequency following ART. Additional risks include multiple pregnancies, preterm birth, and an increase in birth defects.

At the time Mica was born, the location of the culprit gene was known to be on the short arm of chromosome 11. Less than 1 percent of cases would have been detected by a routine chromosome analysis. However, the signs that Mica manifested were classical and diagnostic. We now know the culprit gene (*CDKN1C*) and its neighbors have complex functions that interfere with gene expression and, frequently, growth. Moreover, complex inheritance patterns are now recognized where, for example, the pair of number 11 chromosomes normally contributed by each parent may in fact originate from one parent only (called uniparental disomy).

Questions

- How and why was the diagnosis of the Beckwith-Wiedemann syndrome missed?
- Did that failure result in the lack of a surveillance plan?

Commentary

There are over two thousand congenital malformation syndromes. Geneticists constantly use major databases when confronted with patients manifesting multiple malformations. It would be unrealistic to expect a family physician or pediatrician to immediately recognize a rare syndrome. It is, however, the expected standard of care for the primary-care doctor, and those caring for infants and children in particular, to note specific and particular signs. Mica had a large tongue (macroglossia), hemihypertrophy, a birthmark on her forehead, and hypoglycemia. The hemihypertrophy alone should have immediately led to a referral to a clinical geneticist. Further departures from the expected standard of care included the failures to either confer or refer to a geneticist and to establish a surveillance program, starting with an ultrasound of Mica's liver and kidneys. Moreover, the required serial alpha-fetoprotein measurement was not made and no arrangement scheduled for the necessary surveillance every three months for both the alpha-fetoprotein level and abdominal ultrasound scanning until the age of eight years. This would have led directly to the early diagnosis and timely treatment of the developing embryonal hepatoblastoma.

The orthopedic surgeon had the responsibility to refer Mica to a geneticist. His duties extended beyond orthotics or a later plan to surgically deal with Mica's leg-length discrepancy.

I have repeatedly emphasized the frequency and importance of diagnostic errors in other chapters and will not reiterate the discussion here. The additional lesson that Mica's case introduces is the critical importance of anticipatory surveillance in the face of a diagnosed genetic disorder.

The Beckwith-Wiedemann syndrome represents only one example where an established schedule of surveillance can be lifesaving. Many other genetic disorders are in this category. For example, in neurofibromatosis (see chapter 27), the realization of the increased risk of a tumor involving the optic nerves in the brain (optic glioma) is important enough to establish surveillance imaging. In another case I have reviewed, failure led to a missed diagnosis of an optic glioma that had resulted in blindness thus far and will eventually lead to death of that patient because of the inability to resect the whole tumor due to its location in the brain. Another commonly inherited genetic disorder called tuberous sclerosis requires imaging surveillance of both the brain (for tumors) and the kidney (for tumors). Awareness of pigmented spots on the lips or genitals, which may signal the future development of colon cancer, should also initiate lifelong attention and surveillance.

Diagnostic failure has immediate and late, often disastrous, consequences.

This case was settled. But once again, neither doctor knew they did not know. After considerable suffering, Mica died.

CULPABILITY

Alice was twenty-five years old and happy to be pregnant at last. She had a history of irregular menses and ovarian cysts, and it had taken over a year to achieve a pregnancy. Other than repeated urinary-tract infections, pregnancy proceeded without other problems. Records did, however, note that Alice had a history of alcohol abuse. Alice's own mother informed the doctor that her drinking was out of control. Alice acknowledged that she had been drinking twenty-four beers per week and an entire case of beer on weekends. She had also had three alcohol-related legal offenses.

Alice's father had a history of petit mal seizures in childhood, intellectual disability, delayed motor development, and a developmental language disorder, for all of which he had required special-education services throughout schooling.

Alice went into labor at forty-one weeks gestation. Because of a failure to progress, arrangements were made to assist delivery by vacuum extraction. When her doctor applied the vacuum extractor in an attempt to pull the baby out, he used such force as to cause the vacuum extractor to break in two. Undaunted, he applied a second vacuum extractor but without success. Incredulously, he asked for a third vacuum extractor, which, in addition to the first two, also lost suction and popped off the scalp. Approximately, one hour was spent in the failed attempts to extract the baby out of the birth canal. Almost another hour went by waiting for a specialist obstetrician to appear, at which time the decision was made for Cesarean section. At this time, the monitor strips of the fetal heart were nonreassuring.

Abby was born smeared with meconium (the first stool) but with a lusty cry. She weighed eight pounds twelve ounces and had a normal head circumference and length. There was a prominent bulge at the site where the suction cup had been placed (a cephalhematoma). Her Apgar scores were eight and eight at one and five minutes, respectively, indicating normal heart rate, respiration, color, reflexes, and tone.

However, some four hours after delivery, she suddenly had an episode of rhythmic movements that progressed into a grand mal seizure. She had a few more seizures as well as some significant periods of apnea (not breathing). An immediate CT scan of her brain revealed a very small subdural hemorrhage.

A few seizures later, her oxygen saturation diminished as a consequence of episodes of respiratory distress. She was intubated, attached to a ventilator, and transferred to a teaching hospital. During her first two weeks of life in hospital, she was also noted to have a urinary-tract infection and reflux of urine back up the ureters toward the kidneys (vesicoureteral reflux). Due to a maternal history of herpes viral infection, Abby was started on prophylactic antiviral medication (acyclovir). She was also started on intravenous antibiotics because of possible urinary-tract infection.

By three months of age, strabismus (cross-eyes) was noted, and the growth rate of her brain had slowed resulting in a head circumference in the tenth percentile. At one year of age, it was clear that she had significant psychomotor delay. At twenty-one months of age, her head circumference had lagged further to the fifth percentile with a note that she had just begun taking her first steps at twenty months of age. She also had episodes of screaming during the night and day. A neuropsychological evaluation at two years three months of age documented significant delays across multiple domains, including adaptive behaviors and language, cognitive, and motor functioning. Brain imaging at the time showed thinning of the corpus callosum (the bundle of neurons that connects the two hemispheres).

At two years of age, Abby's head circumference was in the third percentile. She had midface underdevelopment (hypoplasia); a comma-shaped fold in the corner of each eye (epicanthal folds); short palpebral fissures (measurements from the inner to outer corner of each eye); drooping eyelids; a broad, flat bridge to her nose; a thin upper lip; a long, flat philtrum (the midline indentation of the skin below the nose); a small jaw; a high-arched palate; and low-set ears. Her fifth fingers and fifth toes curved inward (clinodactyly), and her toenails were underdeveloped. On formal testing and screening, her verbal performance and full-scale IQ were below the third percentile. At twenty-one months, brain imaging by

MRI showed tiny, scattered areas of brain damage (encephalomalacia) as well as microcephaly (small brain).

Alice and her husband sued her family doctor (who was board certified in obstetrics) and the hospital for their negligence in causing the irremediable brain damage to Abby, for their failure to perform a timely Cesarean section, for allowing the use of the vacuum extractor incorrectly and when not appropriate for an excessive period of time and with excessive force, and for failing to recognize that Abby's head was too large for the birth canal (cephalopelvic disproportion).

Pertinent Medical Facts

The use of the vacuum extractor with repeat pop-offs was not in line with guidelines from the American College of Obstetrics and Gynecology. The initial brain-imaging findings of both subdural (under the outer cover—the dura that envelopes the brain) and subgaleal (under the tight membrane that covers the bones of the skull) hemorrhage were consistent with injury due to excessive force in the attempts made by the vacuum extractor. Later imaging showing multifocal encephalomalacia confirmed more extensive brain damage. Encephalomalacia occurs when blood flow, and hence oxygen, ceases entirely in tiny capillaries, resulting in the death of brain tissue in the tiny areas supplied by the capillary. The brain tissue dies, and the dead tissue is resorbed, forming tiny cysts; hence, the term "cystic encephalomalacia," which Abby sustained.

A study of 5,036 women focused on maternal alcohol consumption was reported from the Vanderbilt University Medical Center in Nashville, Tennessee. The researchers noted that 55 percent of these participants reported using alcohol in the first three months of pregnancy. The US Centers for Disease Control has similar figures for women imbibing alcohol and again stresses the fact that more than half of all pregnancies in the United States are unplanned.

The Centers for Disease Control and Prevention has established guidelines for the diagnosis of fetal

alcohol syndrome. In essence, children are assigned an alcohol-exposure-related diagnosis based on their

criteria:

- Growth restriction with current or past weight and height less than the tenth percentile

- Abnormal facial features that include a smooth philtrum, thin upper lip (narrow vermillion

   border), and short palpebral fissures (length between inner to outer corners of the eye)

- Central nervous system abnormalities that show structural, functional, or neurological deficits

   evidenced by a head circumference below the tenth percentile; structural changes on brain

   imaging; functional deficits reflected by global cognitive delays with performance below the third

   percentile; and standardized tests of cognitive, executive, motor, attentional, and social skills or

   sensory function more than two standard deviations below the mean.

Children who have confirmed exposure and meet criteria for the abnormal facial features mentioned,

together with neurodevelopmental deficits, but have normal growth patterns are diagnosed with partial

fetal alcohol syndrome. Clearly, Abby had confirmed alcohol exposure, very significant functional deficits,

global cognitive delays, seizures, esotropia (one eye turned inward), and the vesicoureteral reflux related to

the fetal alcohol exposure. Her growth, however, was normal, giving her the designation of partial fetal

alcohol syndrome. There was, however, thinning of the corpus callosum, a finding consistent with alcohol

exposure.

Fetal alcohol spectrum disorders (FASDs) rank as the most important cause of preventable developmental

deficits and disabilities *in the world*. The prevalence of all forms of FASD ranges between 2.4 and 4.8

percent in the US population. These staggering figures represent one in forty-two to one in twenty-one

individuals affected in some significant way by maternal alcohol consumption. The American Academy

of Pediatrics has clearly stated that no amount of alcohol intake at any time during pregnancy can be

considered safe and that binge drinking is especially risky.

Questions

- Was Abby's claimed brain damage due to the vacuum extractor or her mother's alcoholism?

Commentary

I have been saddened by the hundreds (actually more than a thousand) of cases I have reviewed for either plaintiffs or defense of claims of brain damage due to alleged obstetrical negligence. My role has not been to comment on the standards of expected obstetrical care but rather to determine if a genetic or other basis existed for claims made could be substantiated. I have learned about the almost-invariable multifactorial causation in all of these cases. Inevitably, in the face of an adverse pregnancy outcome, there is frequently an effort to blame the obstetrician or midwife who provided the necessary care.

Cases included prolonged labor, malfunction of the electronic fetal monitor, problems related to vacuum use, the long decision-to-incision time for Cesarean section, lack of the availability of the obstetrician or anesthesiologist, absence of a pediatrician available for newborn resuscitation, the noncaring attitude of the attending staff, and on and on. However, not infrequently, other factors besides outright neurogenetic disorders impact the outcome. These on occasion may include chromosomal abnormalities, microdeletion or microduplication abnormalities in the genome (see chapter 38), maternal gestational diabetes, fetal alcohol exposure, medications that cause birth defects, and maternal genetic disorders. There are many more factors.

It is startling how often a prospective mother is careless about her own health (obesity, alcohol, drugs, no or late prenatal care) only to blame her doctor for an adverse outcome to pregnancy. While the care rendered in this case fell well below the expected standard of care, it is all but certain that Abby was also irreparably brain damaged by her mother's alcoholism. The small subdural and subgaleal bleeds caused by the vacuum did not affect brain tissue, as confirmed by imaging. The defense was weakened by the doctor's incorrect use of the vacuum and the observation of encephalomalacia.

I have noticed over and over again that babies with various genetic disorders or birth defects often don't do well during labor and delivery. Babies who seem normal at birth (with normal Apgar scores), but after a difficult and prolonged labor and delivery, not infrequently are found later to have a genetic disorder, such as a microdeletion or microduplication (see chapter 38). That diagnosis surprisingly is often made during the course of litigation.

In this case, Alice also had a family history of a grandfather with narcolepsy (a disorder with excessive sleep) and a father who had had seizures in childhood and who had a borderline IQ.

It didn't help much that in this case, the obstetrician had some years earlier entered a plea of guilty to a federal felony crime that he knowingly and intentionally possessed cocaine with the intent to distribute. He had also been sentenced to serve a term of incarceration for one year and one day and was fined $15,000 following his plea of guilty. His license to practice medicine had been suspended. Some years later, his letter requesting his reinstatement was approved.

Not unexpectedly, the case was settled.

A BINDER VERSION

Marian was startled when the ultrasound technician suddenly announced that the fetus was lying in the breech position. This study was being done at thirty-two weeks of pregnancy, with three previous ultrasound studies of that pregnancy showing normal results and the fetus in vertex (head first) position. The obstetrician quickly came in and reassured Marian that all would be well and that he would either reposition the fetus so as to achieve a vaginal delivery head first or, if really necessary, perform a Cesarean section. He also said that it was additionally comforting to know that there were no abnormalities seen on the ultrasound study.

At thirty-eight weeks, yet another ultrasound confirmed the breech position. The obstetrician decided to turn the fetus around, which he proceeded to do with a known maneuver (external podalic version). The fetus immediately somersaulted back to the breech position. Undaunted, the obstetrician called his partner, and together they repeated the external podalic version, holding the fetus in the vertex position by wrapping a tight binder around Marian's belly. The binder remained in place for another week until she went in to labor and delivered her first son, Abe. It was immediately obvious at birth that Abe was paralyzed from the nipple line downward.

At birth, Abe weighed seven pounds ten ounces, had a normal head circumference, and had a good heart rate of 120 beats per minute. He had good color and tone of his upper limbs but completely flaccid legs. Initially, he had respiratory difficulty and required oxygen by bag and mask. Dismay filled the labor ward. Wild speculation filled the air, with suggestions of a spinal tumor, a spinal fracture during delivery, or some rare genetic disorder affecting the spine. Other than the obstetrician in attendance, no one in the labor ward knew about the external podalic version and the use of the binder.

Needless to say, Marian and her husband were horrified at the outcome of what was an otherwise uneventful pregnancy, except for the breech position. It did not take long for them to consult a lawyer even as they confronted the enormous challenges ahead caring for Abe with his high-level spinal-cord paralysis. An MRI of Abe's spine revealed an infarction (tissue death from inadequate blood supply) of his spinal cord, extending from thoracic vertebra one to the fourth thoracic vertebra.

Marian and her husband sued the obstetrician and the birthing hospital for the irreversible, irremediable injury Abe sustained in utero from the binder used to keep him in a vertex position.

<u>Pertinent Medical Facts</u>

About 3–4 percent of all pregnant women have a fetus at term lying in breech. All babies with a breech birth have an increased risk of complications during or following pregnancy. Babies born feet first in the breech position and delivered vaginally are likely to have more cognitive problems than those born head first. The likely reason is the possibility of some delay in delivering the head still in the birth canal as well as some potential pressure to the umbilical cord squished by the head as it passes through the birth canal. Published evidence shows that external podalic version after thirty-seven weeks of pregnancy reduces not only the number of babies in the breech position but also the number of Cesarean sections that would otherwise be required. However, delivery of the baby in the breech position requires solid training and experience. Many obstetricians today are likely to recommend a Cesarean section given a fetus in the breech position. Attempts at external podalic version in the thirty-three- to thirty-five-week period are associated with an increased risk of preterm delivery.

Certainly for the single fetus in the breech position, Cesarean section has been regarded as safer for the fetus than vaginal birth. It is important to remember that Cesarean section is associated with an increased incidence of maternal morbidity as well as mortality.

Unfortunately, external podalic version is often unsuccessful, as was the case in Marian's pregnancy. What was particularly unusual in this pregnancy was the unorthodox use of a binder to maintain the fetus in a vertex position after the podalic version.

Specific guidelines for external podalic version include the following conditions:

- The presenting part of the fetus must not be engaged in the pelvis.

- The abdominal muscles and the uterine muscles must not be highly irritable and contracting.

- There has to be a sufficient volume of amniotic fluid.

- Continuous monitoring of the fetal heart with ultrasound is required.

- An ultrasound study immediately after the procedure is important to confirm that all is well with the fetus.

- Anesthesia should not be used in order to avoid undue force being used while performing the version.

Complications of this procedure include entanglement of the umbilical cord, thereby cutting off or interfering with the oxygen supply to the fetus, peeling of the placenta off the uterine wall (abruptio placenta), precipitating preterm labor, premature rupture of the membranes, and on occasion having the mother experience considerable pain. Complication rates over time have been less than 2 percent.

An additional risk for the baby born from a breech position is a slight increase in the frequency of birth defects. Instead of a 3–4 percent average background risk for all couples having a baby with a birth defect, intellectual disability, or genetic disorder, children born from a breech position have risks that approximate 6 percent. Why that is the case is speculative. Possibly, the condition affecting the baby may influence the movement inside the womb and limit the self-repositioning to a vertex position.

Question

- Did the use of the binder cause the spinal-cord infarction that paralyzed Abe?

Commentary

The use of the binder was clearly not the standard of care. Adopting an unorthodox method, without recent precedent and evidence of safety, introduced a risk for the patient and liability for the doctor. But how, you might ask, could a binder around Marian's belly interfere with the blood supply to one small portion of the spinal cord? Infarction of any tissue implies interruption of blood flow, and hence oxygen, to the tissue in question. How could there be an interruption of blood supply to this small portion of the body without any other tissue or organ involvement? One could theorize that the binder squeezed Abe in the womb, thereby interfering with the blood returning from the rest of his body via the largest vein in the body (the inferior vena cava that enters the heart) and thereby interrupting the blood flow to that region of the spinal cord. The additional information needed to support that theory is that in the affected region, there was a vascular watershed. That is, a congenital abnormal arrangement of the blood vessels at that spot represented an inborn vulnerability that threatened the viability of the spinal cord if the blood pressure dropped or the oxygen supply suddenly decreased.

So much for theory!

Further liability attached when it became clear that Marian had not provided informed consent for the unorthodox use of the binder, nor had there been any explanation of potential risk.

Given the unorthodox use of the binder and the lack of informed consent for use of that method, the case was readily settled.

A few years later, a published report from Japan in an American obstetrics journal reported an almost identical spinal-cord infarction in a pregnancy that had neither the fetus in breech nor the use of a binder!

WHO'S ON FIRST?

For those with long memories, this must evoke a smile. But in this case, this baseball metaphor applies to a tragic circumstance.

Marta and Henrique's first son was ten years of age when they decided to try and have another child. Their son, Ricardo, was diagnosed with Duchenne muscular dystrophy when he was five years of age. His ascending muscle weakness had progressed, resulting in him being confined to a wheelchair. I discussed this X-linked disorder in chapter 7 and outlined the awful progression of the disorder. A DNA test that demonstrated a duplication in the *Duchenne muscular dystrophy* (*DMD*) gene originally established Ricardo's diagnosis. At that time, the family was referred to a genetic counselor in the muscular dystrophy clinic in the teaching hospital.

Genetic counseling was provided, and genetic testing for Marta was recommended. In addition, recommendations were made, but without referral, about the need for cardiac surveillance, as carriers have risks of heart arrhythmias and even heart failure. The family, beset with the deteriorating status of Ricardo, did not pursue further testing.

About two years later, Marta and Henrique decided to try and have another child. Marta was in contact with the genetic counselor, who sent her the requisition to be taken to her primary-care doctor. This apparently was necessary because her insurance coverage required her primary-care doctor to sign any laboratory requisition. This was done, and a blood sample was sent to a major reference laboratory for analysis of the *DMD* gene. That laboratory sent a phlebotomist directly to Marta's home to draw the blood. In due time, the laboratory-test result came back to the signatory of the requisition form, the primary-care doctor.

In her deposition, the primary-care doctor stated that she simply looked at the name of the patient on the lab report and had it sent directly to Marta. This doctor stated that she wouldn't have read the laboratory report because of her inability to understand the complex nature of the genetic test results. She did, however, acknowledge that, as the ordering physician, she would receive the result. She stated that she sent the laboratory report to the mother (who could hardly speak English, let alone read) so that she could "do due diligence" and take the report to the muscular-dystrophy clinic for a proper explanation. The genetic counselor's name and contact information were also on the requisition form, but she did not receive a copy of the report.

No further communication occurred until some four months later, when the neurologist in the muscular-dystrophy clinic informed the genetic counselor by e-mail that the carrier-test result for Marta was negative. The genetic counselor called Marta to discuss the good news that she was not a muscular-dystrophy carrier.

Fourteen months passed when Marta returned to the muscular-dystrophy clinic for a visit with her first son. She was twenty-nine weeks along in her second pregnancy. That pregnancy went uneventfully to term.

For almost two years, their second son, Arturo, did reasonably well, except for walking rather late at fifteen months of age. However, a few months later, just prior to his second birthday, it was clear that he too was affected by Duchenne muscular dystrophy.

Only after Arturo was diagnosed did the neurologist and the genetic counselor discover the error in their communication based on their failure to actually see the laboratory report that clearly stated Marta was a carrier of a *DMD* gene mutation. By the time this error about Marta's true carrier status had been communicated, Arturo was already three years of age.

A letter of apology was written by the clinical geneticist, who had the responsibility of overseeing the genetic counselor.

The primary-care doctor was in private practice, and the muscular-dystrophy clinic was in the teaching hospital that employed the neurologist, the clinical geneticist, and the genetic counselor.

Marta and Henrique sued all the physicians, the associated university, and the hospital for the negligent care that resulted in the birth of Arturo with an irreversible, irremediable, fatal genetic disorder.

Pertinent Medical Facts

In chapter 7, I outlined the symptoms and signs that characterize Duchenne muscular dystrophy. The responsibilities in this case are clear.

The primary-care doctor who signed the order form and understood that she would get the result had the primary responsibility of communicating the extremely important report of Marta's carrier status directly to the patient. If, for any reason, she was unable to understand the report that clearly stated that Marta was a carrier, she had the responsibility to contact the patient and direct her to immediately see a clinical geneticist. Sending a technical report with genetic sequencing information to a patient, who spoke little English in the first place, was highly irresponsible and demonstrated a profound lack of knowledge and a pathetic lack of understanding and professionalism.

The genetic counselor whose name was also on the requisition form had the responsibility of obtaining the report and explaining the information to Marta. This genetic counselor, it turned out, was working without a license.

The neurologist in the muscular-dystrophy clinic made the error of confusing Marta with another patient's results, compounding all errors by informing the genetic counselor that Marta was not a carrier even without seeing the report.

The clinical geneticist had the responsibility of overseeing the genetic counselor.

Questions

- How did three physicians and a genetic counselor fail to provide proper care and treatment to a patient at high risk of having a second child with muscular dystrophy?

Commentary

This is yet another instance of appalling care by multiple doctors caring for the same patient. The sheer ignorance of the primary-care doctor about the most common form of muscular dystrophy in childhood leaves one speechless. This was a doctor who had been *recertified*. What hopeless exercise does that recertification represent? She stated, under oath, that she knew very little about muscular dystrophy. Compounding her ignorance was the complete lack of her awareness of her responsibility to inform the patient face-to-face about an extremely important laboratory result that had life-threatening consequences. If she did not understand the laboratory report that clearly stated that Marta was a carrier, she should have made sure in Spanish (which she spoke) that the patient understood the critical importance of immediately seeing a clinical geneticist or the genetic counselor. Incredulously, she maintained in her deposition that she did not even look at the report, which she would not be able to understand, but simply forwarded it on to the patient by mail, expecting her to "do due diligence and take the report to the muscular dystrophy clinic." Her actions were the proximate cause of a series of management errors by others involved in Marta's care.

The neurologist was aware that a carrier test had been done. She neither saw nor sought the laboratory report. After being away for a few days, she returned to her office and sent an e-mail to the genetic counselor, stating that Marta was not a carrier of the *DMD* gene mutation, and quoted in that e-mail a completely different mutation to what Marta already had. Long after she eventually got to know the true positive test result, she instructed the genetic counselor to inform the mother of the failure in communication rather than do that herself. She also blamed the victim, Marta, who she thought would either call for the result or seek the advice of the neurologist who was treating her son once she received the copy of the laboratory report. She acknowledged that Marta, who hardly spoke English, would not be able to interpret the result and would hardly be able to understand the implications.

The genetic counselor, working in the teaching hospital, did not have a license! She never received a copy of the laboratory report even though her name and contact information were on the laboratory requisition form, nor did she bother either to look for it or to request a copy. She also had no pending test-result list. She did receive the e-mail from the neurologist in the muscular-dystrophy clinic and was aware of the specific mutation causing the DMD in Marta's first son. She failed to recognize the error in the neurologist's e-mail that stated a completely different mutation in a *DMD* gene, which clearly belonged to another patient. Based on the neurologist's e-mail, she let Marta know that she was "not a carrier."

Only after Ricardo was diagnosed at two years of age did the search begin for Marta's original carrier-test report. At that time, the report was found in the medical chart. After it became clear that Marta had been wrongly informed about her carrier status, the neurologist instructed the genetic counselor to inform Marta. The genetic counselor called the patient, left a message, and received no return call. A full seven months then elapsed before Marta was informed of the error. No good explanation of why it took so long was given.

The genetic counselor was placed on "administrative leave."

The senior clinical geneticist who had the responsibility for overseeing the genetic counselor appeared to exercise very limited and inadequate control over her activities. She was vested with the responsibility of writing a letter of apology, which she sent by certified mail to Marta some seven months after the error had been discovered.

After their first son had been diagnosed with DMD, Marta and Henrique had received genetic counseling, were informed of the 50 percent risk of having another affected boy, and were told that a carrier test was recommended for Marta. For all of the five years after their first son was diagnosed, Marta and Henrique coped with the anguish having their child in a wheelchair, destined to die, and postponed their decision to have another child. Because of the miserable insurance system they were subject to, Marta first saw the genetic counselor, who provided the requisition form for the test. This form, she had to take to the primary-care doctor on a second trip in order for the form to be signed. Thus began the awful series of events with an ultimately catastrophic ending.

As an aside, and a further indicator of poor care, it took some five years for a diagnosis to be made in their first son.

It was also a highly irregular practice for a commercial laboratory to send a phlebotomist to a patient's house to draw blood for genetic testing.

Yet again, this sad case reflects administrative and system shambles. There was inadequate or no oversight of an unlicensed genetic counselor, who failed to obtain a critically important laboratory report and failed to timely contact the patient. The neurologist communicated the wrong result, pointing to the fallibility of people, despite the electronic medical record. Conjoined errors in this case included ignorance, communication failure, lack of judgment, and absent oversight.

Here once again was a family who suffered "loss of chance," the doctrine that deprived them of the opportunity to avoid, in this case, a fatal genetic disorder. Beyond the disorganization that this case represents, there is one single predominant problem. No one cared about the family, let alone to do their job properly. Careless, thoughtless, and insensitive management continues to plague medical care. This was a case where all of the involved caregivers should have known that failure of simple communications could result in such devastating consequences. Shame on them!

THE LONG AND THE SHORT

Tanya and Marvin fell in love during their junior year in college. They found that they had many interests in common, except for Marvin who enjoyed long-distance marathon-like runs. Both were tall and good looking, and they were both in good health. Tanya did have a history of having fainted twice in the past when she was twelve and thirteen years of age. Her parents ascribed both of those unexpected events to dehydration on hot days. On both occasions, they took her to her pediatrician, who upon a thorough physical examination found no abnormalities and reassured them that all was well. He did not take a family history.

When Tanya and Marvin returned from their spring break, tensions between them began to emerge. On a bright spring day, the tensions culminated in a fierce argument, with Marvin storming out of her dorm room, shouting that he was done with their relationship. Distraught, Tanya picked up the phone and called her mother, sobbing. She was drowsy and irritable from the antihistamine that she had been taking for her spring allergies. While speaking to her mother, she looked out of the window to see Marvin striding toward his car. Crying, she rushed out of her room and raced down three flights of stairs, shouting out to him to stop. Some thirty yards from the exit, and still shouting for Marvin to wait, Tanya fell down, dead.

The mandatory autopsy revealed no obvious cause of death.

The coroner could only speculate that Tanya had had a sudden fatal arrhythmia that caused her death.

Many months later, her mother came to see me with the concern about what happened to Tanya and whether her two other children were at risk. This was especially concerning given that two of her brothers died suddenly, one in his twenties and one in his thirties, without an established diagnosis in either case.

I suggested that a sample of tissue that the coroner would have collected and kept from his autopsy of Tanya be obtained so that we could perform specific DNA tests for at least one or more genetic disorders associated with cardiac arrhythmias and sudden death. The sample was duly obtained, and we determined a precise mutation in a gene that results in a disorder called the long QT syndrome (LQTS). The family history was typical, with a history of fainting and sudden death in family members. We went on to show that Tanya's mother also had this genetic mutation.

She had been considering a lawsuit against her pediatrician but eventually did not pursue litigation.

Cardiologists have generally not been as fortunate. Closed claims of medical professional-liability risk were analyzed in cases against 781 cardiologists. Some 13.6 percent resulted in an indemnity payment. More than 50 percent of all claims involved a patient's death. Acute coronary syndrome was the most frequent condition.

***

Tanya's case was sadly reminiscent of a legal case for which I was consulted.

Linda, in anticipation of her marriage scheduled in four weeks' time, decided to have her wisdom teeth out while she was still on her parent's insurance. Her longtime dentist did the extraction using a precisely focused local anesthetic. Literally moments after the extraction, Linda twitched briefly and appeared to lose consciousness. Actually, she had stopped breathing and had died in the dentist's chair. The horrified dentist and his assistant simply looked on aghast and shocked, without knowing what to do. They had no protocol to follow and no emergency kit to use, and it took some five minutes before realizing that she actually had died. They tried CPR, first in the dental chair and then lifting her down to the floor while a call was made to emergency services. The first responders arrived within ten minutes, only to confirm that Linda had died.

Linda's parents sued this dentist whose total unpreparedness deprived Linda of the chance of survival.

Pertinent Medical Facts

Much has been learned about the long QT syndrome (LQTS) since its first description in 1957. We now know that a rhythm disturbance of the heart (arrhythmia) that can prove fatal can occur when there is interference with the normal nervous-system-generated currents that keep our hearts beating normally. These generated currents spread like an electric wave through the heart muscle and are controlled by complex neurophysiological mechanisms. These involve the movement of potassium, sodium, and calcium through ion channels, whose structure and function in turn are controlled by proteins from specific genes. The LQTS is therefore regarded as a "channelopathy," one of many genetic disorders that are so categorized.

From a study of forty-five thousand newborns, the determination was made that the LQTS occurs in between one in two thousand and one in twenty-five hundred people. The LQTS is for the most part an inherited autosomal dominant disorder caused by abnormalities in those cardiac ion channels. An affected person has a 50 percent risk of transmitting the disorder to each of his or her offspring. Just as in all autosomal dominantly inherited disorders, new mutations do occur but are thereafter transmissible to offspring.

There are instances, however, of acquired forms of LQTS. A family history, therefore, provides the very first potential warning of this condition. Specifically, a history of someone mostly under forty years of age, who was otherwise healthy, dying suddenly, always raises the question of the possible LQTS. A history of unexplained fainting is generally the most common first indication of this disorder and reflects extremely rapid sudden-onset escalation of the heart rate (ventricular tachycardia). Spontaneous cessation allows a person to get up and resume his or her activities, but the tachycardia may morph into fatal ventricular fibrillation. About 50 percent of those affected experience their first cardiac event by the age of twelve (usually fainting) and 90 percent by the age of forty. The cause of sudden infant death syndrome (SIDS) is thought to be due to the LQTS in about 10 percent of cases.

Remarkably, specific triggers of arrhythmias in the LQTS are well recognized. Among the most important are physical exertion, especially swimming, emotional stress, or a sudden loud noise such as an alarm clock or telephone (typically upon waking). A history of a major seizure (epilepsy) occurring without explanation and accompanied by no findings on a physical examination or on brain imaging also raises the question of the LQTS. An electrocardiogram should then be added to the evaluation. Curiously, hormones also have some effect, with increased risks recognized in mothers in the weeks after birth, and the fact that males have an increased risk prepuberty, with females more commonly affected after puberty, as well as postmenopause.

The peaks and valleys of the squiggles seen when an electrocardiogram is done are named by letters (*P, Q, R, S, T*). Extremely precise measurements are made of the spaces between the peaks. Knowing the precise normal range, for example, between the Q and T peaks in milliseconds, and computed by well-known formulas, enables the detection of a prolonged interval between Q and T (the long QT syndrome) or a very short interval (the short QT syndrome).

Thus far at least fifteen genes and their mutations can cause LQTS. These mutated genes and the resulting abnormal proteins interfere with the structure and function of the ion channels causing the LQTS. Some of the more common LQTS genes and their mutations are known to more likely trigger arrhythmias that occur during swimming or emotional events. The longer the QT interval is, the greater the likelihood of an arrhythmia.

QT prolongation may even be noted in affected infants. We published our genetic findings in 2005 of the LQTS in eight infants ranging in age from one day to one year. The LQTS has also been diagnosed prenatally with the electronic fetal monitor in the third trimester of pregnancy or as early as eleven weeks of pregnancy by precise gene-mutation analysis. Knowing the exact mutation would allow an affected person the opportunity to utilize preimplantation genetic diagnosis to avoid transmitting this disorder to future offspring or to have prenatal genetic diagnosis.

Once diagnosed, and hopefully before any cardiac rhythm abnormalities, treatment with a beta-blocker has proven to be very effective in preventing arrhythmias. On occasion, when beta-blockers are contraindicated, surgery can be considered to interrupt the sympathetic nerve chain aiming to cut the nerve-driven stimulation of the heart. Many affected individuals have chosen to have an implantable cardioverter-defibrillator inserted in their chest wall. This device shocks the heart automatically should there be a cardiac arrest. Survival after cardiac arrest on medical treatment, or not, is a clear indication for this device, which should also be used to resolve continuing episodes of fainting while on medical treatment. Another indication is the finding of two different mutations in the same patient who is experiencing syncope while taking a beta-blocker. The usual recommendation to someone with the LQTS is to desist from competitive sports and similar activities but especially swimming.

Questions

- Why did Tanya's family not know that some of their members harbored a mutation in one of the LQTS genes?

- What triggered the arrhythmia that caused Tanya's death?

- Why did the dentist not have the required protocol and necessary measures to resuscitate Linda?

Commentary

Gene studies in Tanya's family revealed a mutation in the most common LQTS gene. It was the one in which physical exertion and emotional stress play a significant role as a trigger. However, there are other precipitating factors.

A whole range of drugs are known that have the potential to prolong the QT interval and may induce ventricular tachycardia or even ventricular fibrillation. An awesome list of drugs to be avoided if possible by anyone with LQTS can be found at www.azcert.org or www.torsades.org. On that list are antihistamines, including the one taken by Tanya! There is evidence of a genetic susceptibility to drug-induced QT-interval prolongation. We can anticipate that pharmacogenetic tests already reported will eventually be offered prior to starting a specific medication that risks QT prolongation.

Unexpected death during anesthesia has made additional protocols prior to, during, and after surgery necessary, with special attention to the QT interval.

There is a rare autosomal recessive type of LQTS that is associated with deafness and webbed fingers and toes. For recessive disorders, both parents of an affected person are carriers of a mutation in the same gene, causing the LQTS. There are also some other rare forms of the LQTS with additional signs that include periodic paralysis, a bone abnormality or defect, immune deficiency, intellectual disability, and even autism.

While a very prolonged QT interval bodes trouble and potential disaster if not treated, a very short QT interval also invites potentially fatal arrhythmias. Fortunately, the short QT syndrome is rare. The therapeutic approach is, however, similar to the LQTS treatment protocols.

Tanya's two maternal uncles lived far apart and of course had different doctors. After the second uncle died years later, no one focused on the family history. Even though the family history is vital to the maintenance of a family's health, physicians systematically fail to maintain a carefully drawn family pedigree to which they could add life events at the time of the annual checkup, such as births, deaths, and specific diseases. Few appear to have the time or the inclination to do this simple but time-consuming task. Knowledge of these deaths by Tanya's pediatrician who was confronted with her fainting twice should have initiated an order for an electrocardiogram. Tanya's life almost certainly would have been saved by attention to this simple test. Needless to say, ignorance of the LQTS being heralded by fainting episodes is a further disturbing realization. Unfortunately, Tanya had multiple triggers for her arrhythmia that included a gene mutation, emotional distress, physical exertion, and the antihistamine.

Another unexpected error in this new era of precision medicine came to light in the *Boston Globe*. The report, commented on by an expert on the LQTS, Michael Ackerman, MD, of the Mayo Clinic, described a patient who had an implanted heart defibrillator. The commercial laboratory report had indicated the presence of a mutation in a LQTS gene, which led to the recommendation of the implantable cardiac defibrillator. Reanalysis by Dr. Ackerman revealed that the reported change in the gene was a harmless variant!

The dentist who cared for Linda was stunned into semiparalysis when she lost consciousness. It appeared that he could not promptly determine that she had had a cardiac arrest. Apparently, no stethoscope was available, and Linda's pulse could not be obtained. It took some five minutes for cardiopulmonary resuscitation to begin in earnest.

Professor Morton Rosenburg at Tufts University School of Dental Medicine has drawn attention to the fact that every dentist can be expected to be involved in this type of medical emergency over the course of clinical practice. He has emphasized that dentists should be able to diagnose medical problems that include fainting, hyperventilation, anaphylactic shock, and, of course, cardiac arrest. Every dentist is expected to have basic emergency drugs, equipment, and supplies as well as trained personnel with an established protocol to deal with unexpected emergencies. Critically important is the availability of lifesaving equipment that include a portable oxygen cylinder, nasal cannulae, bag and valve mask devices, Magill forceps to extract foreign objects stuck in the throat during dental treatment, an external cardiac defibrillator, and emergency drug kits that include epinephrine, an antihistamine, nitroglycerin, bronchodilator, glucose, aspirin, aromatic ammonia, and an anticonvulsant. State Boards of Registration in Dentistry have rather limited standard protocols for emergencies in the dental office. Sadly, Linda attended a dentist fully unprepared to act immediately and appropriately in a way that could have saved her life. This dentist had no idea that he didn't know, he didn't know.

The fact that this case was settled did not make up for the anguish Linda's family felt from losing their daughter, never mind the wedding plans.

EPILOGUE

The avoidable deaths and harm in the families described represent a small fraction of the many that I have encountered. I selected cases that taught lessons and that would enable future avoidance and prevention of tragedy. While my involvement has invariably been about genetic issues at all ages, the lessons learned are truly generic and applicable to all specialties. Errors know no boundaries and ignore no medical discipline.

My discussion in this epilogue is addressed to all who are or will become patients. That is almost all of us, including physicians and nurses, who will also become patients. There are also very clear lessons and alerts for physicians and nurses. As patients and caregivers, we need to be watchful joint partners in our care. Awareness of potential pitfalls and where, when, and how errors occur empowers protective thought and action. If your doctor takes umbrage to your questions, concerns, or requests for a second opinion, seek another physician. Each of our lives and those of our loved ones are precious. Some 250,000 annually no longer have a say in saving their own lives!

Most errors are made by good doctors. Slips, lapses, fumbles, distraction, preoccupation, inattention, laziness, carelessness, and thoughtlessness dominate the error spectrum. These errors, often seemingly simple, however, may have catastrophic consequences. Errors are invariably unintentional and hence hard to prevent or control. Deaths and lifetime harm often occur from desperately simple omissions.

Major events leading to tragic outcomes are, to an important extent, avoidable and preventable. I place failure to care above the usually top-ranked error, diagnostic failure. Where proper care is delivered, greater effort is made that includes conferring, referring, testing, and following up. On the heels of diagnostic error comes failures of oversight and supervision, incompetence, lack of skill, and system errors. In my experience, a lack of knowledge, though real, has not been a common major factor. Nor has misguided ineffective leadership (not uncommon) been a major contributor to the genesis of error.

Failures in rational decision making under circumstances of uncertainty, urgency, and pressure have featured largely in the obstetrics and emergency-medicine arenas. Much greater attention will be necessary in teaching about the need for situational awareness and orderly thinking without mental blinders.

A profound sense of sadness envelopes me when I confront the reality of all the thousands of families who have endured deaths and injuries of loved ones due to medical negligence. Many decades in the practice of medicine have taught me much about the complexities and challenges that we physicians constantly face. Learning from failure is an unpleasant experience and, when crowned by a lawsuit, is both devastating and demoralizing. Nevertheless, the legal cases I have selected do convey important messages about medical practice, systems issues, and being a doctor. I will discuss these in turn, recognizing inevitable overlap. My recommendations stem directly from the painful and poignant litigated cases described and from my extensive equal involvement for both plaintiff and defense.

Medical Practice

Experience is replete with simple examples in practice that end with disastrous consequences. The moment potential life-threatening or life-changing situations are recognized, both physicians and patients should be on full alert. Warning signals are often banal. For example, this could be as simple as a recommended key appointment not kept, a crucial referral not made, or a timely communication not sent or received. The physician initiating the appointment or crucial referral must ensure that the staff confirm to him or her personally that arrangements have indeed been made. No dependence on a fax should be permissible. Where the information is important, the physician is expected to be in direct *verbal* contact with the other caregivers. Who would otherwise have expected that death and life-destroying consequences would flow from failure to attend to such simple matters? Patients should make no assumptions. "I didn't hear from my doctor, so I assumed the test results were OK."

Important laboratory, imaging, pathology, or special test results should be communicated directly to the patient by the physician to ensure that there is no misunderstanding about the implications and immediate recommendations. Where any uncertainty exists about a technical report, the physician should personally call the laboratory. Test results should never be reinterpreted. The communications made should be documented and dated, even briefly.

In multiphysician practices (especially obstetrics) where a patient will be seen for continuing care from a different doctor for each visit, for example, during a pregnancy, or patients seen over years, one physician should be vested with overall responsibility, lest a critical piece of information be overlooked by another doctor who has not delved into a thick medical record or extensive electronic medical record. Dr. Donald Berwick, president emeritus of the Institute for Healthcare Improvement, has emphasized that "where responsibility is diffused, it is not clearly owned; with too many in charge, no one is."

Contemporary medical care very often has a patient being cared for by at least two specialists. There is a cogent need for intercommunication, especially, but not only, about medications. Pregnancy is a special case in this regard. Patients need to ensure their doctors are in communication (preferably by letter) about their shared care.

In this golden era of human genetics, every primary-care doctor's medical chart or electronic medical record should begin with a three-generation family pedigree, recording details about ethnicity, diseases, birth defects, births, and deaths. This pedigree should be updated at the time of each annual medical checkup. Now that over five thousand genes and their disease-causing mutations have been identified, opportunities abound for avoidance and prevention of serious to fatal genetic disease via carrier detection, prenatal diagnosis, and preimplantation genetic diagnosis. There are over seven thousand rare genetic disorders, and about one in twelve individuals are affected, knowingly or not. Gene discovery continues at a remarkable pace. Families with genetic disorders whose culprit genes have yet to be identified are advised to consult a geneticist annually.

If a physician is uncertain about the need to refer to a clinical geneticist, a phone call to confer is wise. The absence of a geneticist in the same town or area is no longer an excuse for failure to confer or refer. Blood samples for DNA studies can easily be sent to laboratories distantly located. At our Center for Human Genetics in Cambridge, Massachusetts, for example, we receive samples from forty-five countries!

The physician who signs a requisition for a laboratory test or whose name is affixed to it bears the responsibility of seeing (or seeking, if necessary) the result and ensuring that the patient at risk is informed. Over and over, I have noted disastrous consequences when physicians have not bothered to get an important result and neither cared nor communicated it. Patients cannot and should not assume that their result is normal, having not heard anything to the contrary. Needless to say, sending a complex laboratory report that has serious implications to a patient with the hope that they will "do due diligence" is a travesty and is outright negligent (chapter 46).

In hospitals, laboratory tests are usually ordered by residents in training, albeit under the watchful eyes of the attending resident. So often, after that, the resident rotates off the service or actually leaves the hospital, having completed training, and no one sees, seeks, or communicates the result to the patient or parent. I have repeatedly seen a lifetime of disability (and one death) as a consequence of failure to see or seek a critical laboratory result. Attending physicians with oversight of residents are expected to be aware of pending results and have the responsibility to obtain and communicate them and document that action. Resident handoffs represent a particularly vulnerable juncture in care, involving, as it often does, fatigue and haste, even in the face of the seriously ill.

In medical practice, an absolute strict rule should be in place that no laboratory report can be filed without being seen and initialed by the ordering physician. Unfortunately, completion of a requisition form by an assistant may result in the order of the wrong test (chapter 6). A simple glance by the physician in that case would have avoided a shortened lifetime of chronic illness. Where and when the test being ordered is unusual, uncommon, or particular in some way, the physician should personally contact the laboratory, radiologist, or a specific responsible individual. Deaths and lifetime handicaps have been the consequences of failures to perform this simple act (chapter 28).

Serious disorders that occur before the age of fifty should be considered as genetic until proven otherwise. Molecular tests are now often available to help resolve such questions. This turns out to be important, since there is a legally recognized "duty to warn" (chapter 14).

Notwithstanding the overall improvements, strict adherence to required checklists, and shout-outs in the surgical setting, serious errors continue to occur. "Never events" should surely be never (chapter 21). Obvious as it might seem, information checklists completed by patients should be carefully scrutinized (chapter 2).

Since to err is unfortunately human, we need to have the foresight of fallibility and be able to anticipate and plan prospectively for inevitable missteps. This calls for detailed, in-hospital, and in-practice meetings to recognize potential vulnerabilities and to discuss and plan both preventive and backup responses. Why wait for meetings to discuss root-cause analysis following a catastrophe?

I have discussed a wide range of errors and negligence in this book. Sadly, this subject is endless, and my selection has not included the common missed diagnoses of heart attacks and other diseases or the complications and harms due to iatrogenic catheter-associated urinary-tract infections, central-line bloodstream infections, venous clots (emboli) to the lungs, fall injuries, and pressure ulcers. Also not included are the myriad orthopedic and other surgical snafus (such as a cut brachial nerve) and obstetrical mishaps, including skull fractures at birth, hysterectomy with an undiagnosed fetus, and hundreds of infants' brains damaged by a lack of oxygen during delivery and whose files I have reviewed.

Remedial System Changes

Equipment failures aside, systems errors are people bound and therefore possibly remedial. The problems encountered that add to the carnage are deeply entrenched and not easily changed. The first problem area is poor leadership and management. Relevant to this discussion is the working atmosphere in which physicians, nurses, and other caregivers labor. The tone set by the CEO, surprisingly often unknown by the board of trustees of a hospital, may breed retaliatory consequences to expressed concerns and complaints (chapter 17). This attitude, as noted in an egregious case described, results in conscientious physicians not reporting colleagues perpetrating serous malpractice, dangerous consequences, or drug and alcohol addiction (chapter 22).

Underlying the second but related problem is greed, not necessarily personal but institutional. The dreadful example of the Swedish Cherry Hill Hospital saga (chapter 17) serves as a prime example for both problems. Why do boards of trustees who have fiduciary responsibilities so frequently appear oblivious to awful realities, only to rid institutions of errant leaders when it is often too late?

While mundane but equally critical for saving lives, detailed organizational oversight is essential. This would include attention to how urgent test results (laboratory, radiology, pathology, etc.) are received from inside the hospital or from elsewhere, how intensive-care units and neonatal intensive-care units are equipped and staffed, and how hospital pharmacies are managed to avoid errors. An institutional climate that fosters a caring atmosphere encourages both physicians to report negligent colleagues, aberrant behavior, drug and alcohol use, and nurses to break rank and report malpractice or behavioral aberrations without fear of retaliation or dismissal.

One hopes that reiteration of the grave concerns expressed in the introduction is not necessary here. There is an urgent and compelling need for state Boards of Registration in Medicine, accreditation agencies, state and federal governments, and professional colleges and societies to recognize the carnage and the crisis. One would hope that public indignation, anger, and dismay would lead to change. Surely impetus to such action could originate from the hundreds of thousands of families who have lost loved ones from medical negligence and the many more than that who have been harmed. Or are you waiting to swell the numbers?

Doctoring and Negligence

Let me emphasize again that the overwhelming majority of physicians are good, caring, and conscientious. Nevertheless, negligent acts obviously continue to occur at an alarming rate. Foresight and caring would go a long way to preventing catastrophes, especially if combined with planning and in anticipation of human limitations.

Diagnostic errors loom large on the horizon of negligence. Limited time in a busy practice is a constant and serious threat to the diagnostic effort. Remaining up to date, given huge advances in medicine, is a long-term challenge frequently foiled by fatigue. One would have hoped that recertification would go a long way to solving the problem of the out-of-date physician. Clearly, this is not always the case (chapter 46).

The categories of negligent failures I have personally noted in the many litigated cases that I have reviewed or testified in constitute a grim, dishonor roll, which I will briefly summarize. The failures listed are not rank ordered, and all have axiomatic and self-evident necessary remedies.

- Failure to care

- Failure to make a diagnosis of a serious or fatal disorder

- Communication failures

- Failure to render an expected standard of newborn care

- Making a preconceived diagnosis without establishing a meaningful differential diagnosis

- Decision failures in the face of uncertainty

- Failure to establish or use checklists

- Failure to apologize

- Failure to recognize infection in the newborn

- Failure in the preparation of intravenous medications or infusions

- Failure to recognize genetic causation

- Making erroneous assumptions about causation

- Failure to correctly interpret genetic test results

- Failure to observe and act on incidental findings

- Failure to obtain informed consent

- Failure to graph measurements

- Failure in reporting incorrect laboratory results

- Assuming omniscient power over patients' destinies

- Failure to carefully hand off patient care to a colleague

- Failure to discipline or fire errant physicians

- Failure to provide honest letters of reference

- Failure to recognize and warn of genetic risk

- Careless, thoughtless, callous handling of a patient, or failure to establish rapport

- Misleading trainees with false assumption of knowledge

- Visiting personal dictates of conscience on a patient

- Failure to consult, confer, or refer

- Incompetence and lack of skill

- Failure to check the execution of an order given to an assistant

- Not communicating with other physicians sharing the care of the same patient

- Blaming others for personal failures

- Depending on others without checking that necessary action was taken

- Failure to appreciate consequences of actions taken or not

- Failure to seek, see, and properly communicate reports vital for patient safety

- Lack of knowledge

- Failure to carefully listen to a patient

- Failure to recognize the genetic implications of ethnicity

- Failure to recognize imminent catastrophe

- Failure to report alcoholism or drug addiction resulting in dangerous care by caregivers

- Failure to discipline surgeons following "never events"

- Failure of oversight

- Laboratory mix-ups resulting in catastrophes

- Failure to heed warnings from nurses

- Failure to recognize the teratogenic effects of certain medications

- Ignorance, arrogance, and hubris

We all recognize the characteristics of the good doctor and one whom we would hope would care for us or our families—someone who is warm, empathic, kind, sensitive, and knowledgeable. All of us wish for a physician who is caring and concerned, engenders trust, is attentive, and actually looks at one instead of at a computer. We all need someone who listens and doesn't immediately interrupt (one often-quoted study revealed that it takes, on average, only eighteen seconds for a physician to interrupt a patient). One hopes that over time, when getting to know your physician, you may find that he or she refers and confers, willingly suggests another opinion, admits when he or she does not know, and is a decent human being.

We all hope we will not encounter arrogance, thoughtlessness, carelessness, hubris, and lack of knowledge in the physician we chose or were assigned to our care. Later we may discover that he or she is disheveled, robotic, insensitive, uncaring, and even angry. All of these epithets I have encountered in cases that have ended up in litigation, with specific reference to the failure of physicians to establish rapport and, unsurprisingly, to apologize. The latter two characteristics have frequently driven litigants to lawyers, often to discover what actually happened.

The number of deaths due to medical negligence every week of the year exceeds the losses on 9/11. Why has there been no mass uprising, no public indignation? Two hundred and fifty thousand dead from medical negligence! Many more than that harmed! A silent press, asleep. Federal and state-government agencies, accreditation agencies, professional colleges and societies, deans of medical schools, all recognizing no urgency. No crisis. No epidemic. It is time for all of us patients to become proactive and urge those in responsible positions to end the carnage.

Is the failure to recognize this ongoing tragedy due to our overwhelming need to believe in our doctors? Does our anxiety that we will not be cared for when in need trump any concern about harm to unknown others, dispersed across a nation, until it is a loved one? To know is to care. Now you know!

REFERENCE SOURCES*

Introduction

- Balogh EP, Miller BT, Ball JR. Improving diagnosis in health care. Washington, DC: The National Academies Press. 2015.
- Bell SK, Mann KJ, Truog R, et al. Should We Tell Parents When We've Made an Error? Pediatrics 2015;135;159.
- Burkle CM. Medical Malpractice: Can We Rescue a Decaying System? Mayo Clin Proc. 2011;86(4):326.
- Classen DC, Resar R, Griffin F et al. 'Global Trigger Tool' Shows That Adverse Events In Hospitals May Be Ten Times Greater Than Previously Measured. Health Affairs 2011;30:581.
- Faigman DL. Judges as "Amateur Scientists." B.U L. Rev. 2006, 86;5:1207.
- Gawande A. The Checklist Manifesto. New York, NY: Henry Holt and Co; 2009.
- Gluck P. Patient safety: Some progress and many challenges. Obstet Gynecol. 2012;120(5):1149.
- He F, Li L, Bynum J, et al. Medical Malpractice in Wuhan, China: A 10-Year Autopsy-Based Single-Study Center. Medicine (Baltimore) 2015 Nov;94(45):e2026.
- Institute of Medicine of the National Academies 2011 Update report: the learning health system and its innovation collaboratives, roundtable on value, and science-driven health care. Washington DC: Institute of Medicine: 2011.
- Kachalia A, Little A, Isavoran M, et al. Greatest Impact Of Safe Harbor Rule May Be To Improve Patient Safety, Not Reduce Liability Claims Paid By Physicians. Health Affairs 2014;33:59.
- Leape LL, Berwick DM. Counting deaths due to medical errors [letter]. JAMA 2002;288(19):2405.
- Leape LL, Berwick DM. Five Years After *To Err is Human*. JAMA 2005;293:2384.
- Makary MA, Daniel M. Medical error—the third leading cause of death in the US. BMJ 2016;353:i2139.
- McGlynn EA, McDonald KM, Cassel CK. Measurement Is Essential for Improving Diagnosis and Reducing Diagnostic Error. JAMA 2015;314:2501.
- Mello MM, Studdert DM, Kachalia A. The Medical Liability Climate and Prospects for Reform. JAMA 2014:312(20)2146.
- Nahed BV, Babu MA, Smith TR, et al. Malpractice liability and defensive medicine: a national survey of neurosurgeons. PLos One 2012;7(6):e39237.
- Newman-Toker DE, Pronovost PJ. Diagnostic Errors-The Next Frontier for Patient Safety. JAMA 2009;301(10):1060.
- Parekh A, Hoagland GW. Medical Liability Reform in a New Political Environment. JAMA 2017;317:1311.
- Pronovost P, Colantuoi E. Measuring preventable harm. JAMA 2009;301:1273.
- Pronovost P, Needham D, Berenholtz et al. An intervention to decrease catheter-related bloodstream infections in the ICU. N Engl J Med 2006;355:2725.
- Pronovost P, Vohr E. Smart Patients, Smart Hospitals. New York, NY: Hudson Street Press; 2010.
- Raine JE. An analysis of successful litigation claims in children in England. Arch Dis Child 2011;96:838.
- Reason JT. Beyond the organisational accident: the need for "error wisdom" on the frontline. Qual Saf Health Care 2004;13:ii28.
- Reason JT. Human Error. Cambridge University Press. Cambridge, 1990.

---

*Listed references represent only a selected fraction of sources that form the basis of this text. References are listed only once, although are applicable to other chapters too.

- Reason JT. Understanding adverse events: human factors. Quality in Health Care 1995;4:80.
- Reason JT, Carthey J, de Leval MR. Diagnosing "vulnerable system syndrome": an essential prerequisite to effective risk management. Quality in Health Care 2001;10:ii21.
- Saber Tehrani AS, Lee H, Mathews SC, et al. 25-Year summary of US malpractice claims for diagnostic errors 1986-2010: an analysis from the National Practitioner Data Bank. BMJ Qual Saf. 2013 Aug;22(8):672.
- Schulz K. Being Wrong: Adventures in the Margin of Error. New York: NY: Harper Collins Publishers; 2010.
- Shojania KG, Burton EC, McDonald KM, et al. Changes in rates of autopsy-detected diagnostic errors over time: a systematic review. JAMA 2003;289(21):2849.
- Thaler RH, Sunstein CR. Nudge. New Haven, CT: Yale University Press; 2008.

Chapter 1

- Milunsky A, Milunsky JM. Genetic Disorders and the Fetus: Diagnosis, Prevention and Treatment. 2015. Wiley: UK.
- Yandell DW, Campbell TA, Dayton SH, et al. Oncogenic Point Mutations in the Human Retinoblastoma Gene: Their Application to Genetic Counseling. N Eng J Med 1989;321(25):1689.

Chapter 2

- Grady MF. Why are people negligent? Technology, nondurable precautions, and the medical malpractice explosion. Northwestern Law Review 82;2:293.

Chapter 3

- Alpert, JS. What's In a Word? Using Words Carefully. Amer J Med 2015;128:1045.
- Hakonen AH, Davidzon G, Salemi R, et al. Abundance of the POLG disease mutations in Europe, Australia, New Zealand, and the United States explained by single ancient European founders. Eur J Hum Genet 2007;15:779.
- Milunsky A and Annas GG. Genetics and the Law III. Plenum Press, New York , 1984.
- Rajakulenran S, Pitceathly RDS, Taanman JW, et al. A Clinical, Neuropathological and Genetic Study of Homozygous A467T POLG-Related Mitochondrial Disease. PLoS ONE 2016;11(1):e0145500.

Chapter 4

- Casassus B. France bans sodium valproate use in case of pregnancy. 2017;390:217.
- Friend SH, Bernards R, Rogelj S, et al. A human DNA segment with properties of the gene that predisposes to retinoblastoma and osteosarcoma. Nature 1986;323(16);643.
- Herzog AG, Mandle HB, Cahill KE, et al. Predictors of unintended pregnancy in women with epilepsy. Neurology 2017;89:728.
- Lawn BA, Gareis K, Kormos W, et al. Communicate, don't litigate: The Schwartz Center Connections Program. J Healthcare Risk Man 2013;33(1):3.
- Meador KJ, Lindhour D. Epilepsy and unintended pregnancies. Neurology 2017;88:724.
- Milunsky A, Jick H, Jick SS, et al. Multivitamin/folic acid supplementation in the earliest weeks of pregnancy reduces the prevalence of neural tube defects. JAMA 1989;262:2847.

Chapter 5

- Annas GJ. Scientific evidence in the courtroom: The death of the Frye rule. N Eng J Med 1994;330:1018.
- Gold JA, Zaremski MJ, Lev ER, et al. Daubert v Merrell Dow: The Supreme Court Tackles Scientific Evidence in the Courtroom. JAMA 1993;270(24):2964.
- Masten J, Strzelczyk J. Admissibility of Scientific Evidence Post-*Daubert*. Health Phys 2001;81(6):678.

Chapter 6

- College of American Pathology. General Checklists and Patient Safety Plan,
- Milunsky A, Annas G. Genetics and the Law: Vol I. Plenum Press, NY. 1976.

Chapter 7

- Hendriksen JG, Vles JS. Neuropsychiatric disorders in males with Duchenne muscular dystrophy: frequency rate of attention-deficit hyperactivity disorder (ADHD), autism spectrum disorder, and obsessive-compulsive disorder. J Child Neurol 2008;23:477.
- Kieny P, Chollet S, Delalande P, et al. Evolution of life expectancy of patients with Duchenne muscular dystrophy at AFM Yolaine de Kepper centre between 1981 and 2011. Ann Phys Rehabil Med 2013;56:443.
- Pane M, Messina S, Bruno C, et al. Duchenne muscular dystrophy and epilepsy. Neuromuscul Disord 2013;23:313.
- Papa R, Madia F, Bartolomeo D, et al. Genetic and Early Childhood Clinical Manifestations of Females Heterozygous for Duchenne/Becker Muscular Dystrophy. Pediatr Neurol 2016;55:58.
- Sarrazin E, von der Hagen M, Schara U, et al. Growth and psychomotor development of patients with Duchenne muscular dystrophy. Eur J Paediatr Neurol 2014;18:38.

Chapter 8

- Javid B, Said-Al-Naief N. Craniofacial manifestations of β-thalassemia major. Oral Surgery, Oral Medicine, Oral Pathology and Oral Radiology 2015;119(1):e33.
- Committee on Genetics. Counseling About Genetic Testing and Communication of Genetic Test Results. Obstet Gynecol 2017;129:e96.

Chapter 9

- Cook JR, Carta L, Galatioto J, et al. Cardiovascular manifestations in Marfan syndrome and related diseases; multiple genes causing similar phenotypes. Clin Genet 2015;87:11.
- Solomon RA, Connolly ES. Arteriovenous Malformations of the Brain. N Engl J Med. 2017; 376:1859.
- Stapf C, Parides MK, Mohr JP. Arteriovenous Malformations of the Brain. N Engl J Med. 2017; 377:497.

Chapter 10

- Milunsky A, Milunsky JM. Genetic Disorders and the Fetus: Diagnosis, Prevention and Treatment. 2015. Wiley: UK.

Chapter 11

- Groopman J. How Doctors Think. Houghton Mifflin, Boston. 2007.
- Mauksch LB. Questioning a Taboo: Physicians' Interruptions During Interactions With Patients. JAMA 2017;317:1021.

Chapter 12

- Milunsky A. Your Genes, Your Health: A Critical Guide that could Save Your Life. Oxford University Press, NY. 2012.

Chapter 13

- Biancalana V, Glaesar D, McQuaid S, et al. EMQN best practice guidelines for the molecular genetic testing and reporting of fragile X syndrome and other fragile X-associated disorders. Eur J Hum Genet 2015;23:417.
- Burke T, Rosenbaum S. *Molloy v Meier* and the Expanding Standard of Medical Care: Implications for Public Health Policy and Practice. Public Health Reports 2005;120:209.
- Hallberg M, McClain TF. *Molloy v. Meier* Extends Genetic Counseling Duty of Care to Biological Parents and Establishes that Legal Damages Must Occur Before a Wrongful Conception Action Accrues for Statute of Limitations Purposes. William Mitchell Law Review. 2005;31:939.
- Krause J. *Molloy v. Meier* – The Supreme Court of Minnesota Finds a Duty to Warn Parents Regarding a Child's Genetic Testing and Diagnosis. Health Law Perspectives. August 27, 2004.
- Lacroix M, Nycum G, Godard B, et al. Should physicians warn patients' relatives of genetic risks? CMAJ 2008 Feb;178(5):593.
- Lucassen A, Parker M. Confidentiality and sharing genetic information with relatives. Lancet. 2010;375:1507.
- Molloy v. Meier. Court of Appeals of Minnesota. May 6, 2003.
- Mor P, Oberle K. Ethical issues related to BRCA gene testing in orthodox Jewish women. Nurs Ethics. 2008;15(4):512.
- Nguyen, TD. The concept of loss of chance: A major evolution in the definition of damage or how to prevent litigation for loss of chance?. Cancer Radiother. 2016 Jul;20(5):411.
- Sulmasy DP. On Warning Families about Genetic Risk: The Ghost of Tarasoff. Am J Med. 2000;109:738.

Chapter 14

- Court Decision Ignores The Patient's Right to Privacy in Gene Testing. Cancer Network. May 01, 1998.
- Ferris LE, Barkun H, Carlisle J, et al. Defining the physician's duty to warn: consensus statement of Ontario's Medical Expert Panel on Duty to Inform. CMAJ 1998;158:1473.
- Florida recognizes duty to warn patient of transmissibility of genetic disease to child – Pate v. Threlkel, 661 So.2d 278 (Fla. 1995), rehearing denied (Oct 10, 1995). The Law, Science & Public Health Law Site.
- Garwin MJ. Risk creation, loss of chance, and legal liability. Hematol Oncol Clin N Am 2002;16:1351.
- Keeling SL. Duty to warn of genetic harm in breach of patient confidentiality. J Law Med 2004;12:235.

- Kovalesky, ML. To disclose or not to disclose: Determining the scope and exercise of a physician's duty to warn third parties of genetically transmissible conditions. University of Cincinnati Law Review. 2008;78:1019.
- Marchant GE, Lindor RA. Personalized medicine and genetic malpractice. Genetics in Medicine 2013;15:921.
- Offit K, Groeger E, Turner S, et al. The "duty to warn" a patient's family members about hereditary disease risks. JAMA 2004;292:1469.
- Safer v. Estate of Pack. Superior Court of New Jersey, Appellate Division. July 11, 1996.
- Safer v. Estate of Pack. Superior Court of New Jersey, Appellate Division. September 01, 1998.
- Storm C, Agarwal R, Offit K. Ethical and Legal Implications of Cancer Genetic Testing: Do Physicians Have a Duty to Warn Patients' Relatives About Possible Genetic Risks? J Oncol Pract 2008;4:229.
- Sudell A. To tell or not to tell: The scope of physician-patient confidentiality when relatives are at risk of genetic disease. J Contemp Health Law and Policy 2001;18:273.

Chapter 15

- Kilgannon JH, Jones AE, Shapiro NI, et al. Association Between Arterial Hyperoxia Following Resuscitation From Cardiac Arrest and In-Hospital Mortality. JAMA 2010;303(21):2165.
- Raghuraman N, Temming LA, Stout MJ, et al. Intrauterine Hyperoxemia and Risk of Neonatal Morbidity. Obstet Gynecol 2017;129:676.

Chapter 16

- Carroll AE, Buddenbaum JL. Malpractice claims involving paediatricians: epidemiology and etiology. Pediatrics 2007;120:10.
- Chudova D.J., Schnert A.J. Copy-Number Variation and False Positive Prenatal Screening Results. N Eng J Med 375;1:97.
- Cummings J.J. The Well-Appearing Newborn at Risk for Early-Onset Sepsis: We Can Do Better. Pediatrics 2017;139:e20164211.
- Fernandez CV, Gillis-Ring J. Strategies for the prevention of medical error in pediatrics. J Pediatr 2003;143:155.
- Hershey T.B., Kahn J.M. State Sepsis Mandates—A New Era for Regulation of Hospital Quality. N Eng J Med 376;24:2311.
- McAbee GN, Donn SM, Mendelson RA, et al. Medical Diagnoses Commonly Associated With Pediatric Malpractice Lawsuits in the United States. Pediatrics 2008;122:e1282.
- Mukhopadhyay S, Taylor JA, Von Kohorn I, et al. Variation in Sepsis Evaluation Across a National Network of Nurseries. Pediatrics 2017;139:e20162845.
- Najaf-Zadeh A, Dubos F, Aurel M, et al. Epidemiology of malpractice lawsuits in pediatrics. Acta Paediatrica 2008;97:1486.
- Schiff GD, Puopolo AL, Huben-Kearney A, et al. Primary care closed claims experience of Massachusetts malpractice insurers. JAMA Intern Med. 2013; 173(22):2063.

Chapter 17

- Baker M., Mayo J. High Volume, Big Dollars, Rising Tension. The Seattle Times. February 10, 2017. Response by Veritas9 on February 25, 2017.
- Pascall E, Trehane SJ, Georgiou A, et al. Litigation associated with intensive care unit treatment in England: an analysis of NHSLA data 1995-2012. Br J Anaesth, 2015 Oct;114(4):601.
- Sappideen C. Medical teams and the standard of care in negligence. J Law Med 2015 Sep;23(1)69.

Chapter 18

- American Academy of Pediatrics Committee on Fetus and Newborn. The Apgar Score. Pediatrics 2015;136:819.
- Andreasen S, Backe B, Øian P. Claims for compensation after alleged birth asphyxia: a nationwide study covering 15 years. Acta Obstetricia et Gynecologica Scandinavica 2014 Feb;93(2):152.
- Berglund S, Grunewald C, Pettersson H, et al. Severe asphyxia due to delivery-related malpractice in Sweden 1990-2005. BJOG 2008;115:316.
- Bernstein PS, Combs CA, Shields LE, et al. The development and implementation of checklists in obstetrics. Am J Obstet Gynecol 2017;217:B2.
- Clark SL, Belfort MA, Dildy GA, et al. Reducing Obstetric Litigation Through Alterations in Practice Patterns. Obstet Gynecol 2008;112:1279-1283.
- Cohen WR, Friedman EA. Perils of the new labor management guidelines. Am J Obstet Gynecol 2015;212:420.
- Glaser LM, Alvi FA, Milad MP. Trends in malpractice claims for obstetric and gynecologic procedures, 2005 through 2014. Am J Obstet Gynecol 2017;217:340.
- Kadar N. Peer review of medical practices: missed opportunities to learn. Amer J Obstet Gynecol 2014;211:596.
- Kahneman, Daniel. Thinking Fast and Slow. Farrar, Straus and Giroux. New York, 2011.
- Maurice A. Jackson v. Rashonda Pollion, et al. United States Court of Appeals for the Seventh Circuit No 12-2682. October 28, 2013.
- Mickleborough T. Intuition in medical practice: A reflection on Donald Schon's reflective practitioner. Medical Teacher 2015, 37:889.
- Scott I. Errors in clinical reasoning: causes and remedial strategies. BMJ 2009:339:22.

Chapter 19

- Horwitz LI. Does Improving Handoffs Reduce Medical Error Rates? JAMA 310:21:2255.
- Joint Commission Center for Transforming Healthcare Releases Targeted Solutions Tool for Hand-off Communications. Jt Comm Perspect 2012;32:1.
- Kachalia A, Studdert DM. Professional Liability Issues in Graduate Medical Education. JAMA 2004;292:1051.
- McAbee GN, Deitschel C, Berger J, et al. Pediatric Medicolegal Education in the 21st Century. Pediatrics 2006;117;1790.
- Reid A. Identifying medical students at risk of subsequent misconduct. BMJ 2010;340:c2169.
- Sadhu J. Transition in House Staff Care and Patient Mortality. JAMA 2017;317:1178.
- Schenarts PJ, Langenfeld S. The Fundamentals of Resident Dismissal. Am Surg 2017 Feb 1;83(2):119.
- Singh H, Thomas EJ, Petersen LA, et al. Medical Errors Involving Trainees. Arch Intern Med 2007;167: 2030.

- Yates J, James D. Risk factors at medical school for subsequent professional misconduct: multicenter retrospective case-control study. BMJ 2010:340:c2040.

Chapter 20

- ACMG Board of Directors. Direct-to-consumer genetic testing: a revised position statement of the American College of Medical Genetics and Genomics. Genet Med 2016;18(2):207.
- Committee on Genetics. Carrier Screening for Genetic Conditions. Obstet Gynecol 2017;129:e41.
- Grody WW. Where to Draw the Boundaries for Prenatal Carrier Screening. JAMA 2016;316:717.
- Norton ME. Expanded Carrier Screening: A Rational Approach to Screening for Rare Diseases. Obstet Gynecol 2017;130:260.
- Shi L, Webb BD, Birch AH, et al. Comprehensive population screening in the Ashkenazi Jewish population for recurrent disease-causing variants. Clin Genet 2017;91:599.
- Stevens B, Krstic N, Jones M, et al. Finding Middle Ground in Constructing a Clinically Useful Expanded Carrier Screening Panel. Obstet Gynecol 2017;130:279-84.
- Tingle JH. Do guidelines have legal implications? Arch Dis Child 2002;86(6):387.

Chapter 21

- Ahuja N, Zhao W, Xiang H. Medical Errors in US Pediatric Inpatients With Chronic Conditions. Pediatrics 2012;130(4):e786.
- Barthel ER, Stabile BE, Plurad D, et al. Surgical malpractice in California: res judicata. Am Surg 2014;80:1007.
- Bonifield J. Ohio family: Hospital 'botched' transplant, threw out kidney. CNN Report. August 30, 2013.
- Cima, RR, Kollengode A, Garnatz J, et al. Incidence and characteristics of potential and actual retained foreign object events in surgical patients. J Am Coll Surg. 2008;207:80.
- Cuschieri A. Nature of Human Error: Implications for Surgical Practice. Ann Surg 2006;244:642.
- De Vries EN, Eikens-Jansen MP, Hamersma AM, et al. Prevention of surgical malpractice claims by use of a surgical safety checklist. Ann Surg 2011 Mar;253(3):624.
- Donovan L. World audience told of mastectomy error. Saint Paul Pioneer Press. January 21, 2003.
- Duvall A. One in Five U.S. Hospitals Fail to Adopt Crucial "Never Events" Policies. Castlight Heath 2016.
- Eliminating Serious, Preventable, and Costly Medical Errors – Never Events. Centers for Medicare and Medicaid Services 2006.
- Factsheet: Never Events. The Leapfrog Group 2016.
- Frable WJ. Error reduction and risk management in cytopathology. Seminars in Diagnostic Pathology 2007;24:77.
- Gawande A. Complications: A Surgeon's Notes on an Imperfect Science. Henry Holt and Company. New York, 2002.
- Gawande A. Better: A Surgeon's Notes on Performance. Henry Holt and Company. New York, 2007.
- Gawande AA, Studdert DM, Orav EJ, et al. Risk factors for retained instruments and sponges after surgery. N Engl J Med. 2003;348:229.
- Greenberg CC, Gawande AA .Retained foreign bodies. Adv Surg. 2008;42:183.

- Groff MW, Heller JE, Potts EA, et al. A survey-based study of wrong-level lumbar spine surgery : the scope of the problem and current practices in place to help avoid these errors. World Neurosurg 2013;79(3-4):585.
- Groves B. "Wrong lung" doc wants his license back. The Jersey Journal. July 8, 2008.
- Hospital cited in death of boy placed under heating blanket. The Boston Globe. August 24, 2017
- Hospital Repeats Wrong-Sided Brain Surgery. ABC News. November 28, 2007.
- Jaslow R. Wrong kidney removed at Mount Sinai Medical Center in New York City. CBS New York. May 10. 2013.
- The Joint Commission. Sentinel Event Policy and Procedures. 2013. Retrieved from http://www.jointcommission.org/Sentinel_Event_Policy_and_Procedures/
- Kohn L, Corrigan J, Donaldson M. To Err is Human: Building a Safer Health system. National Academy Press, Washington D.C, 1999.
- Kopp C. Anatomy of a Mistake. CBS News. March 16 2003.
- Kowalczyk L. Hospital faulted over medical error. The Boston Globe. October 14, 2016.
- Kowalczyk L. Medical mishaps: what to expect if one happens to you. The Boston Globe. September 1, 2014.
- Kowalcyzk L. Mistaken identity. The Boston Globe. November 21, 2016.
- Kwaan MR, Studdert DM, Zinner MJ, et al. Incidence, patterns, and prevention of wrong-site surgery. Arch Surg. 2006;141:353 (discussion 7–8).
- Landrigan CP, Parry GJ, Bones CB, et al. Temporal Trends in Rates of Patient Harm Resulting from Medical Care. N Engl J Med 2010;363:2124.
- Lincourt AE, Harrell A, Cristiano J, et al. Retained foreign bodies after surgery. J Surg Res. 2007;138:170.
- List of Serious Reportable Events. National Quality Forum.2002.
- Marshall M, Heath I, Sweeney K. Clinical practice: when things go wrong. Lancet 2010;375:1491.
- Mastectomy Mistake Patient: 'I Was in Shock'. CNNAccess January 20, 2003.
- Mehta SP, Bhananker SM, Posner KL, et al. Operating room fires: a closed claims analysis. Anesthesiology, 2013;118(5):1133.
- Mehtsun WT, Ibrahim AM, Diener-West M, et al. Surgical Never Events in the United States. Surgery 2013;153:465.
- Michaels RK, Makary MA, Dahab Y, et al, Achieving the National Quality Forum's "Never Events": Prevention of Wrong Site, Wrong procedure, and wrong patient operations. Ann Surg. 2007;245:526.
- Moritz O. Docs unscathed in double mastectomy mixup. Daily News (New York). January 21, 2003.
- Never Events: Data By Hospital on Nationally Standardized Metrics. Castlight Health 2016.
- Never Events. Patient Safety Network 2016.
- Ohio Hospital somehow loses infant's remains. The Boston Globe. September 29, 2015.
- Patient at Halifax Hospital has surgery on wrong leg. Orlando Sentinel. August 15, 2013.
- Patient gets needless mastectomy after hospital mix-up. CBC News Aug 12, 2013.
- Pecci AW. Never Event Frequency "Troubling,' Standards Lacking. Health Leaders Media 2015.
- Pregnant woman dies after ovary removed by mistake. The Telegraph. April 15, 2014.
- Pronovost PJ. Safe Patients, Smart Hospitals: How One Doctor's Checklist Can Help Us Change Health Care From the Inside Out. New York: Hudson Street Press. 2010.
- Pronovost PJ, Bo-Linn GW. Preventing Patient Harms though Systems of Care. JAMA 2012;308:769.
- Pronovost PJ, Dang D, Dorman T, et al. Intensive care unit nurse staffing and the risk for complications after abdominal aortic surgery. Eff Clin Pract. 2001;4(5):199.

- Pronovost PJ, Murphy DJ, Needham DM. The science of translating research into practice in intensive care. Am J Respir Crit Care Med. 2010;182(12):1463.
- Reason J. Human Error: Models and Management. BMH 2000;320:768.
- Reason J. Understanding adverse events: human factors. Qual Health Care. 1995;4:80.
- Saltzman J. VA chief outs 3rd official at N.H. hospital. The Boston Globe. August 5, 2017.
- Seiden SC, Barach P. Wrong-side/wrong-site, wrong-procedure, and wrong-patient adverse events: are they preventable?. Arch Surg. 2006;141:931.
- Smetzer J, Baker C, Byrne FD, et al. Shaping Systems for Better Behavioral Choices: Lessons Learned from a Fatal Medication Error. Jt Comm J Qual Patient Saf 2010;36:152.
- St. Paul: Breasts removed in error. Saint Paul Pioneer Press. January 19, 2003.
- St. Vincent Hospital blames mistaken kidney removal on outside physician. MassLive. August 11, 2016.
- Stahel PF, Sabel AL, Victoroff MS, et al, Wrong-site and wrong-patient procedures in the universal protocol era: analysis of a prospective database of physician self-reported occurrences. Arch Surg. 2010;145:978.
- Steinhauer J. Surgeon Treated Wrong Side of Two Brains, Albany Says. The New York Times. March 1, 2000.
- Thiels CA, Lal TM, Nienow JM, et al. Surgical Never Events and Contributing Human Facts. Surgery 2015;158:515.
- Toolan CC, Cartwright-Terry M, Scurr JR, et al. Causes of successful medico-legal claims following amputation. Vascular 2014;22:346.
- Wagar EA, Stankovic AK, Raab S, et al. Specimen labeling errors: a Q-probes analysis of 147 clinical laboratories. Arch Pathol Lab Med 2008;132(10):1617.
- West, J.C. Surgical "never events": how common are adverse occurrences? J Health Care Risk Mgmt. 2006;26:15.
- Wick MR. Medicolegal liability in surgical pathology: a consideration of underlying causes and selected pertinent concepts. Seminars in Diagnostic Pathology 2007;24:89.
- Woman Has Needless Double Mastectomy, Sues. CBS News October 4, 2017.

Chapter 22

- Committee on Patient Safety and Quality Improvement. Behavior That Undermines a Culture of Safety. Obstet Gynecol 2017;129:e1.
- Dyer C. Doctor and two nurses charged with manslaughter over death of boy at Leicester Royal Infirmary. BMJ 2014;349:g7755.
- Dyer C. Doctor gets suspended prison sentence for not giving priority to "very sick boy." BMJ 2015;351:h6832.
- Dyer C. Doctor who injected adrenaline against advice found guilty of manslaughter. BMJ 2009;338:b545.
- Dyer C. Paediatrician found guilty of manslaughter after boy's death from septic shock. BMJ 2015;351:h5969.
- Dyer C. Urologist who was jailed for manslaughter is allowed back to work. BMJ 2014;349:g4931.
- Emery E, Balossier A, Mertens P. Is the medicolegal issue avoidable in neurosurgery? A retrospective survey of a series of 115 medicolegal cases from public hospitals. World Neurosurg 2014;81(2):218.
- Fargen KM, Friedman WA. The Science of Medical Decision Making: Neurosurgery, Errors, and Personal Cognitive Strategies for Improving Quality of Care. World Neurosurgery 2014;82:E21.
- Goodman M. Dr. Death. D Magazine Health & Medicine 2016.

- Houston Chronicle. In Texas, a bad doctor can wreak havoc for decades with impunity, harming patients and making millions in the process. December 29, 2004.
- Jiam NT, Cooper MA, Lyu HG, et al. Surgical malpractice claims in the United States. J Healthc Risk Manag 2014;33:29.
- Katz JD. The impaired and/or disabled anesthesiologist. Curr Opin Anaesthesiol 2017;30:217.
- Klaas PB, Berge KH, Klaas KM, et al. When Patients Are Harmed, But Are Not Wronged: Ethics, Law, and History. Mayo Clin Proc 2014;89(9):1279.
- Lyons B. Medical manslaughter. Ir Med J 2013;106:26.
- Mukherjee S, Pringle C, Crocker M. A nine-year review of medicolegal claims in neurosurgery. Ann R Coll Surg Engl 2014;96(4):266.
- Rovit RL, Simon AS, Drew J, et al. Neurosurgical experience with malpractice litigation: an analysis of closed claims against neurosurgeons in New York State, 1999 through 2003. J Neurosurg 2007;106(6):1108.
- Sachs, BP. A 38-Year-Old Woman With Fetal Loss and Hysterectomy. JAMA 2005;294:833.
- Steele L, Mukherjee S, Stratton-Powell A, et al. Extent of medicolegal burden in neurosurgery – An analysis of the National Health Litigation Authority Database. Br J Neurosurg. 2015;29(5):622.
- White P. More doctors charged with manslaughter are being convicted, shows analysis. BMJ 2015;351:h4402.
- Wu KH, Cheng SY, Yen YL, et al. An analysis of causative factors in closed criminal medical malpractice cases of the Taiwan Supreme Court: 2000-2014. Leg Med (Tokyo) 2016;23:71.

Chapter 23

- Bruix J, Sherman M, American Association for the Study of Liver Diseases. Management of Hepatocellular Carcinoma: An Update. Hepatology 2011;53:1020.
- Gordon EJ, Mullee J, Skaro A, et al. Live liver donors' information needs: A qualitative study of practical implications for informed consent. Surgery. 2016;160:671.
- Kotloff RM, Blosser S, Fulda GJ, et al. Management of the Potential Organ Donor in the ICU: Society of Critical Care medicine/American College of Chest Physicians/Association of Organ Procurement Organizations Consensus Statement. Crit Care Med. 2015;43(6):1291.
- Lee SG. A Complete Treatment of Adult Living Donor Liver Transplantation: A Review of Surgical Technique and Current Challenges to Expand Indication of Patients. Am J Transplant 2015;15:17.
- Main BG, McNair A, Blazeby JM. Informed Consent and the Reasonable-Patient Standard. JAMA 2016;316:992.
- Marrero JA, Ahn J, Rajender RK, et al. ACG Clinical Guideline: The Diagnosis and Management of Focal Liver Lesions. Am J Gastroenterol 2014;109:1328.
- Rogers AC, Chalasani S, Ryan AG, et al. The Twin Evils of Concomitant Rare Pathology with Variant Anatomy: Superior Mesenteric Artery Aneurysm and a Replaced Right Hepatic Artery. Ann Vasc Surg 2017;38:318.e1.
- Rude MK, Crippin JS. Liver Transplantation for Hepatocellular Carcinoma. Curr Gastroenterol Rep 2015;17:11.
- Sangiovanni A and Colombo M. Treatment of Hepatocellular Carcinoma: Beyond International Guidelines. Liver Int 2016;36(S1):124.
- Spatz ES, Krumholz HM, Moulton BW. The New Era of Informed Consent: Getting to a Reasonable-Patient Standard Through Shared Decision Making. JAMA 2016;315:2063.

- Tabrizian P, Roayaie S, Schwatz ME. Current Management of Hepatocellular Carcinoma. World J Gastroenterol 2014;20:10223.

Chapter 24

- Batchelor JS. USP report blasts radiology medication errors. AuntMinnie. January 19, 2006.
- Berland LL, Silverman SG, Gore RM, et al. Managing Incidental Findings on Abdominal CT: White paper of the ACR Incidental Findings Committee. J Am Coll Radiol 2010;7:754.
- Berlin L. Malpractice Issues in Radiology: 2nd edition. American Roentgen Ray Society. Leesburg, Virginia. 2003.
- Berlin L. Communicating radiology results. Lancet 2006;367:373.
- Berlin L. The incidentaloma: a medicolegal dilemma. Radiol Clin North Am 2011;49:245.
- Berlin L. How do you solve a problem like incidentalomas? Appl Radiol 2013;42:10.
- Berlin L. Malpractice and Ethical Issues in Radiology. AJR Am J Roentgenol 2016;207:W133.
- Berlin L. Malpractice and Ethical Issues in Radiology. AJR Am J Roentgenol 2017;208:W54.
- Berlin L. Malpractice and Ethical Issues in Radiology: The Incidentaloma. AJR 2013;200:W91.
- Berlin L. Malpractice and Ethical Issues in Radiology: Judging the Competency of a Radiologist Colleague. AJR 2016;206:W29.
- Berlin L. Malpractice Issues in Radiology: The Miasmatic Expert Witness. AJR 2003;181:29.
- Berlin L, Murphy DR, Singh H. Breakdowns in communication of radiological findings: an ethical and medico-legal conundrum. Diagnosis (Berl) 2014;1:263.
- Commonwealth of Massachusetts Board of Registration in Medicine. Incidental Findings Advisory. Quality and Patient Safety Division. August 2016.
- Frank L, Quint LE. Chest CT incidentalomas: thyroid lesions, enlarged mediastinal lymph nodes, and lung nodules. Cancer Imaging 2012;12:41.
- Fujikawa T, Tamamoto S, Sekine Y, et al. Operative Results and Clinical Features of Chronic Stanford Type B Aortic Dissection: Examination of 234 Patients Over 6 Years. Eur J Vasc Endovasc Surg 2015;50:738.
- Grandval P, Fabre AJ, Béroud C, et al. Consideration surrounding incidental findings throughout multigene panel testing in cancer genetics. Clin Genet 2016;89;267.
- Harvey HB, Tomov E, Babayan A, et al. Radiology Malpractice Claims in the United States From 2008 to 2012: Characteristics and Implications. J Am Coll Radiol 2016;13:124.
- Hitzeman N, Cotton E. Incidentalomas: Initial Management. AFP 2014;90:784.
- Iafrancesco M, Ranasinghe AM, Claridge MW, et al. Current Results of Endovascular Repair of Thoraco-Abdominal Aneurysms. Eur J Cardiothorac Surg 2014;46:981.
- Icenhower M. Incidentalomas: Managing the Risk of the Incidental Finding. Coverys Risk Management. June 2017.
- Isselbacher EM, Bonaca MP, Di Eusanio M, et al. Recurrent Aortic Dissection: Observations from the International Registry of Aortic Dissection. Circulation 2016;134:1013.
- Kella DK, Desai R, Rubinsztein L, et al. An Incidentaloma in the Cardiology Clinic. Am J Med 2016;130:e140.
- Lee CS, Nagy PG, Weaver SJ, et al. Cognitive and system factors contributing to diagnostic errors in radiology. AJR Am J Roentgenol 2013;201:611.
- Luijtgaarden KM, Heijsman D, Maugeri A, et al. First Genetic Analysis of Aneurysm Genes in Familial and Sporadic Abdominal Aortic Aneurysm. Human Genet 2015;134:881.
- Miner GH, Faries PL, Costa KD, et al. An Update on the Etiology of Abdominal Aortic Aneurysms: Implications for Future Diagnostic Testing. Expert Rev Cardiovasc Ther 2015;13:1079.

- Salata K, Katznelson R, Beattie WS, et al. Endovascular Versus Open Approach to Aortic Aneurysm Repair Surgery: Rates of Postoperative Delirium. Can J Anaesth 2012;59:556.
- Santosa F, Schrader S, Nowak T, et al. Thoracal, Abdominal, and Thoracoabdominal Aortic Aneurysm. Int Angiol 2013;32:501.
- Todo S, Furukawa H. Living Donor Liver Transplantation for the Treatment of Small Hepatocellular Carcinomas in Patients with Cirrhosis. Ann Surg 2004;240:451.
- Waite S, Scott J, Gale B, et al. Interpretive Error in Radiology. AJR Am J Roentgenol 2016;27:1.
- Whang JS, Baker SR, Patel R, et al. The causes of medical malpractice suits against radiologists in the United States. Radiology 2013;266:548.
- Yu SJ. A Concise Review of Updated Guidelines Regarding the Management of Hepatocellular Carcinoma Around the World: 2010-2016. Clin Mol Hepatol 2016;22:7.

Chapter 25

- Black C, Craft A. The competent doctor: a paper for discussion. Clinical Medicine 2004;4:527.
- Carabuena JM, Mitani AM, Liu X, et al. The Learning Curve Associated with the Epidural Technique Using the Episure™ AutoDetect™ Versus Conventional Glass Syringe: An Open-Label, Randomized, Controlled, Crossover Trial of Experienced Anesthesiologists in Obstetric Patients.
- Chin M, Lagasse RS. Assessment of competence: developing trends and ethical considerations. Curr Opin Anaesthesiol. 2017;30(2):236.
- Cohen AW. Competency. AJOG 2016:215:4.
- Drake EJ, Coghill J, Sneyd JR. Defining competence in obstetric epidural anaesthesia for inexperienced trainees. Brit J Anaesth 2015;114:951.
- Ranum D, Ma J, Shapiro FE, et al. Analysis of patient injury based on anesthesiology closed claims data from a major malpractice insurer. J Healthcare Risk Manag 2014;34(2):31.
- Stone, NJ. Clinical Confidence and the Three C's: Caring, Communicating, and Competence. Am J Med 2006;119:1.
- Wakeford R. Commentary: Criteria, competencies, and confidence tricks. BMJ 2006:332:233.

Chapter 26

- Flannery FT, Parikh PD, Oetgen WJ. Characteristics of Medical Professional Liability Claims in Patients Treated by Family Medicine Physicians. JABFM 2010;23(6):753.
- Pagon, Roberta. GeneReviews https://www.ncbi.nlm.nih.gov/books/NBK1116/

Chapter 27

- Cook LA, Van Vliet HA, Lopez LM, et al. Vasectomy occlusion techniques for male sterilization. Cochrane Database Syst Rev. 2014 Mar 30;(33):CD003991.
- DeRosa R, Lustik MB, Stackhouse DA, et al. Impact of the 2012 American Urological Association Vasectomy Guidelines on Postvasectomy Outcomes in a Military Population. Urology 2015;85:505.
- Hancock P, Woodward BJ, Munner A, et al. 2016 Laboratory guidelines for postvasectomy semen analysis: Association of Biomedical Andrologists, the British Andrology Society and the British Association of Urological Surgeons. J Clin Pathol 2016;69:655.

- Rayala BZ, Viera AJ. Common Questions About Vasectomy. Am Fam Physician 2013;88:757.

Chapter 28

- Gale BD, Bissett-Siegel DP, Davidson SJ, et al. Failure to notify reportable test results: significance in medical malpractice. J Am Coll Radiol. 2011;8(11):776.
- Laroia R. The Power of a Laboratory—Are We Taking Full Ownership as Hospitalists? Hosp Pediatr. 2014;4(2):119.
- Ostrom, CM. $50M awarded over birth defect; test said baby would be OK. The Seattle Times. December 10, 2013.

Chapter 29

- Ahmed AA Zhang L, Reddivalla N, Hetherington M. Neuroblastoma in children: Update on clinicopathologic and genetic prognostic factors. Pediatr Hematol Oncol. 2017: 34" 165-185.
- Schulte JH, Eggert A. Neuroblastoma. Crit Rev Oncog. 20: 20: 245-70.

Chapter 30

- Kaplan M, Hammerman C, Bhutani VK. The preterm Infant: A high-risk situation for neonatal hyperbilirubinemia due to Glucose-6-Phosphate Dehydrogenase Deficiency. Clin Perinatol.2016; 43: 325-40.
- Luzzatto L, Nannelli C, Notaro R. Glucose-6-Phosphate Dehydrogenase Deficiency. Hematol Oncol Clin North Am. 2016; 31: 373-93.

Chapter 31

- Horani A, Ferkol TW. Primary ciliary dyskinesia and associated sensory ciliopathies. Expert Rev Respir Med. 2016;10(5): 569.
- Paterick BB, Waterhouse BE, Paterick TE, et al. Liability of physicians supervising nonphysician clinicians. J Med Pract Manage. 2014;29(5):309.
- Reinhart K, Daniels R, Kissoon N, et al. Recognizing Sepsis as a Global Health Priority—A WHO Resolution. N Engl J Med 377;5:414.
- Tammelleo AD. Nurses Followed Dr.'s DNR Order on Patient. Nurs Law Regan Rep 2010;51(4):1.
- The Thin Line Between Care and Error: A Risk Management Case Study. Coverys Risk Management. August 2013.

Chapter 32

- Centers for Disease Control and Prevention. 2010 guidelines for the prevention of perinatal group B streptococcal disease. Available at https://www.cdc.gov/groupbstrep/guildelines/index.html
- Gaschignard J, Levy C, Romain O, et al. Neonatal bacterial meningitis: 444 cases in 7 years. Pediatr Inec dis J. 2011;30(3):212.
- Jena AB, Chandra A, Seabury SA. Malpractice Risk Among US Pediatricians. Pediatrics 2013;131:1148.
- Khullar D, Jha AK, Jena JB. Reducing Diagnostic Errors—Why Now? N Engl J Med 373;26:2491.
- Ku LC, Boggess KA, Cohen-Wolkowiez M. Bacterial meningitis in infants. Clin Perinatal. 2015;41(1):29.

- Marcovitch H. When are paediatricians negligent? Arch Dis Child 2011;96:117.
- Stensvold HJ, Klingenberg C, Stoen R, et al. Neonatal Morbidity and 1-Year Survival of Extremely Preterm Infants. Pediatrics 2017;139:e20161821.
- Sudduth CL, Overton EC, Lyu PF, et al. Filtering authentic sepsis arising in the ICU using administrative codes coupled to a SIRS screening protocol. J Crit Care 2017 Jun;39:220.

Chapter 33

- Kahle KT, Kulkarni AV, Limbrick DD Jr, Warf BC, Hydrocephalus in children. Lancet 2016; 387. 788-799.
- Kousi M, Katsanic N. The genetic basis of hydrocephalus. Annu Rev Neurosci. 2016; 39: 409-35.
-

Chapter 34

- Finkelstein JE, Hauser ER, Leonard CO, et al. Late-onset ornithine transcarbamylase deficiency in male patients. J Pediatrics. 1990;117:897.
- Harada E, Nishiyori A, Tokunaga et al. Late-onset ornithine transcarbamylase deficiency in male patients: prognostic factors and characteristics of plasma amino acid profile. Pediatr Int 2006;48(2):105.
- Milunsky A. Lies, Damned Lies, and Medical Experts: The Abrogation of Responsibility by Specialty Organizations and a Call for Action. J Child Neurol 2003;18:413.
- Nendaz M, Perrier A. Diagnostic errors and flaws in clinical reasoning: mechanisms and prevention in practice. Swiss Med Wkly 2012;142:w13706.
- Rimoin DL, Connor JM, Korf B. Principles and Practice of Medical Genetics. 5th Edition. Academic Press. 2007.
- Schulz CM, Burden A, Posner KL. Frequency and Type of Situational Awareness Errors Contributing to Death and Brain Damage. Anesthesiology 2017;127:326.

Chapter 35

- Kar SP. Addressing underlying causes of violence against doctors in India. Lancet 2017;389:1979.
- Ligi I, Millet V, Sartor C, et al. Iatrogenic Events in Neonates: Beneficial Effects of Prevention Strategies and Continuous Monitoring. Pediatrics 2010;126:e1461.

Chapter 36

- Adamkin DH. Neonatal hypoglycemia. Seminars in Fetal & Neonatal Medicine 2017;22:36.
- Asadollahi R, Oneda B, Joset P, et al. The clinical significance of small copy number variants in neurodevelopmental disorders. J Med Genet. 2014;51(10):677.
- Burns CM, Rutherford MA, Boardman JP, et al. Patterns of Cerebral Injury and Neurodevelopmental Outcomes After Symptomatic Neonatal Hypoglycemia. Pediatrics 112:1:65.
- De Lonlay P, Fournet J. Heterogeneity of persistent hyperinsulinaemic hypoglycaemia. A series of 175 cases. Eur J Pediatr 2002;161:37.
- Hawdon JM, Beer J, Sharp D, et al. Neonatal hypoglycaemia: learning from claims. Arch Dis Child Fetal Neonatal Ed. 2017;102(2):F110.
- Inder, T. How Low Can I Go? The Impact of Hypoglycemia on the Immune Brain. Pediatrics 122:2:440.

- Mahajan G, Mukhopadhyay K, Attri S, et al. Neurodevelopmental Outcome of Asymptomatic Hypoglycemia Compared With Symptomatic Hypoglycemia and Euglycemia in High-Risk Neonates. Pediatr Neurol 2017;74:74.
- Schattner A, Simon SR. Diminishing Patient Face Time in Residencies and Patient-Centered Care. Am J Med 2017;130:387.
- Thompson-Branch A, Havranek T. Neonatal Hypoglycemia. Pediatrics in Review 38:4:147.
- Topazian RJ, Hook CC, Mueller PS. Duty to Speak Up in the Health Care Setting A Professionalism and Ethics Analysis. Minnesota Medicine 2013;96(11):40.

Chapter 37

- Jarjour IT. Neurodevelopmental Outcome After Extreme Prematurity: A Review of the Literature. Pediatr Neurol 2015;52:143.
- Kruszka P, Porras AR, Addissie YA, et al. Noonan Syndrome in Diverse Populations. AJOG 2017;173:2323.

Chapter 38

- Alabdullatif MA, Al Dhaibani MA, Khassawneh MY, et al. Chromosomal microarray in a highly consanguineous population: diagnostic yield, utility of regions of homozygosity, and novel mutations. Clinical Genetics 2017;91:616.
- Asadollahi R, Oneda B, Joset P, et al. The clinical significance of small copy number variants in neurodevelopmental disorders. BMJ 2014;51:677.
- Conrad DF, Pinto D, Redon R, et al. Origins and functional impact of copy number variation in the human genome. Nature 2010;464(7289):704.
- Florentino F, Napoletano S, Caiazzo F, et al. Chromosomal microarray analysis as a first-line test in pregnancies with a priori low risk for the detection of submicroscopic chromosomal abnormalities. Eur J Hum Genet. 2013 Jul; 21(7): 725.
- Forthun I, Wilcox AJ, Strandberg-Larsen K, et al. Maternal Prepregnancy BMI and Risk of Cerebral Palsy in Offspring. Pediatrics 2016;138(4):e20160874.
- Mannik K, Magi R, Mace A, et al. Copy Number Variations and Cognitive Phenotypes in Unselected Populations. JAMA 2015;313(20):2044.
- Stark Z, Behrsin J, Burgess T, et al. SNP microarray abnormalities in a cohort of 28 infants with congenital diaphragmatic hernia. Am J Med Genet A 2015; 167A(10):2319.
- Watson CT, Marques-Bonet T, Sharp AJ, et al. The Genetics of Microdeletion and Microduplication Syndromes : An Update. Annu Rev Genom Hum Genet 2014.15:215.

Chapter 39

- Indo Y. Congenital Insensitivity to Pain with Anhidrosis. In: Adam MP, Ardinger HH, Pagon RA, et al., editors. GeneReviews® [Internet]. Seattle (WA): University of Washington, Seattle; 1993-2007.

Chapter 40

- Carmichael SL, Rasmussen SA, et al. Prepregnancy Obesity: A Complex Risk Factor for Selected Birth Defects. Birth Defects Research (Part A): Clinical and Molecular Teratology 2010;88:804.
- Gestational Diabetes. ACOG Practice Bulletin No. 30. American College of Obstetricians and Gynecologists. Obstet Gynecol 2001;98:525.

- Lipschuetz M, Cohen SM, Ein-Mor E, et al. A large head circumference is more strongly associated with unplanned cesarean or instrumental delivery and neonatal complications than high birthweight. Am J Obstet Gynecol. 2015;213(6):833.e1-833.e12.
- Nevo Y, Kramer U, Shinnar S, et al. Macrocephaly in Children with Developmental Disabilities. Pediatr Neurol 2002;27:363.
- Villamor E, Tedroff K, Peterson M, et al. Association Between Maternal Body Mass Index in Early Pregnancy and Incidence of Cerebral Palsy. JAMA. 2017;317(9):925.

Chapter 41

- Doherty C, McDonnell C. Tenfold Medication Errors: 5 Years at a University-Affiliated Pediatric Hospital. Pediatrics 2012;129:916.
- Gates JE. $4M award upheld in malpractice case. Clarion-Ledger. October 25, 2008.
- Godspiel B, Hoffman JM, Griffith NL, et al. ASHP Guidelines on Preventing Medication Errors with Chemotherapy and Biotherapy. Am J Health-Sys Pharm. 2015;72:e6.
- Haga SB, Burke W, Ginsburg GS, et al. Primary care physicians' knowledge of and experience with pharmacogenetic testing. Clinical Genetics 2012;82:388.
- Howlett M, Curtin M, Doherty D, et al. Paediatric Standardised Concentration Infusions – A National Solution. Arch Dis Child 206;10:A1.
- Hughes CF. Medication errors in hospitals: what can be done? Med J Aust 2008;188:267.
- Aspden P, Wolcott JA, Palugod RL, et al. Preventing Medication Errors. Institute of Medicine of the National Academies. 2006.
- McCool WF, Guidera M, Griffinger E, et al. Closed Claims Analysis of Medical Malpractice Lawsuits Involving Midwives: Lessons Learned Regarding Safe Practices and the Avoidance of Litigation. J Midwifery Womens Health 2015;60:437.
- Nichols P, Copeland T, Craib IA, et al. Learning from error : identifying contributory causes of medication errors in an Australian hospital. Med J Aust 2008;188:276.
- Otero P, Leyton A, Mariani G, et al. Medication Errors in Pediatric Inpatients: Prevalence and Results of a Prevention Program. Pediatrics 122:3:737.
- Rashed AN, Tomlin S, Aguado V, et al. Sources and magnitude of error in preparing morphine infusions for nurse-patient controlled analgesia in a UK paediatric hospital. Int J Clin Pharm. 2016 Oct;38(5):1069.
- Sawer P. Diana doctor's failures led to banker's death. The Telegraph 25 June 2017.
- Smetzer J, Baker C, Byme FD, et al. Shaping systems for better behavioral choices: lessons learned from a fatal medication error. Jt Comm J Qual Patient Saf. 2010;36(4):152.
- Wittich CM, Burkle CM, Lanier WL. Medication Errors: An Overview for Clinicians. Mayo Clin Proc 2014;89:1116.

Chapter 42

- Benders MJ, Groenendaal F, De Vries LS. Preterm arterial ischemic stroke. Semin Fetal Neonatal Med. 2009;14:272.
- Li C, Miao JK, Xu Y, et al. Prenatal, perinatal and neonatal risk factors for perinatal arterial ischaemic stroke: a systematic review and meta-analysis. Eur J Neurol 2017;24:1006.
- O'Brien SH. Perinatal thrombosis: implications for mothers and neonates. Hematology Am Soc Hematol Edu Program 2015;2015:48.

Chapter 43

- Brzezinksi J, Shuman C, Choufani S, et al. Wilms tumour in Beckwith-Wiedemann Syndrome and loss of methylation at imprinting centre 2: revisiting tumour surveillance guidelines. Eur J Hum Genet 2017;25:1031.
- Mussa A, Molinatto C, Cerrato F, et al. Assisted Reproductive Techniques and Risk of Beckwith-Wiedemann Syndrome. Pediatrics 2017;140(1):e20164311.
- Pappas JG. The Clinical Course of an Overgrowth Syndrome, From Diagnosis in Infancy Through Adulthood: The Case of Beckwith-Wiedemann Syndrome. Curr Probl Pediatr Adolesc Health Care 2015;45:112.
- Udayakumaran S, Onyia CU. Beckwith-Wiedemann syndrome and Chiari I malformation—a case-based review of central nervous system involvement in hemihypertrophy syndromes. Childs Nerv Syst. 2015;31(5):637.

Chapter 44

- Hoyme HE, Kalberg WO, Elliott AJ, et al. Updated Clinical Guidelines for Diagnosing Fetal Alcohol Spectrum Disorders. Pediatrics 2016;138:e20154256.
- Pryor J, Patrick SW, Sundermann AC, et al. Pregnancy Intention and Maternal Alcohol Consumption. Obstet Gynecol 2017;129:727.

Chapter 45

- Hofmeyr GJ. Effect of external cephalic version in late pregnancy on breech presentation and caesarean section rate: a controlled trial. Br J Obstet Gynaecol 1983;90:392.
- Van Dorsten JP. Safe and effective external cephalic version with tocolysis. Contemp Ob/Gyn 1982;19:44.

Chapter 46

- Chen Y, Bartanus J, Liang D, et al. Characterization of chromosomal abnormalities in pregnancy losses reveals critical genes and loci for human early development. Hum Mutat 2017;38:669.
- Cukovic-Bagic I, Hrvatin S, Jelicic J, et al. General dentists' awareness of how to cope with medical emergencies in paediatric dental patients. Int Dent J 2017;67:238.
- Gray B, Vandergrift J, Lipner RS, et al. Comparison of Content on the American Board of Internal Medicine maintenance of Certification Examination with Conditions Seen in Practice by General Internists. JAMA 2017;317(22):2317.
- Massachusetts Court System. 234 CMR: Board of Registration in Dentistry. 5.15-5.16.
- Nichols DG. Maintenance of Certification and the Challenge of Professionalism. Pediatrics 2017;139:e20164371.

Chapter 47

- Abrams DJ, MacRae CA. Long QT Syndrome. Circulation. 2014;129:1524.
- Fazio G, Vernuccio F, Grutta G, et al. Drugs to be avoided in patients with long QT syndrome: Focus on the anaesthesiological management. World J Cardiol 2013;5(4):87.
- Mangalmurti S, Seabury SA, Chandra A, et al. Medical professional liability risk among US cardiologists. Am Heart J. 2014;167(5):690.
- Mizusawa Y, Horie M, Wilde AA. Genetic and Clinical Advances in Congenital Long QT Syndrome. Circ J. 2014;78(12):2827.

- Nakano Y, Shimizu W. Genetics of long-QT syndrome. J Hum Genet. 2016:61:51.
- Precision medicine isn't always precise. STAT. October 31, 2016.
- Rosenberg M. Preparing for medical emergencies: The essential drugs and equipment for the dental office. JADA 2010;141:14S.
- Strauss DG, Vincente J, Johannesen L. Common Genetic Variant Risk Score Is Associated With Drug-Induced QT Prolongation and Torsade de Pointes Risk. Circulation. 2017;135:1300.

Epilogue

- Bernstein PS, Martin JN, Barton JR, et al. National Partnership for Maternal Safety: Consensus Bundle on Severe Hypertension During Pregnancy and the Postpartum Period. Obstet Gynec 2017;130:347.
- Carranza L, Lyerly AD, Lipira L, et al. Delivering the Truth: Challenges and Opportunities for Error Disclosure in Obstetrics. Obstet Gynecol 2014;123:656.
- Clinton HR, Obama B. Making Patient Safety the Centerpiece of Medical Liability Reform. N Engl J Med 2006;354:2205.
- Cohen JR. Advising Clients to Apologize. Southern California Law Review 1999;72:1009.
- Delbanco T, Bell SK. Guilty, Afraid, and Alone – Struggling with Medical Error. N Eng J Med 2007:357;1682.
- Hawkes N. Serious errors and neglect in the NHS should be a criminal offense, says safety expert. BMJ 2013;347:f4973.
- Hobgood C, Tamayo-Sarver JH, Elms A, et al. Parental Preferences for Error Disclosure, Reporting, and Legal Action After Medical Error in the Care of Their Children. Pediatrics 2005;116:1276.
- Kachalia A, Bates DW. Disclosing medical errors: The view from the USA. The Surgeon 2014;12:64.
- Meyer G, Lewin DI, Eisenberg J. To Err Is Preventable: Medical Errors and Academic Medicine. Am J of Med 2001;110(7):597.
- Rehm PH, Beatty DR. Legal Consequences of Apologizing. J Dispute Resolution 1996;1:115.
- Vincent C. Principles of Risk and Safety. Acta Neurochir 2001;78:

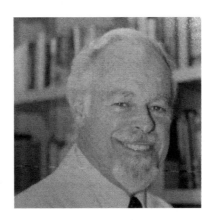

ABOUT THE AUTHOR
Aubrey Milunsky, MD, D.Sc., FRCP, FACMG, DCH

Dr. Aubrey Milunsky is the founder of the non-profit Center for Human Genetics, now in its 35th year. He is a Co-Director with his son and is an adjunct Professor of Obstetrics and Gynecology at Tufts University School of Medicine. He was Professor of Human Genetics, Pediatrics, Obstetrics and Gynecology, and Pathology at Boston University School of Medicine. Boston University named the **AUBREY MILUNSKY CHAIR IN HUMAN GENETICS.**

He was born and educated in Johannesburg, South Africa and is triple board-certified in Pediatrics, Genetics, and Internal Medicine. He served as a medical geneticist at Harvard Medical School and the Massachusetts General Hospital for 12 years before his professorial appointments at Boston University School of Medicine. The Center's laboratories are a major International Referral Center for molecular diagnostics and for prenatal genetic diagnosis, now located in Cambridge, Massachusetts.

He is the author and/or editor of 25 books, including all seven editions of his major reference work, *Genetic Disorders and the Fetus: Diagnosis, Prevention, and Treatment* (2015), now co-edited with his son, Jeff, who was Professor of Pediatrics and Genetics and Genomics at Boston University School of Medicine. This book received the "Highly Commended" Award Certificate in 2010 from the British Medical Association. He has published five books for the lay public, the last being *Your Genes, Your Health: A Critical Family Guide That Could Save Your Life*. An earlier book (*Know Your Genes*) appeared in nine languages. His is the author or co-author of over 450 scientific communications.

He has given hundreds of invited lectures in 35 countries and the Vatican.
In 1982, he was honored by election as a Fellow of the Royal College of Physicians of England. In that year, his alma mater, the University of the Witwatersrand School of Medicine, conferred the D.Sc. degree for his work on the prenatal detection of genetic disorders. He is an elected member of the Society for Pediatric Research and the American Pediatric Society and a Founding Fellow of the American College of Medical Genetics. He has been listed repeatedly in the "Guide to America's Top Pediatricians" and listed in "Top Doctors" in Genetics in Boston.

He has led the teams that first located the gene for X-linked Lymphoproliferative disease, first cloned the PAX3 gene for Waardenburg syndrome, demonstrated the 70% avoidance rate for spina bifida due to folic acid supplementation, and determined newly recognized genes for Chronic Intestinal Pseudo-Obstruction. He and his coworkers have made the first prenatal diagnosis of various genetic disorders, including tuberous sclerosis.

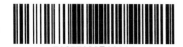
Made in the USA
Middletown, DE
13 April 2018